Practicing Mindfulness:
An Introduction to Meditation

Mark W. Muesse, Ph.D.

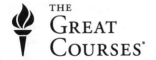

THE
GREAT
COURSES®

PUBLISHED BY:

THE GREAT COURSES
Corporate Headquarters
4840 Westfields Boulevard, Suite 500
Chantilly, Virginia 20151-2299
Phone: 1-800-832-2412
Fax: 703-378-3819
www.thegreatcourses.com

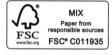

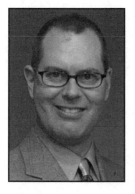

Mark W. Muesse, Ph.D.

W. J. Millard Professor of Religious Studies
and Director of the Asian Studies Program
Rhodes College

Professor Mark W. Muesse is the W. J. Millard Professor of Religious Studies and Director of the Asian Studies and Life: Then and Now programs at Rhodes College. He earned his bachelor of arts degree summa cum laude in English from Baylor University and a master of theological studies, a master of arts, and a doctor of philosophy in The Study of Religion from Harvard University. He has traveled extensively throughout Asia and has studied at the International Buddhist Meditation Centre in Wat Mahathat, Bangkok, Thailand; the Himalayan Yogic Institute in Kathmandu, Nepal; the Subodhi Institute in Piliyandala, Sri Lanka; and the Middle East Technical University in Ankara, Turkey.

Professor Muesse has taught at Harvard College, Harvard Divinity School, and the University of Southern Maine, where he also served as Associate Dean of the College of Arts and Sciences. In 1988, he became Assistant Professor of Religious Studies at Rhodes College. In 1995, he became Associate Professor, and he served as Chair of the Department of Religious Studies from 2004 to 2008. He teaches courses in world religion and philosophy, modern theology, and spirituality. Professor Muesse has also been Visiting Professor of Theology at the Tamilnadu Theological Seminary in Madurai, India.

Professor Muesse has produced three of The Great Courses: *Great World Religions: Hinduism*; *Religions of the Axial Age: An Approach to the World's Religions*; and *Confucius, Buddha, Jesus, and Muhammad*. He is the author of many articles and reviews on comparative religion and theology. His most recent book is *The Hindu Traditions: A Concise Introduction*.

In 2007, Professor Muesse received Fortress Press's Undergraduate Teaching Award at the American Academy of Religion's annual meeting.

i

In 2008, he received the Clarence Day Award for Outstanding Teaching, Rhodes College's highest honor for a member of its faculty. Known for his experiential teaching style, Professor Muesse was honored for his "effective use of imaginative and creative pedagogy" as well as his ability to motivate his students toward lifelong study.

Professor Muesse's wife, Dhammika, is a native of Sri Lanka and teaches in the Rhodes College Chemistry Department. They have a daughter, Ariyana, who attends St. Mary's Episcopal School. ∎

Table of Contents

Table of Contents

Table of Contents

Practicing Mindfulness: An Introduction to Meditation

Scope:

Mindfulness is the skill of being deliberately attentive to one's experience as it unfolds—without the superimposition of our usual commentary and conceptualizing. The capacity to be mindful provides a wholesome way to attend to our experiences and helps us overcome the unskillful habits of mind that cause us to suffer needlessly. This course is a practical guide to developing the skill of mindfulness and applying it to every aspect of daily life.

The foundational technique for cultivating mindfulness is the practice of meditation. Meditation is a form of physical and mental exercise that serves to strengthen the natural ability to bring moment-by-moment awareness to our lives. Since mindfulness is the skill of opening ourselves to reality without judgment, it is important that we approach the practice of meditation in this spirit, relinquishing preconceptions and expectations about the discipline. It is also essential to provide a spiritual and physical context conducive to meditation. Using the Five Precepts of Buddhism, we will consider the interconnections of ethical behavior with the development of mindfulness and the shaping of personal character. Then, we'll study the most effective postures for sitting meditation. Beginning the actual practice of meditation starts with focusing attention on the breath and observing when the mind strays. By noticing when attention has wandered away from its focal point and then gently returning it to the breath, we gradually strengthen our capacities for concentration and awareness.

Practicing mindfulness over time reveals and develops the qualities of wisdom and compassion, the twin virtues of the discipline. Wisdom means seeing clearly into the fundamental nature of reality. Through meditative practice, we can deeply recognize the eternal arising and passing away of all phenomena and see the unsatisfactory quality of ordinary human experience that derives from the illusion of the self as an entity separate from the rest of reality.

Practice is the key to mindfulness. Mindfulness techniques are skills that anyone can develop and apply to the simplest aspects of living: breathing, sensing, feeling, eating, walking, speaking, and even driving. When we've covered the fundamental aspects of mindfulness practice, we'll work on more challenging things: cultivating compassion for ourselves and others; developing a life of generosity; accepting our mortality; and coping with physical pain, grief, and anger. We'll explore difficulties often encountered in meditation and ways of working with these impediments to strengthen concentration and to counter frustration and discouragement.

Compassion—the desire to alleviate suffering—is an essential component of our nature as human beings. Mindfulness practices such as metta meditation allow us to cultivate compassion and develop empathy for others, deeply recognizing their inner experience. *Dana* (sharing with others) reveals the life-giving effects of generosity on both the giver and the receiver and helps us understand our attachment to "things." We'll also consider the ways in which both inner experience and outward action are influenced by our use of language, reflecting on four Buddhist principles of skillful communication.

Finding compassion for ourselves is more challenging for many of us, particularly the perfectionists among us; mindfulness techniques can help us embrace and accept both imperfection and perfectionism as an opening to freedom and deeper humanity. The skills of mindfulness also offer powerful means to work with physical discomfort—through understanding the crucial distinction between pain and suffering—as it directly affects our perceptions.

Reflecting on the universality of loss, we'll take a deeper look at the notion of impermanence. By learning to embrace life's transience and to center our focus in the present moment, we are able to experience loss and even grief without fear or aversion. In the mindfulness tradition, the practice of reflecting on death is considered to be both liberating and essential to living a full and satisfying life. We'll examine the ways in which our culture conditions us to avoid and deny death, and we'll learn meditations that deepen both the awareness of life's transience and our ability to live freely.

Finally, we'll reflect on the capacity of mindfulness practice to profoundly alter our perceptions of ourselves, the world, and our place in it. ■

Mindlessness—The Default Setting

Lecture 1

This course is predicated on the conviction that it is not necessary to live at the mercy of an untamed mind. By coming to understand the way our minds work, we can learn to shape our mental functions in ways that will remove the frantic, driven, distracted, semiconscious qualities from our lives. We'll learn to use mindfulness meditations and exercises to enhance our awareness of everyday experiences—such as breathing, eating, and walking—and to help us cope with the more challenging aspects of life—such as pain, grief, and anger.

Mindlessness as a Mental Condition

- Most of the time, our minds function by generating a constant swirl of remarks and judgments that create a barrier of words and images that separate us from our own lives. This mental condition of **mindlessness** makes it difficult to be mindful, or attentive, to the experiences of our lives.

- The very dynamics that lead to mindlessness can be gently redirected through meditation to cultivate the quality of mindfulness and to develop the mind in ways that will be conducive to our happiness and to the happiness of others.

- The mind is a notoriously elusive concept. We all have an intuitive idea of what we mean by it, but trying to define it concretely seems almost impossible.

- Throughout the centuries, theologians, philosophers, psychologists, and other thinkers have offered various ways of conceiving of the mind and trying to bring some specificity to the notion.

- The mind has been associated with such functions as consciousness, thought, perception, memory, emotion, willing, reasoning, and imagination—and with various combinations thereof. In this course, the mind will refer to all of these mental processes.

- In short, we'll remain content with a rather vague conception of the mind. As we proceed, we'll begin to see the value of allowing this concept to remain broad and inclusive.

Owners of Our Minds

- We ordinarily think of our minds as our own—as something belonging to ourselves and to no one else. No one can "read" our minds, but they may infer our mental states by becoming familiar with facial expressions or other gestures that coordinate with particular forms of our subjectivity.

- Scientists may be able to analyze certain brain activity using sophisticated imaging techniques, but they cannot perceive what our minds are thinking.

- We basically think of ourselves as in control of our own thought processes. Our minds are in fact our most private domains. Most people will more readily regard their minds as the locus of their true or real selves—rather than, say, their bodies.

- We usually experience our minds as somehow connected to our bodies. Specifically, the mind seems to work within the same space occupied by the head, suggesting a close relationship between mind and brain. However, specifying the exact nature of the relationship between mind and body has bedeviled thinkers for millennia.

- Despite the obvious importance that we accord the mind and the intimacy it has with our physical natures, we do not really understand it or use it very well. We pay some attention to the content of our mind, but we have little awareness of how our mind functions.

- Most of us simply have not taken the time to observe the operation of our mind. In general, we pay about as much attention to our minds as we do to the rest of our lives, which is to say, of course, not very much.

Attending to the Present

- Most of our daily lives are essentially governed by routine. The great value of these habits is that they free our minds to do other things; we do these things without having to expend precious energy trying to make up our minds.

- Unfortunately, the freedom such routines afford the mind is not well used. If they find a moment when complete attentiveness to the present is not demanded, our minds tend to gravitate to one of two places: the past or the future.

- Your thoughts may even alternate between past and future, but they will tend to avoid the present as much as possible. If you pay attention to your ordinary thought processes, you will discover that you probably spend very little time living in the present.

- Even when we find ourselves attending to the present, we may discover that what our minds churn out is fairly worthless. Most of us are constantly making instantaneous judgments about what we experience. If you allow these trains of thought to continue, you may find them leading to other thoughts and judgments that do not have any real substance.

Controlling the Mind

- We're not ordinarily in control of our minds, despite what we may think. We can't turn them off, and we can't always make them do what we want. Judgments, thoughts, and emotions seem to arise unbidden and often unwelcome.

- Rather than being in control of our minds, our minds seem to control us—compelling us, driving us, urging us in the directions it deems fit.

- Mindlessness comes at a very high cost: Living with a mind that we don't know very well, that is often out of control and semiconscious much of the time, causes us and others to suffer greatly—probably far more than we realize.

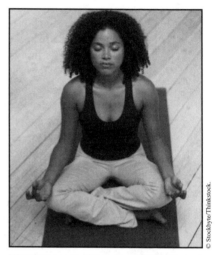

- The Buddha, an individual who knew the mind far better than most of us, put it this way: "Whatever an enemy might do to an enemy, or a foe to a foe, the ill-directed mind can do to you even worse."

- Is it any wonder we so frequently attempt to silence or alter our minds with drugs, amusements, and other forms of distraction? Fortunately, most of us don't reach a mind-driven point of despair, but we nonetheless endure the consequences of an immensely powerful but unruly mind.

Mindfulness is the power of heightened awareness and sensitivity to ourselves and our world.

- We find ourselves entertaining thoughts that serve no wholesome value in our lives. We make snap judgments about individuals based on the slimmest and most trivial of evidence. We spin out falsehoods that we ourselves come to believe. We're constantly comparing ourselves to others, a practice that inevitably leads to pain. All of this, and more, drives us to lead frenzied lives—often on the verge of misery.

- This sense of dissatisfaction, of which we are more or less conscious at different times in our lives, impels us to find something—anything—to bring relief. Unfortunately, our minds have been conditioned to seek solutions to its torment in the most unhelpful ways.

- The beliefs that compel us to keep looking somewhere else for something to bring us relief are so common that we rarely consider that it might be time to try another approach. Rather than seek happiness through the usual ineffective and often counterproductive means, this course will offer you a different way.

- It's possible to cultivate a wholesome mind that will produce thoughts that contribute to our well-being and to the well-being of the whole world. We can shape our mental functions in ways that will remove the frantic, driven, distracted, semiconscious qualities from our lives—but it will not be easy.

Conditioning the Mind

- Our minds are malleable realities; they are plastic and can be reshaped in ways that we choose. The mind, in other words, is a conditioned phenomenon.

- Perhaps we are born with certain dispositions to act and think in particular ways. Many Hindus, Buddhists, and Jains think that **karma**—our thoughts, deeds, and words from previous lives—profoundly influences the mental states we have at birth.

- Essentially, the idea of karma suggests that the way we are now is the consequence of the ways we have thought and acted up to this point. In short, we have been conditioned by ourselves and by others—whether we believe the conditioning process began in former lifetimes or whether it simply began in this lifetime.

- The term **conditioning** is a very useful one for describing this process. Habitual thinking significantly determines what we think, feel, and perceive. The more we entertain a particular thought or a particular kind of thought, the more our minds are prone to generate thoughts of that nature.

- The process of mental conditioning is so powerful that it may seem at times that our whole cerebral function is entirely determined by the factors of our biological makeup or our upbringing. However, we have a small but extremely important capacity to redirect our mind in ways that allow us to recondition it.

- In traditional philosophical terms, we are largely determined but we have a modicum of free will. In this sense, free will is not just a feature of our makeup; instead, it is something that must be exercised and developed. Without cultivation, we are vulnerable to losing the ability to act and think freely altogether.

The Mind as an Instrument

- This course will be unlike most other courses you've ever taken, in which your mind is deliberately stimulated. Stimulating the mind is valuable for many things, but it is not what this course is about. This course is for people whose minds are overstimulated and need a respite from too much thinking.

- In this course, you'll learn to think of the mind not as the center of your personality but as an instrument or tool that you can use for your happiness. Like any instrument, it's essential to learn how to use it properly and to practice using it until the skill becomes second nature.

- Throughout this course, there will be sitting meditations, guided meditations, and other exercises to do. You will need to carve out a time and place to practice them.

- Whether or not this course makes you happy or improves the quality of your life is entirely up to you. Throughout the ages, individuals who have seriously employed the methods we'll discuss have claimed to have discovered something deep and enriching by using them.

- The Buddha, who warned of the tremendously harmful potential of the undisciplined mind, also proclaimed the tremendous benefits of a well-trained mind: "Whatever a mother, father or other relative might do for you, the well-directed mind can do for you even better."

Important Terms

conditioning: The process of habitual thinking that significantly determines what people think, feel, and perceive. The more people entertain a particular thought or a particular kind of thought, the more their minds are prone to generate thoughts of that nature.

karma: The belief of many Hindus, Buddhists, and Jains that thoughts, deeds, and words from people's previous lives profoundly influence the mental states they have at birth.

mindlessness: A mental state in which the mind generates a constant swirl of remarks and judgments that create a barrier of words and images that separate people from their lives. This condition makes it difficult to be mindful—or attentive—to life's experiences.

Questions to Consider

1. How would you characterize your relationship to your mind? Is the mind something you possess, something you are, or something else?

2. Throughout your day, pay attention to your internal dialogue. Ask yourself as many times as you can remember, "What am I thinking?" Are there patterns of thought that correlate to the state of mindlessness?

Mindlessness—The Default Setting
Lecture 1—Transcript

Several years ago, I rented a movie on DVD that sounded very interesting. With great anticipation, I took it home and turned it on. One of the extra features on this film was a commentary by the director and the producer, who conversed between themselves about various aspects of the film as it was being played on screen. This little dialogue was fine, and at first I found it interesting to learn why the director took a certain angle on this particular shot or why this scene was juxtaposed to that one. Initially, I thought the conversation was just part of the opening of the film and that after a few minutes the director and producer would become silent and let the movie proceed without the incessant commentary.

What I soon realized, however, was that the DVD was stuck in this commentarial mode. No matter what I tried, I couldn't turn it off. The only way to watch the film at all was to view it as these two individuals were discussing it. Naturally, I couldn't enjoy the movie because I couldn't really hear it over the fore-grounded conversation.

Later, I realized that this defective DVD had actually provided me with a profound insight into the operation of my own mind. My whole life was like a movie playing out before me, but I couldn't understand or enjoy it because in my head were voices commenting on everything as it happened. Even worse, unlike the DVD, my mind was full of voices, not just a dialogue between two reasonably intelligent persons. It was like a committee meeting with a dozen points of view all vying to be heard. And just like the DVD, I couldn't turn the commentary off.

This, I suggest, is how our minds function most of the time, generating a constant swirl of remarks and judgments that create a barrier of words and images that separate us from our very lives. We end up attending more to the internal cacophony than we do to the world around us. I call this mental condition "mindlessness," not because the mind is uninvolved but because we find it difficult to be mindful—or attentive—to the experiences of our lives. The very dynamics that lead to mindlessness, I contend, can be gently redirected through meditation to cultivate the quality of mindfulness and to develop the mind in ways that will be conducive to our happiness and the happiness of others. That is what this course about.

"Mind" is a notoriously elusive concept. We all have an intuitive idea about what we mean by the word, but trying to define it concretely seems almost impossible. Throughout the centuries, theologians, philosophers, psychologists, and other thinkers, have offered various ways of conceiving of the mind and trying to bring some specificity to the notion. Mind has been identified or associated with such functions as consciousness, thought, perception, memory, emotion, willing, reasoning, and imagination, and with various combinations thereof. None of these proposals, needless to say, has gained universal acceptance. For our purposes, these many fine distinctions need not detain us. In this course, the mind will refer to all of these mental processes. At times, we'll focus on one or two or three to the exclusion of others, but we will always think of the mind as a "society," to use an image suggested by cognitive scientist Marvin Minsky, a society comprised of all of these processes. In short, we'll remain content with a rather vague conception of the mind. As we proceed, we'll begin to see the value of allowing this concept to remain broad and inclusive. With this general definition as our basis, let us now consider how we experience our minds.

Perhaps the first and most obvious thing we can say is that we ordinarily think of our minds as our own. My mind is mine. It does not belong to you or to anyone else. Likewise, I suspect you experience your mind in the same way, as something belonging to you and no one else. No one else, apparently, has access to our minds. No one really knows what goes on in our minds, unless we tell them. No one can "read" our minds, but they may infer our mental states by becoming familiar with facial expressions or other gestures that coordinate with particular forms of our subjectivity.

Scientists may be able to analyze certain brain activity using sophisticated imaging techniques, but they cannot perceive what our minds are thinking or feeling. While our minds may in fact be controlled by demonic beings, alien life-forms, or sentient machines, as in the film *The Matrix*, our ordinary mental experience does not suggest this. We basically think of ourselves in control of our own thought processes. Our minds are in fact our most private domains. So important are they that we tend to identify with our minds by thinking of them as the center of our personality. Most people will more readily regard their minds—or some aspect of it, such as intellect or consciousness—as the locus of their true or real selves—rather than, say, their bodies. To such people, mind isn't just what they possess; it is who they are.

Yet, we usually experience our minds as somehow connected to our bodies. As I stand here in my body, or perhaps as a body, I experience my mind as functioning within the same space my body occupies. Even more specifically, my mind seems to work within the same space occupied by my head, suggesting a close relation between my mind and my brain.

When I move my body to another location, my mind seems to follow it. Wherever my body goes, my mind appears to go with it. This is ordinary experience, of course. If I were under the influence of mystical ecstasy or single-malt whisky, my experience of the relationship between body and mind might be altered. But even the fact that a dram of whisky can affect the functioning of my mind in this way attests to an intimate relationship between these two components of my being. However, specifying the exact nature of that relationship has bedeviled thinkers for millennia.

Despite the obvious importance that we accord the mind and the intimacy it has with our physical natures, we do not really understand it or use it very well. Most of us simply have not taken the time to observe the operation of our mind. We pay some attention to the content of our mind, but we have little awareness of how our mind functions. Consider for a moment where your thoughts come from. Do you know why you have particular thoughts or thoughts that continuously recur? Can you explain why one moment you are contemplating the sobering fact that you may die at any minute and two seconds later you're wondering what's on TV tonight? Most of us cannot give satisfactory answers to these questions.

Our faltering ability to provide good answers derives from inattentiveness. In general, we pay about as much attention to our minds as we do to the rest of our lives, which is to say, of course, not very much. Reflect on the passage of an average day in your life. For how much of those 24 hours are you really there? If you are like most of us, your daily life is essentially governed by routine. You wake up, you get dressed, you have breakfast, you go to work or you do whatever is you do, and your existence is driven along pretty much by well-established habits. The great value of these habits is that they free our minds to do other things. It's not necessary to go through a lengthy intellectual process of trying to decide whether or not to take a shower or reflecting on the pros and cons of brushing our teeth. We just do these things without having to expend precious energy trying to make up our minds.

Unfortunately, the freedom such routines afford the mind is not well used. If they find a moment when complete attentiveness to the present is not demanded, our minds tend to gravitate to one of two places: either the past or the future. If this claim does not have the ring of truth for you, I invite to perform this experiment at your convenience. Simply stop whatever you are doing, sit quietly in a chair, and allow your mind to go wherever it wishes. Try to pay attention to the flow of your thinking. If you are like the vast majority of human beings, you will soon find yourself dwelling on a past event—perhaps a conversation you had that didn't go as well as you would have liked—or a future event you are anticipating, like what's for dinner tonight. Your thoughts may even alternate between past and future, but they will tend to avoid the present as much as possible. If you pay attention to your ordinary thought processes, you will discover that you probably spend very little time living in the present.

Even when we find ourselves attending to the present, we may discover that what our minds churn out is fairly worthless. Most of us are constantly making instantaneous judgments about what we experience. Imagine sitting in a committee meeting. Somehow you've avoided drifting into the past or racing ahead to the future, and you are actually paying attention to what is being said. Well, to some extent. If you watch your mind carefully, you'll probably note that it's only half attentive, if that much. The rest of the time it's feverishly assessing and evaluating, not just the content of what is being said, but the most trivial, insignificant things about how it's said and by whom. You may find yourself looking at the new haircut of the woman across the table and thinking it doesn't fit her face at all. You may notice one of the men wearing a tie that seems to go well with his eyes.

Then you observe that the person running the meeting has a raspy voice that you're always finding irritating. Suddenly you become aware that you haven't said anything in awhile, and you desperately try to think of something that will impress the others or at least make them laugh. If you allow these trains of thought to continue on, you may find them leading to other thoughts and judgments. Your difficulty in coming up with something intelligent to say brings you back to that familiar anxiety you have about not being as competent as others. To avoid that unpleasant thought, you focus on someone else in the room. Strangely, seeing the woman with the odd haircut temporarily soothes your fears of incompetence. At least you don't look hideous—or wait, do you? Well, you certainly don't have an irritating voice, and you can glad for that. You quietly sneak a glance at your watch, wondering how much longer you'll have to endure this ordeal. The whole meeting has become irritating. Wonder what's on TV tonight.

As this scenario suggests, we're not ordinarily in control of our minds, despite what we may care to think. We can't turn them off, and we can't always make them do what we want. Judgments, thoughts, and emotions seem to arise unbidden and often unwelcome. Rather than we controlling our minds, our minds seem to control us: compelling us, driving us, urging us in the directions it deems fit. The image I often conjure when I ponder this situation derives from my childhood, when I attended the annual Heart of Texas Fair and Rodeo. There, I watched seemingly hapless cowboys strapped by a single hand to a bucking bronco or a wild bull and hanging on for dear life as the powerful animal was released into the arena. Years later, I came to think of my relationship to my mind in much the same way: I was like a hapless cowboy strapped to a potent beast of the mind and bound to go in the direction of its choosing, and enduring the inevitable ups and downs of back-cracking bucks.

Mindlessness comes at a very high cost, a cost that I hope you'll agree is too high. To put it in its most general terms, living with a mind that we don't know very well, that is often out of control and semiconscious much of the time, causes us and others to suffer greatly, probably far more than we realize.

The Buddha, an individual who knew the mind far better than most of us, put it this way: "Whatever an enemy might do to an enemy, or a foe to a foe, the ill-directed mind can do to you even worse."

Is it any wonder we so frequently attempt to silence or alter our minds with drugs, amusements, or other forms of distraction? It's probably no coincidence that individuals who choose to end their lives by gunshot almost always put the bullet through their heads.

Fortunately, most of us don't reach this mind-driven point of despair, but we nonetheless endure the consequences of an immensely powerful but unruly mind. We find ourselves entertaining thoughts that serve no wholesome value in our lives. We make snap judgments about individuals based the slimmest and most trivial of evidence. We spin out falsehoods that we ourselves come to believe. We're constantly comparing ourselves to others, a practice that inevitably leads to pain whether we measure up favorably or unfavorably. All of this, and more, drives us to lead frenzied lives, often on the verge of misery.

This sense of dissatisfaction, of which we are more or less conscious at different times in our lives, impels us to find something—anything—to bring relief. Unfortunately, our minds have been conditioned to seek solutions to its torment in the most unhelpful ways. For most of us brought up in the modern West, we look for solace through intoxicating substances and entertainments, incredibly busy lives, over devotion to work, shopping and acquisition, and hours on the Internet. Vast sectors of our entire culture have become refuges for individuals searching for ways to bring contentment to their lives. So far, I have never met a single individual who has professed to find genuine satisfaction in any of these ways. Yet the search rages on.

The beliefs that compel us to keep looking somewhere else for something to bring us relief are so common that we rarely consider that it might be time to try another approach. Rather than seek happiness through the usual ineffective and often counterproductive means, this course will offer you a different way.

Practicing Mindfulness is predicated on the conviction that it is not necessary to live at the mercy of an untamed mind. It's possible to cultivate a wholesome mind that will produce thoughts that contribute to our well-being and the well-being of the whole world. We can actually shape our mental functions in ways that will remove the frantic, driven, distracted, semiconscious qualities from our lives. But it will not be easy.

This conviction is founded on the belief that our minds are malleable realities. They are plastic, and they can be reshaped in ways that we choose. The mind, in other words, is a conditioned phenomenon.

How did our minds get into this sorry state that many of us find them? Perhaps we were born with certain dispositions to act and think in particular ways. Many Hindus, Buddhists, and Jains think that karma—our thoughts, words, and deeds from previous lives—profoundly influences the mental states we have at birth. But you need not accept the theory of rebirth to accept the underlying principle of karma. Essentially, the idea of karma suggests that the way we are now is the consequence of the ways we have thought and acted up to this point. In short, we have been conditioned by ourselves and by others, whether we believe the conditioning process began eons ago in former lifetimes or whether it simply began in this lifetime, at birth or even conception.

The term "conditioning" is a very useful one for describing this process. Think of it in exactly the same way you might think of going to the gym for strength or aerobic conditioning. Each time you lift weights or walk the treadmill, your body responds in a way that makes it slightly easier to manage the same action a few days later. The more you train, the easier these actions become, until they almost seem effortless. Gradually, over time, habitual strength and aerobic conditioning can significantly transform your body. The same process happens with the mind. Habitual thinking significantly determines what we think, feel, and perceive. The more we entertain a particular thought or a particular kind of the thought, the more our minds are prone to generate thoughts of that nature.

The process of mental conditioning is so powerful that it may seem at times that our whole cerebral function is entirely determined by the factors of our biological makeup or our upbringing. But in this course, I take the position that we have a small but extremely important capacity to redirect our minds in ways that allow us to recondition it. Our minds have been considerably influenced, but they are not completely destined by the past.

To put this stance in traditional philosophical terms: We are largely determined but we have a modicum of free will. But free will in this sense is not just a given; it is not a just a feature of our makeup. Free will is something that we must exercise and develop. Without cultivation, we are vulnerable to losing the ability to act and think freely altogether. Ultimately, the goal of this course is to assist you to increase your freedom by practicing it.

This course will be unlike most other courses you've ever taken, in which your mind is deliberately stimulated. Stimulating the mind is valuable for many things, but it is not what this course is about. This course is for people whose minds are over-stimulated and need a respite from too much thinking. As the course title implies, our approach will be eminently practical. We'll be less concerned with theory than practice. In this course, there will be homework and tests, but none of these things will be written. All work will be inscribed by and on your own life. The final grade for the course will be self-assessed, and only you will have access to it. The insights you gain will be principally those you discover on your own.

There will be meditations and other exercises to do. You'll need to carve out a time and place to focus on them. For certain periods of time, you'll have to disregard the TV, the Internet, the telephone, and other distractions. You'll learn to think of the mind not as the center of your personality but as an instrument or tool that you can use for your happiness. Like any instrument, it's essential to learn how to use it properly and to practice using it until the skill becomes second nature. At first, like learning to play the piano or violin, rehearsing the motions will seem awkward and wooden. Over time, the artificiality of the practice will dissipate.

Beginning with the next lecture, I'll introduce you to the concept of mindfulness. I'll tell you more about what mindfulness is and the sorts of benefits and advantages it confers. Then I'll tell you about the basic procedures for becoming more attentive to your mind and for redirecting your attention in ways that will engage you more fully with your life. I hope to remove any aura of exoticism or strangeness about these methods. They are nothing extraordinary. They are skills that anyone can develop. We'll discuss the simplest aspects of living: breathing, sensing, feeling, eating, walking, and standing. When we've covered the fundamental aspects of mindfulness practice, we'll work on more challenging things: cultivating compassion for ourselves and others, developing a life of generosity, accepting our mortality, and coping with physical pain, grief, and anger. We'll talk about how to be more mindful of your speech, your work, and even your driving.

I cannot promise that listening to this course will make you happy or will improve the quality of your life. Whether or not it does is entirely up to you. I can say that throughout the ages, individuals who have seriously employed the very methods that we'll discuss have claimed to have discovered something deep and enriching by using them.

The Buddha, who warned us earlier of the tremendously harmful potential of the undisciplined mind, also proclaimed the tremendous benefits of a mind well trained: "Whatever a mother, father, or other relative might do for you, the well-directed mind can do for you even better."

Mindfulness—The Power of Awareness
Lecture 2

Mindfulness can be defined in a variety of ways, but virtually all definitions understand it as a particular kind of awareness. At its most basic level, mindfulness is a deliberate way of paying attention to what is occurring within oneself as it is happening. Mindfulness is more than just awareness, however; it is paying attention without judgment or evaluation. In recent years, mindfulness has become an especially prominent concept in contemporary psychology and medicine, where it is frequently used in connection with stress reduction and wellness.

Mindfulness and Awareness

- Most of the time, most of us exist in mindlessness, a state of semiawareness governed by habit and inattention. Mindlessness causes us to suffer—probably more than we're even aware. This ordinary mental condition is not inevitable; there is a cure for it, and it's called mindfulness, a skill that anyone can learn.

- **Mindfulness** is moment-by-moment awareness; it is the process of attentively observing your experience as it unfolds. Mindfulness allows us to become keen observers of ourselves and gradually transform the way our minds operate. With sustained practice, mindfulness can make us more attentive to our experience and less captive to the whims that drive our minds around.

- The process of mindfulness is devoid of the constant comparing and assessing that ordinarily occupies our mental functioning. When we're being mindful, we are simply being mentally alert without the overlay of our usual commentary and conceptualizing.

- Because we're not judging our experiences as right or wrong or good or bad, mindfulness is also characterized by a high degree of openness, receptivity, and inquisitiveness. With this open and attentive attitude, we're able to perceive ourselves more clearly, observing the dynamics and details that often escape our notice.

- Mindfulness is not about removing thoughts from our minds—even judgmental thoughts. It is about knowing when we're thinking and recognizing thoughts as momentary events that float through our minds.

- Because mindfulness is based on the universal human faculty of awareness, we've all had experiences very close to mindfulness. Try to recall some time in your in life when you felt especially attentive, perhaps so rapt that your usual internal dialogue was suspended as you became fully present to your experience.

- For example, people often report a heightened sense of awareness whenever their lives are endangered. The perception of slowed time in these instances is related to the sharpening of one's conscious activity as the mind marshals its resources to prevent itself from perishing. The lucid memories of these occasions are based on the same heightened awareness that characterizes mindfulness.

- When we practice mindfulness, we are doing so deliberately. We are taking the same mental functioning found within extraordinary experiences and purposefully developing and applying it to our ordinary lives. In short, we are taking a natural capacity that we usually use only on special occasions and extending its usage to every aspect of our existence.

Mindfulness and Religion

- Because it is innate to human beings, the power of mindfulness has been available to us for tens of thousands of years—but the concept of mindfulness is more recent. The historical evidence suggests that mindfulness was first widely taught 2,500 years ago by the individual known today as the Buddha.

- In his teachings, the Buddha spoke extensively of *sati*, a special form of heightened awareness that promoted the end of suffering and fostered happiness and well-being for all. *Sati* is the Buddha's word that we now translate into English as "mindfulness." According to the Buddha's teachings, mindfulness is essential to eliminating delusion and seeing the world and ourselves as they truly are.

- Although Buddhism has devoted more energy to the study and practice of mindfulness than any other religion, every major religious tradition prescribes something akin to it. These practices are not always as prominent in other religions as they are in Buddhism, but they can often be found within a religion's contemplative and esoteric dimensions.

- Mindfulness is not a discipline that is limited to religion. Forms of mindfulness practice can be found in many schools of secular philosophy in both the East and West.

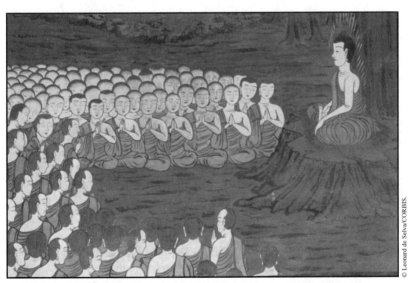

Historical evidence suggests that mindfulness was first widely taught 2,500 years ago by the Buddha.

- In Buddhism, mindfulness is a component of the **Eightfold Path** that leads to enlightenment and freedom from the cycle of continual rebirth. Mindfulness thus serves the purpose of advancing one's quest for **nirvana**.

- In the Christian traditions, mindfulness is often understood to bring one closer to God and to a life of greater holiness, but it has never been regarded as essential to salvation because Christianity grounds redemption on belief and doctrine.

- In Hinduism, mindfulness is said to peel away the many layers of illusion that veil our clear perception of the ultimate reality.

- In Confucianism, mindfulness is part of moral self-cultivation, the regimen that enables individuals to realize their full humanity.

- In all traditions, mindfulness is seen a means to transform one's life in meaningful and wholesome ways.

Benefits of Mindfulness

- One does not need to regard mindfulness in metaphysical categories to find it an extremely beneficial practice. Without discounting the religious and theological interpretations, it is possible to spell out the very pragmatic value of mindfulness for living a more vital and happier life.

- The chief goal of mindfulness, as its definition implies, is increased awareness. Its other benefits, while considerable and of immense value, are essentially of secondary importance. In other words, everything else you might gain from a mindfulness practice depends on strengthening your faculty of awareness.

- Although it is used for these purposes, mindfulness is not fundamentally about relaxation, stress reduction, or even self-improvement. It is about knowing yourself and your world better and more clearly—the kind of knowing that comes only with experience, with seeing things for yourself.

- With mindfulness, you can see how your mind operates and responds to its world. Because mindfulness requires us to focus attention on what is happening within ourselves and our environment as it is occurring, you can be consciously present for your life.

- We learn in the mindfulness disciplines that there is a lot in the world over which we have no control. Mindfulness teaches this fact not as an abstract idea to which we give assent, but as a concrete and clearly demonstrated reality. At the same time, mindfulness teaches that one of the things that we can change is the operation of our own minds.

- Ordinarily, our responses to the elements of life that are out of our control are determined by our conditioning. We tend to act out of habit—without much thought—unaware that we can be more deliberate about the way we allow events beyond our power to affect us.

- Practicing mindfulness can give us a mental spaciousness that offers us greater freedom to shape the kind of person we will become. Mental spaciousness is of immense value in helping us manage the seemingly incessant colloquy of judgments and commentary that constitutes the mindless state. It allows us to recognize the patterns of thinking that are detrimental to the well-being of ourselves and others and enables us to relinquish them and render them harmless.

- Likewise, mindfulness helps us work with difficult emotional states such as anger, greed, and fear, providing us with the resources to act on these states in ways that are beneficial rather than damaging. With dedicated practice you can really learn to handle your anger effectively, to want less, and to be courageous and compassionate.

Mindfulness and Health

- Mindfulness is not only about the mind; it is an invaluable tool in helping us cope with our bodies. Medical science in the last quarter century has amassed an impressive collection of evidence that conclusively demonstrates that mindfulness practice has a salutary effect on health.

- One study recently presented to the American Heart Association showed that patients who practiced mindfulness regularly reduced by half their risk of heart attacks, strokes, and death from all causes as compared with similar patients who were only given education about healthy living and diet.

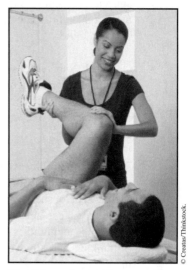

- In addition, a recent meta-analysis—a study of the scientific quality of these studies of mindfulness—concluded that the proposition that mindfulness practices are beneficial to health is a legitimate and empirically verifiable claim.

- Although it is clear that mindfulness offers valuable and even amazing contributions to our physical and psychological well-being,

Mindfulness is used in connection with stress reduction and wellness in contemporary medicine.

it is still unable to stave off the inevitable demise of our bodies. No matter how healthy we have been, each of us will die, and the practice of mindfulness cannot change that reality.

- Mindfulness can help us accept the reality of death and prepare us for the moment when we draw our last breath. One of the essential lessons these practices reveal to us is that life is ephemeral, and denying that only causes great suffering and unhappiness. Genuinely accepting the impermanence of life, however, is liberating and allows us to be happy.

- Just as we learn to accept the loss of our bodies to death, mindfulness practice helps us to accept the loss of everything. Life is such that every one of us must bear a tremendous measure of grief. Mindfulness teaches us to prepare for the inevitability of death and to accept it—not with stoic resignation, but with joy and contentment.

- The acceptance of loss actually helps us relax and be less anxious. The majority of our actions suggest that we believe acquiring and holding on to the people and things that give us pleasure will put our lives at ease. However, it is only by relinquishing our attachment to everything we think will make us happy that we can actually be happy. Mindfulness allows us to see this truth and empowers us to act on it.

Important Terms

Eightfold Path: In Buddhism, mindfulness is a component of this path, which leads to enlightenment and freedom from the cycle of continual rebirth.

mindfulness: The process of attentively observing an experience as it unfolds in a moment-by-moment awareness; it is devoid of the constant comparing and assessing that ordinarily occupies our mental functioning.

nirvana: A state of bliss; in Buddhism, it transcends suffering and karma.

sati: A special form of heightened awareness that promotes the end of suffering and fosteres happiness and well-being for all; it is the Buddha's word that is translated into English as "mindfulness."

1. Can you recall moments in which you have become fully aware of your ordinary experience without the imposition of judgments or other thoughts?

2. Try to notice the times when you suddenly become aware of what is going on around you. It may feel as if you have been pulled out of a dream into a wakening moment.

3. How could mindfulness training help you as an individual? How would you expect mindfulness to help you the most in your life?

Lecture 2: Mindfulness—The Power of Awareness

Mindfulness—The Power of Awareness
Lecture 2—Transcript

Most of the time, most of us exist in mindlessness, a state of semi-awareness governed by habit and inattention. Mindlessness causes us to suffer, probably more than we're even aware.

The good news is that this ordinary mental condition is not inevitable. There is a cure for it, and it's called mindfulness, a skill that anyone can learn. Mindfulness allows us to become keen observers of ourselves and gradually transform the way our minds operate. With sustained practice, mindfulness can make us more attentive to our experience and less captive to the whims that drive our minds to and fro.

Mindfulness can be defined in a variety of ways, but virtually all definitions understand it as a particular kind of awareness. At its most basic level, mindfulness is a deliberate way of paying attention to what is occurring within oneself as it is happening. Mindfulness is moment-by-moment awareness. It is the process of attentively observing your experience as it unfolds. Mindfulness is more than just awareness, however; it is paying attention without judgment or evaluation. The process of mindfulness is devoid of the constant comparing and assessing that ordinarily occupies our mental functioning. When we're being mindful, we are simply being mentally alert, without the overlay of our usual commentary and conceptualizing. Because we're not judging our experiences as right or wrong or good or bad, mindfulness is also characterized by a high degree of openness, receptivity, and inquisitiveness. With this open and attentive attitude, we're able to perceive ourselves more clearly, observing the dynamics and details that often escape our notice.

Of course, defining and describing mindfulness is one thing; but knowing it by experience is another. To give you a taste of this experience, I now invite you to participate in a short exercise. There is nothing you need to do to prepare. Just close your eyes and follow my directions. Try to become a dispassionate observer of your own experience, noticing what is occurring to you in each moment as it passes by. Do nothing more than observe. Now, direct your attention to the sound of my voice. Focus on the sensation of hearing. Concentrate your awareness on your experience of what you hear. Notice the various qualities of that sensation. Be aware of the tonal fluctuations that you perceive. Observe how the pitch of my voice rises and falls and rises again. Listen to the variations of volume as my voice gets quieter and then louder. Attend to the moments when my voice goes silent and when it begins again. Now, open your eyes and reflect on your responses.

Were you able to be fully attentive to the sensation of hearing? If you were, you were being mindful. If you were thinking about this experience, or something else, and you got lost in your thoughts, you defaulted to mindlessness. If you started evaluating the character of my voice or this exercise, you slipped back into mindlessness. If you thought, "People with southern accents sound like bumpkins," you were being mindless. If you thought, "This experiment is a total waste of time," you were being mindless. If, however, you were aware that you were thinking "People with southern accents sound like bumpkins," and you were able to recognize that as merely a passing thought, you were being mindful. If you continued on and thought, "It's bad of me to judge people with southern accents so negatively," you were being mindless again. If you simply thought, "I'm judging myself for judging people with southern accents," you were being mindful again.

This exercise should provide you with a sense of what the experience of mindfulness is like. It is directing and maintaining non-judgmental attention to the experience of our bodies and minds in the present moment. It's not about removing thoughts from our minds—even judgmental thoughts. It is about knowing when we're thinking and recognizing thoughts as momentary events that float through our minds like clouds through the sky.

Because mindfulness is based on the universal human faculty of awareness, we've all had experiences very close to mindfulness. Try to recall some time in your in life when you felt especially attentive, perhaps so rapt that your usual internal dialogue was simply suspended as you became fully present to your experience.

Perhaps the most outstanding instance of such an experience in my own recollection came at the birth of my daughter. I remember with great clarity the moment she was placed in my arms in the delivery room and how, just a few minutes later, she opened her eyes for the first time, looking up at me as I held her. My attentiveness in that instant was as sharp as a razor, as I gazed upon her eyes and observed her every feature with intense curiosity and openness. In that moment, the usual chatter in my head became silent, and I became completely aware of the presence of this new being. Of course, the chatter returned eventually, and the serenity of the moment soon yielded to the anxieties that come with being a parent. In that brief expanse of time, however, my entire being, it seemed, was wholly present to the experience.

Experiences similar to this one are not uncommon in our everyday lives. For example, people often report a heightened sense of awareness whenever their lives are endangered. If you have ever been in a car accident, you may have had the widely known phenomenon of observing events in slow-motion. The perception of slowed time in these instances is related to the sharpening of one's conscious activity as the mind marshals its resources to prevent itself from perishing. If you've never had a life-threatening experience, imagine finding yourself trying to walk across a frozen lake when you suddenly discover yourself on thin ice. Think how attentive you'd become to every aspect of your experience as you try carefully to negotiate your way back to safety. Or recall an instance when you received some bad news. You may be able to remember the experience with great vividness. People often talk in dramatic detail about where they were and what they were doing when they first heard of the assassination of President Kennedy or of 9/11. The lucid memories of these occasions are based on the same heightened awareness that characterizes mindfulness.

What distinguishes these several examples from mindfulness is only the quality of intention. In each of the instances I mentioned, the onset of focused awareness was provoked by external circumstances. When we practice mindfulness, however, we are doing so deliberately. We are taking the same mental functioning found within these extraordinary experiences and purposefully developing and applying it to our ordinary lives. In short, we are taking a natural capacity that we usually use only on special occasions and extending its usage to every aspect of our existence.

Because it is innate to human beings, the power of mindfulness has been available to us for tens of thousands of years. But the concept of mindfulness is more recent. The historical evidence suggests that mindfulness was first taught 2,500 years ago by the individual known today as the Buddha.

In his teachings, the Buddha spoke extensively of *sati*, a specialized form of heightened awareness that promoted the end of suffering and fostered happiness and well-being for all. *Sati* is the Buddha's word that we now translate into English as "mindfulness." According to the Buddha's teachings, mindfulness is essential to eliminating delusion and seeing the world and ourselves as they truly are.

Although Buddhism has devoted more energy to the study and practice of mindfulness than any other religion, every major religious tradition prescribes something akin to it. These practices are not always as prominent in other religions as they are in Buddhism, but they can be found, often within a religion's contemplative and esoteric dimensions. Yet, mindfulness is not a discipline that is limited to religion. Forms of mindfulness practice can be found in many schools of secular philosophy in both the East and West. In recent years, mindfulness has also become an especially prominent concept in contemporary psychology and medicine, where it is frequently used in connection with stress reduction and wellness. As I enjoy telling my psychologist-friends, it is gratifying to see that modern science is finally catching up with the Buddha!

Because of the prominence of mindfulness in the Buddhist tradition, many of the resources for this course come from Buddhism. But our reliance on these resources should not obscure the fact that mindfulness disciplines are found in a wide array of religious, philosophical, and psychological traditions, and, wherever it is appropriate, I will draw attention to these other schools and worldviews and use the resources they make available to us. Let me emphasize that nothing in this course presumes or requires Buddhist belief— or religious belief of any sort. Mindfulness is a non-sectarian practice and has little to do with belief, although it has much to do with how we relate to our beliefs.

Because it requires dedicated work, we may well ask ourselves, "Is mindfulness worth the effort? What is the great value in seeking such a high degree of consciousness? Why should we want to become observers of our experiences and refrain from judging and assessing them? Where does mindfulness get us?" Such questions are especially relevant in a world that demands so much of our time and energy.

The traditional answers to these questions have usually depended on the worldview or philosophical perspective under which mindfulness practices have been pursued. In Buddhism, mindfulness is a component of the Eightfold Noble Path that leads to enlightenment and freedom from the cycle of continual rebirth. Mindfulness thus serves the purpose of advancing one's quest for nirvana. In the Christian traditions, the practice is often understood to bring one closer to God and to a life of greater holiness, but it has never been regarded as essential to salvation, since Christianity grounds redemption on belief and doctrine. In Hinduism, it is said to peel away the layers of illusion that veil our clear perception of the ultimate reality. In Confucianism, mindfulness is part of a moral self-cultivation, the regimen that enables individuals to realize their full humanity. In all traditions, it is seen a means to transform one's life in meaningful and wholesome ways.

But one need not regard mindfulness in metaphysical categories to find it an extremely beneficial practice. Without in any way discounting the religious and theological interpretations, it is possible to spell out the very pragmatic value of mindfulness for living a more vital and happier life. The list of benefits is extensive, and there is no way to mention all of them. But even an abbreviated outline should suffice to convince virtually anyone of the tremendous value of a mindfulness practice.

The chief goal of mindfulness, as its very definition implies, is increased awareness. Its other benefits, while considerable and of immense value, are essentially of secondary importance. To put that in a different way, all else you might gain from a mindfulness practice depends upon strengthening your faculty of awareness.

Although it is used for these purposes, mindfulness is not fundamentally about relaxation, stress reduction, or even self-improvement. It is about knowing yourself and your world better and more clearly. The knowledge we speak of is not the abstract conceptual kind that we can discover in books or conversation. It is the kind of knowing that comes only with experience, with seeing things for yourself. With mindfulness, you can see how your mind operates and responds to its world. Mindfulness practice is a way to fulfill the ancient Greek maxim, "Know thyself."

Because mindfulness requires us to focus attention on what is happening within ourselves and our environment as it is occurring, you can be consciously present for your life. As we observed in the first lecture, we spend much of our lives in a semi-conscious state, dwelling on some triviality, planning the future, or reviewing the past. Too often, we live according to habit and routine without making conscious choices about our lives. For me, it would be tragic to come to the end of my days and realize that for most of them, I simply wasn't there. If that image troubles you like it does me, you might discover that a mindfulness practice will offer you a way to show up for your own existence.

We learn in the mindfulness disciplines that there is a lot in world over which we have no control. Mindfulness teaches this fact not as an abstract idea to which we give assent, but as a concrete and clearly demonstrated reality. At the same time, mindfulness teaches that one of the things that we can change is the operation of our own minds. I cannot stop from getting old or from dying; I cannot control what you think of me; I can't change the past that has shaped who I have become. But I can choose how I will respond to getting old and to your opinion of me; I can decide how my past will influence the person I am now and will be in the future. Ordinarily, our responses to the elements of life that are out of our control are determined by our conditioning. They are not so much responses as they are knee-jerk reactions and reflexes. We tend to act out of habit, without much thought, unaware that we can be more deliberate about the way we allow events beyond our power to affect us. Practicing mindfulness can give us a mental spaciousness that offers us greater freedom to shape the kind of person we will become.

Let me offer a personal example of what I mean by mental spaciousness. Some time ago, one of my former students asked me to conduct her wedding ceremony, which of course I was delighted to do. It was a beautiful summer day in the hills of east Tennessee. The wedding was to take place outdoors, overlooking a gorgeous panoramic view. It was late afternoon, as the sun was approaching the horizon. The bride and groom looked lovely, and I was feeling great, thinking I was looking pretty lovely myself. Everything was perfect. Just as I was beginning the recitation of the vows, a bee that had been buzzing around this idyllic setting landed on my cheek and proceeded to crawl up to the space between my eye and glasses. In that moment, my years of mindfulness practice paid some dividends. Resisting the impulse to freak out and disrupt this elegant occasion, I made myself the observer of my own experience. I didn't flinch; I didn't panic.

As I continued with the service, I kept aware of this insect exploring the area surrounding my eye. I had the presence of mind to realize that if I made some sudden motion to shoo it away, I would likely get stung and upset the ceremony with some ugly form of dancing. I also knew that my greatest chance to survive this event with dignity would be to do nothing, and so I did. The little bee hung around until the bride and groom exchanged their vows and then, to my great relief, flew off to enjoy the rest of its day. I acted just like a Buddha—up to the moment of the bee's departure. If I had been a fully realized being, I wouldn't have reacted with such tremendous relief; a Buddha would have responded with equanimity to both a departure and a sting. But for a few brief, shining moments, my mind was like that of a Buddha.

This same mental spaciousness is of immense value in helping us manage the seemingly incessant colloquy of judgments and commentary that constitutes the mindless state. It allows us to recognize the patterns of thinking that are detrimental to the well-being of ourselves and others and enables us to relinquish them and render them harmless.

Likewise, mindfulness helps us work with difficult emotional states such as anger, greed, and fear, providing us with the resources to act on these states in ways that are beneficial rather than damaging. With dedicated practice you can really learn to handle your anger effectively, to want less, and to be courageous. You can become more compassionate towards others and learn to be a true friend.

Mindfulness is not only about the mind; it is an invaluable tool in helping us cope with our bodies. Medical science in the last quarter century has amassed an impressive collection of evidence that conclusively demonstrates that mindfulness practice has a salutary effect on health. Limitations of time prevent me from enumerating all of these studies, so I'll just mention only a few.

One study recently presented to the American Heart Association showed that patients who practiced mindfulness regularly reduced by half their risk of heart attacks, strokes, and death from all causes as compared with similar patients who were only given education about healthy living and diet. The same study concluded that practitioners of mindfulness significantly reduced their blood pressure and were able to remain free from disease longer than those who did not practice. Other research indicates that practicing mindfulness, along with physical exercise and better diet, can actually reverse certain deleterious heart conditions. Mindfulness practice has also been demonstrated to reduce fatigue, pain, and depression among persons with psoriasis, multiple sclerosis, and breast and other cancers. Patients with chronic asthma have learned to breathe easier using mindfulness techniques.

One study showed that the recurrence rate for patients who had experienced three or more bouts of depression was reduced by half through a routine of mindfulness meditation. Researchers at the University of New Mexico found that participation in a similar mindfulness routine helped decrease anxiety and binge eating. A prison that offers mindfulness training for inmates found that those who completed the course showed lower levels of drug use, greater optimism, and better self-control. There is evidence indicating that mindfulness improves the memory, enhances learning, and lessens the incidence of accidents in the home. Some insurance companies have now begun to offer mindfulness CDs to individuals about to undergo surgery, because they have discovered that recovery time was quicker and less expensive by using mindfulness meditation to aid in healing. Finally, a recent meta-analysis—a study of the scientific quality of these studies of meditation—concluded that the proposition that mindfulness practices are beneficial to health is a legitimate and empirically verifiable claim.

Although the evidence is clear that mindfulness offers valuable and even amazing contributions to our physical and psychological well-being, it is still unable to stave off the inevitable demise of our bodies. No matter how healthy we have been, each of us will die, and the practice of mindfulness cannot change that reality. But mindfulness can help us accept the fact and prepare us for the moment when we draw our last breath. One of the essential lessons these practices reveal to us is that life is ephemeral and denying that only causes great suffering and unhappiness. Genuinely accepting the impermanence of life, however, is liberating and allows us to be happy.

Just as we learn to accept the loss of our bodies to death, mindfulness practice helps us to accept the loss of everything. Life is such that every one of us must bear a tremendous measure of grief. In the end, we will be separated from everything we have ever held dear. Throughout our lives, we have to say goodbye to loved ones, to cherished possessions, to our dreams and hopes. Mindfulness teaches us to prepare for that inevitability and to accept it, not with stoic resignation, but with joy and contentment.

It may seem ironic, but the acceptance of loss actually helps us to relax and be less anxious. I say ironic because this idea flies in the face of the way most of us live our lives. The majority of our actions suggest that we believe acquiring and holding on to the persons and things that give us pleasure will put our lives at ease. The irony is that the opposite is true; it is only by relinquishing our attachment to everything we think will make us happy that we can actually be happy. Mindfulness allows us to see this truth and empowers us to act on it.

Much of what I've said in this lecture may sound too good to be true, and I wouldn't be surprised if you greet my claims about the benefits of mindfulness with a healthy dose of skepticism.

In fact, I hope you do. A skeptical attitude was precisely what the Buddha encouraged among his would-be followers. He insisted that they take nothing he said on his authority but test out his teachings on their own. "Ehi passiko," he told them. "Go and see for yourself." Throughout the remainder of the course, this is exactly what we will do.

Expectations—Relinquishing Preconceptions
Lecture 3

Mindfulness is a function of our mental faculties that we all use to a small degree in our everyday life. Our objective in this course is to understand that function better and learn to develop it so that we are able to use it to a greater extent throughout every aspect of our existence. For millennia, individuals throughout the world have been studying mindfulness and cultivating ways to refine its usage, and we'll be relying on their wisdom to guide us.

Mindfulness and Meditation

- The principal instrument for strengthening our capacity for mindfulness is a practice widely known as meditation. Mindfulness and meditation are not synonymous terms, but they appear together so frequently in print and in discourse that one might easily think they were.

- Mindfulness refers to the power of our minds to give close, nonjudgmental attention to our experience as it unfolds. **Meditation** refers to certain exercises that can be used to enlarge and refine mindfulness. Not all forms of meditation, however, intend to cultivate mindfulness.

- Some meditative practices are oriented toward generating transcendent experiences, achieving a trance state, or gaining extraordinary powers, but the particular types of meditation we'll discuss in this course are practices whose central purpose is to make us more mindful.

- Meditation helps us become more mindful by providing us with specific ways to train our awareness. In this sense, meditation gives us a particular context in which to work at putting our minds in better condition.

- Some of the ideas people have about meditation may fit other forms of the disciplines that go by that name, but they may not be correct for mindfulness meditation. Therefore, whatever preconceived ideas you may have about this practice, begin to relinquish them—another exercise in mindfulness.

Preconceptions about Meditation

It's Not Just Thinking

- Meditation usually suggests a form of deep thinking, the kind of mental activity associated with taking a thought or a problem and intensely reflecting on it—mulling it over in the mind.

- This kind of deliberate thought process is a very important mental activity, but it is not the kind of discipline that helps develop mindfulness. In fact, it is quite possible to ruminate or think over an idea without being mindful. Awareness and thinking are two different mental functions.

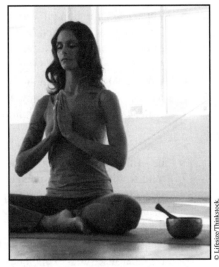

- Interestingly, the tradition on which mindfulness practice is founded does not use the term

Practices like meditation and yoga are rapidly becoming a part of our cultural mainstream.

meditation. Buddhism calls this practice *bhavana*, which is most accurately translated as "cultivation." *Bhavana* does not mean deep thinking but, rather, the awareness and discipline that allow one to shape the mind in ways conducive to happiness and well-being.

- When the Buddha chose this word for the practices that enhance mindfulness, he was selecting an ordinary agricultural metaphor, an image deeply resonant with the common people of his day. He was comparing the process of developing the mind to the way that farmers prepare and care for the land to produce a rich, nourishing crop.

It's Not Exotic

- Meditation is not exotic, at least not in the way that we will study and practice it. Given its early associations with Hindu gurus and Buddhist monks, many in the Western world have come to regard meditation practice as rather strange and foreign.

- For some, the aura of exoticism exerts a compelling attraction. They become interested in meditation precisely because it smacks of the unusual, the mystical, and the esoteric.

- Others, however, might find the aura of exoticism repellant. We have an ingrained tendency to view different practices and beliefs with suspicion, if not outright fear.

- The "other"—as philosophers call people and things different from us—often threatens our sense of identity and security; hence, we tend to discount or disparage the other. Although meditation and yoga are rapidly becoming a part of our cultural mainstream, for many, meditation still retains a sense of otherness.

- Those who are attracted to meditation and those who are repulsed by it because of its exotic quality are both mistaken. Meditation, at least mindfulness meditation, is profoundly ordinary; there is really nothing extraordinary or strange about it.

- If you take up meditation because you think it is exotic or because you want to be pious and deepen your spirituality, your attraction to meditation may simply arise from the ego—the desire to appear other than you actually are.

- It is perfectly fine to begin a mindfulness practice because it seems exotic or because it serves your ego needs in some way. Ultimately, it does not matter why you start, but for mindfulness practice to become truly constructive in your life, your initial motives will have to be relinquished.

It's Not an Extraordinary Experience

- Like the attraction to its exotic trappings, some people take up meditation because they seek certain extraordinary experiences or altered states of consciousness. Again, such motivations are fine at the start, but for mindfulness meditation, they will need to be eventually given up.

- Mindfulness is not about having unusual or transcendent experiences. Strange, fascinating, and mysterious experiences may, in fact, occur while you are meditating; with meditation, it is possible to have any kind of experience imaginable.

- Particular kinds of experiences are not the goal of meditating. Rather, we are seeking to develop a way to relate to all of our experiences, regardless of their quality or content.

It's Not Easy or Fast

- Today especially, many people become interested in meditation because they are attracted to the possibility of reducing the stress in their lives and becoming a more relaxed person. Like beginning meditation to serve one's ego needs, starting a practice to relax and become calmer is perfectly fine.

- Although greater serenity is indeed one of the results of meditation, tranquility is often not realized early in the practice. Consequently, many people have disappointing experiences with their first encounters with meditation. For the vast majority of practitioners, meditation is not easy and its benefits are not quickly realized.

- It makes sense that many people show up to learn meditation thinking that it will be a swift solution to their problems. We live in an impatient culture that has come to expect quick fixes. Mindfulness meditation can teach us to be more patient, but we have to be patient to learn that lesson.

- Particularly in the beginning stages, meditating can also be very difficult. Most of us are not accustomed to sitting still for very long. In addition, being alone with your thoughts can be terrifying, which is why many people avoid it at all costs. Stored in that awesome brain are many dreadful things, as you well know.

It's Not an Escape from Reality

- Some people consider meditation to be an escape from reality, but this is another common misconception. Given its bold intention to attend unflinchingly to all of our experiences without judgment, it is more precise to call mindfulness meditation an escape into reality.

- From the perspective of mindfulness, our lives as we ordinarily live them seem profoundly out of touch with what is real. Few people appear to live in accord with what seem to be sobering truths—that death will overtake us all, that the world is in constant change, that suffering is pervasive.

- Instead, what seem to be escapes from reality include such activities as racing about in hot pursuit of trivial successes, possessions, and pleasures; working and amusing ourselves to death; and filling our minds with useless junk.

It's Not Self-Centered

- Just as meditation has sometimes been criticized as escapist, it has also been charged with being self-centered. The expression "navel-gazing" has entered the English language as a term to refer to both meditation and egotism. In the view of some, both are forms of self-absorption.

- While the practice of mindfulness meditation no doubt begins with turning inward toward one's own experience, the sharp distinction between self and world gradually begins to fade.

- A mindfulness practice reveals the intricate ways our lives are intertwined with one another. As a consequence, meditation begins to awaken our empathy and helps develop our natural sense of compassion.

- In the Buddhist tradition, compassion and wisdom are twin virtues, and both are cultivated by the practice of meditation. It is not possible to have true wisdom without genuine compassion, and vice versa.

- To be wise is to see things clearly—without delusion. Wisdom thus means to recognize the interdependence of our life with the lives of others, and seeing our interdependence with others evokes our compassion. Therefore, a meditation practice that produces only self-satisfaction is not a genuine mindfulness practice.

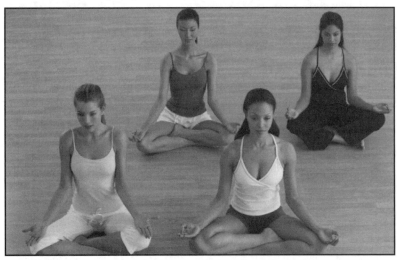

Mindfulness practice is not as easy as it is portrayed to be on the covers of yoga magazines.

It's Not a Success-or-Failure Practice

- Conventional ideas of success and failure may also need to be abandoned when you take up meditation. In fact, you'll probably discover that you have a hard time figuring out what you need to do with your body, how to focus your attention, and what do with your mind. When you're unable to follow the instructions exactly, you may be tempted to judge your effort as a failure—but that would be a mistake.

- In meditation practice, you fail only when you do not pay attention, but even failing to pay attention is not a failure if you realize you're not paying attention. Eventually, you'll see that you cannot fail at meditation, if you just do it. By the same token, you'll see that you cannot succeed at it either.

- Meditation practice is an activity that is best approached with an openness of mind and sincerity of heart. If you can't muster openness and sincerity, that's fine—meditation can teach you that as well.

Important Terms

bhavana: Most accurately translated as "cultivation," this is what Buddhism calls meditation. It does not mean deep thinking but, rather, the awareness and discipline that allow one to shape the mind in ways conducive to happiness and well-being.

meditation: Refers to certain exercises that can be used to enlarge and refine mindfulness. Not all forms of meditation, however, intend to cultivate mindfulness.

1. What preconceptions do you bring to the practice of meditation? Why is it important to relinquish both positive and negative ideas about meditation?

2. Meditation has appeared throughout history in different forms. In your particular faith, philosophy, or practice, is meditation—or something like it—encouraged?

Expectations—Relinquishing Preconceptions
Lecture 3—Transcript

Mindfulness is a function of our mental faculties that we all use to a small degree in our everyday life.

Our objective in this course is to better understand that function better and learn to develop it so that we are able to use it to a greater extent throughout every aspect of our existence. For millennia, individuals throughout the world have been studying mindfulness and cultivating ways to refine its usage. We'll be relying on their wisdom to guide us.

The principal instrument for understanding and strengthening our capacity for mindfulness is a practice widely known as meditation. Mindfulness and meditation are not synonymous terms, although they appear together so frequently in print and discourse that one might easily think they were. Mindfulness refers to the power of our minds to give close, non-judgmental attention to our experience as it unfolds. Meditation refers to certain exercises that can be used to enlarge and refine mindfulness. Not all forms of meditation, however, intend to cultivate mindfulness. Some meditative practices are oriented toward generating transcendent experiences, achieving a trance state, or gaining extraordinary powers. But the particular types of meditation we'll discuss in this course are practices whose central purpose is to make us more mindful. Meditation helps us become more mindful by providing us with specific ways to train our awareness. In this sense, meditation does for mindfulness what going to the gym does for our physical well-being: It us gives a particular context in which to work at putting our minds in better condition. Think of mindfulness meditation as a treadmill for your mind.

In later installments of this series, we will go into great detail about the features of this discipline. But before we begin to explore how it is done, I must say a few words about what mindfulness meditation is not. Since the 1960s, meditation has become somewhat familiar to Westerners. People have a great many ideas about what it is, and many of those preconceptions are not accurate for the practice we'll be studying in this course. Some of the ideas people have about meditation may fit other forms of disciplines that go by that name, but they may not be correct for mindfulness meditation. It's a good idea, therefore, to relax our expectations about meditation. Whatever preconceived ideas you may have about this practice, I ask you to begin to relinquish them. This in fact will be another exercise in mindfulness, for much of mindfulness is becoming aware of the contents of the mind and then letting them go. Relinquishment will be a word you'll hear a lot throughout this series.

To assist in relinquishing our preconceptions about meditation, let's spend some time discussing some of the common ideas many people have about this discipline. Then once we've cleared the ground a bit, I'll begin the more difficult job of describing and demonstrating what mindfulness meditation actually is.

Let's start with the word itself: "Meditation" is an unfortunate choice of terms to designate the kinds of activities we'll study in this course, but because the word is so widely used, we're probably stuck with it. Because it's an unfortunate word, meditation usually suggests a form of deep thinking, the kind of mental activity associated with words like rumination and contemplation.

Such expressions suggest that one takes a thought or a problem and intensely reflects on it, mulling it over in the mind. This kind of deliberate thought process is a very important mental activity, but it is not the kind of discipline that helps develop mindfulness. It is useful for finding solutions and gaining certain insights, but it is not especially valuable in helping us see how the mind itself operates and how best to encourage the mind to function in a more wholesome way. In fact it is quite possible to ruminate, or think over an idea, without being mindful. Awareness and thinking are two different mental functions.

Interestingly, the tradition on which mindfulness practice is founded does not use the term meditation. Buddhism calls this practice *bhavana*, which is most accurately translated as "cultivation." Bhavana does not mean deep thinking, but rather the awareness and discipline that allow one to shape the mind in ways conducive to happiness and well-being. Bhavana is less about thinking intensely than creating the type of mind that provides fertile ground from which skillful thinking arises. When the Buddha chose this word for the practices that enhance mindfulness, he was selecting an ordinary agricultural metaphor, an image deeply resonant with the common people of his day. He was comparing the process of developing the mind to the way that farmers prepare and care for the earth to produce a rich, nourishing crop.

As we proceed, this distinction between contemplation and cultivation will become clearer. For now, I invite you simply to ruminate on this thought: Meditation is not what you think.

Here is another thing that meditation isn't—at least not in the way we will study and practice it here. It is not exotic. Given its early associations with Hindu gurus and Buddhist monks, many in the Western world have come to regard meditation practice as rather strange and foreign. For some, the aura of exoticism exerts a compelling attraction. They become interested in meditation precisely because it smacks of the unusual, the mystical, the esoteric. My first interest in meditation, at the age of 16, was precisely of this sort. As an adolescent trying to establish a sense of identity by distinguishing myself from my parents and peers, meditation was perfect. It wasn't illegal or dangerous like drugs; it fit my pensive, introspective inclinations; and it made me appear deep and thoughtful. Even though it was the early '70s, there were not many meditators in my conservative hometown, so it helped me stand out from the crowd. In short, it was ideally suited to shore up my ego. Unlike my youthful self, however, others might find the aura of exoticism repellant. We have an ingrained tendency to view different practices and beliefs with suspicion, if not outright fear. The "other"—as philosophers call people and things different from us—often threatens our sense of identity and security; hence, we tend to discount or disparage the other. Although practices like meditation and yoga are rapidly becoming a part of our cultural mainstream, for many, meditation still retains that sense of otherness.

Yet those who are attracted to meditation and those who are repulsed by it because of its exotic quality are both mistaken. Meditation, at least mindfulness meditation, is profoundly ordinary. There is really nothing extraordinary or strange about.

Although it may be associated with holy men in robes and long beards or monks with clean shaven heads, meditation has no intrinsic connection with beards or bald skulls. You need not subscribe to an Asian religion to practice it. You don't have to don special clothes, adopt certain beliefs, or give yourself a Tibetan name in order to meditate. You certainly do not have to be holy or even religious. It is quite possible, in fact, that these trappings could impede your meditation practice. If you take up meditation because you think it is exotic or because you want to be pious and deepen your spirituality, your attraction to meditation may simply arise from the ego, the desire to appear other than you actually are.

That is not to say, however, that you should not start to practice meditation because you think it is exotic. It's only to say that like many other preconceptions, this idea is one that will also need to be relaxed sooner or later. It is perfectly all right to begin a mindfulness practice because it seems exotic or because in some way it serves your ego needs. You can begin to meditate for all kinds of bad or semi-appropriate reasons. Ultimately, it does not really matter why you start. But for mindfulness practice to become truly constructive in your life, those initial motives will have to be relinquished.

Like the attraction to its exotic trappings, some people take up meditation because they seek certain extraordinary experiences or altered states of consciousness. Many meditators have adopted the practice in quest of unity with the divine or to gain mystical knowledge of the world. Again, such motivations are fine at the start, but for mindfulness meditation, they too will need to be given up eventually. Mindfulness is not about having unusual or transcendent experiences. Strange, fascinating, and mysterious experiences may in fact occur while you are meditating. You may indeed have a moment that you consider ecstatic communion with God. You may feel yourself at one with the universe or in the presence of the holy. You may have an out-of-body experience as you find your soul hovering over your meditating body, looking down at yourself. With meditation, it is possible to have any kind of experience imaginable.

But particular kinds of experiences are not the goal of meditating. We are not looking to have unusual experiences in mindfulness meditation, although such experiences may and indeed do happen. Rather, we are seeking to develop a way to relate to all of our experiences, regardless of their quality or content.

Let me repeat that: Mindfulness practice is not about having a particular kind of experience; it is about how we relate to all of our experiences. Those experiences may be profoundly extraordinary, or they may be profoundly routine. From a mindfulness perspective, it does not matter one bit. You can gain as much from the experience of boredom as you can from the experience of ecstasy.

Today, especially, many people become interested in meditation because they are attracted to the possibility of reducing the stress in their lives and becoming a more relaxed person. Like beginning meditation to serve one's ego needs, starting a practice to relax and become calmer is perfectly fine. As we discussed in our previous talk, relaxation and stress reduction is a documented benefit of a mindfulness practice. But again, that expectation may have to be relinquished, and in this case sooner is probably better than later. Although greater serenity is indeed one of the results of meditation, tranquility is often not realized early in the practice. Consequently, many people have disappointing experiences with their first encounters with meditation. They're disappointed because they approach the practice with two particular expectations: One, they think meditation is easy, and two, they expect to become blissful rather quickly. So that we may approach the practice with a proper frame of mind, let me say at the outset: For the vast majority of practitioners, meditation is not easy, and its benefits are not quickly realized.

I can understand why many people show up to learn meditation, thinking that it will be a swift solution to their problems. We live in an impatient culture that has become quick to expect fixes rapidly. Our lack of patience, of course, is one of the reasons we experience so much negative stress in our lives, which, in turn, is one of the reasons people seek to practice meditation. It behooves us, therefore, to be aware that we may be harboring this expectation, since it may ultimately sabotage our efforts. Mindfulness meditation can teach us to be more patient, but we have to be patient to learn that lesson!

I'm perplexed, however, as to why some people think that mindfulness practice will be easy. Perhaps it has something do with the popular images of meditators that are found on the covers and insides of yoga and spirituality magazines. You've probably seen them on the rack as you check out of the grocery store. They almost always feature an attractive young woman in a suggestive outfit, with a cheerful look on her face as she sits cross-legged fashion on a white-sandy beach or in a lush meadow. (For some reason, these popular magazines rarely portray meditating men.) Even *Time* magazine used a version of this image for its cover story on meditation in 2003.

Whatever the source of this idea, we might be in for a bit of disappointment if we expect meditation to be easy, especially if we try to make it a daily discipline. Particularly in the beginning stages, meditating can be very difficult. Most of us are not accustomed to sitting still for very long. Your body may begin to ache and itch in places you didn't know existed. You may get bored and think of a hundred others things you'd rather be doing. There are times as you're meditating when washing the dishes may seem like the most important thing in the world for you to do. But perhaps the hardest part of a meditation practice is facing your own mind. Being alone with your thoughts can be terrifying, which is why many people avoid it at all costs. Stored in that awesome brain are many dreadful things, as you well know: a lifetime of regrets and sorrows; memories of unpleasant experiences and unfulfilled hopes; unresolved anger and frustrations; feelings of self-loathing and self-doubt; lurid fantasies, nonsensical images, and haphazard ideas. It's hard to imagine that those cheery magazine meditators are taking a good hard look at these demons.

In the traditional story of the Buddha's awakening while meditating under the Bodhi-tree, his encounter with his own internal demons is represented as a contest with Mara, a tempter figure much like the character of Satan in the New Testament. Just as Satan enticed Jesus to abandon his divine mission during a 40-day fast in the wilderness, so too does Mara try to prevent Siddhattha Gotama from attaining the wisdom that made him the Buddha. Mara attempts to deter Gotama with visions of beautiful women, terrifying thunderstorms and floods, and attacking war-elephants, all efforts to disturb his equanimity. When these visions fail, Mara himself appears and tries to persuade Gotama of his unworthiness to gain enlightenment. Gotama is unmoved by Mara's taunts, of course, and ultimately realizes his goal. Even in its early stages, Buddhism understood Mara and his ministrations as representative of the mind's own inner conflicts. Mara exists not so much as a literal being but as the symbol of all within us that tries to thwart our happiness and fulfillment as human beings. Meditation puts us face-to-face with Mara.

When one considers that mindfulness meditation invites such fiends to appear, it's difficult to understand why some consider the practice to be an escape from reality, another common misconception. Perhaps that idea derives from the belief that meditation is a way to empty your mind of its contents. Or perhaps the notion is related to the fact that in the 1960s and '70s, many of the first Westerners to experiment with meditation also liked to experiment with hallucinogenic drugs.

In any event, it is inaccurate to suggest that mindfulness meditation is somehow an escape from reality. Given its bold intention to attend unflinchingly to all of our experiences without judgment, I think it is more precise to call mindfulness meditation an escape into reality.

Jack Kornfield, now a highly regarded meditation teacher, was one of the first Americans to take ordination in Thailand as a Buddhist monk in the 1960s. Kornfield ultimately left Asia to return to the United States in the early '70s. Shortly after his arrival back in the States, with his head still shaven and still wearing his orange monastic robes, he decided to visit his brother in New York. The plan was to meet his sister-in-law at a ritzy day spa on Fifth Avenue, where she was redeeming a gift certificate for a full day's treatment. When he arrived at the spa, he was greeted with some disbelieving looks by the receptionist and was shown to a lounge to wait for his brother's wife to finish. As he waited, he decided to do what monks do in these situations—meditate. As he sat on a comfortable couch, he crossed his legs, closed his eyes, and began his practice. In his book *A Path with Heart*, he describes the scene that ensued:

> After ten minutes I began to hear laughter and noises. I continued to meditate, but finally I heard a group of voices and a loud exclamation of "Is he for real?" from the hall across the room, which

caused me to open my eyes. I saw eight or ten women dressed in … (gowns) … staring at me, many had their hair in rollers or in other multiple fishing-reel-shaped contraptions. Several had what looked like green avocado smeared on their faces. Others were covered with mud. I looked back at them and wondered what realm I had been born into and heard myself say, "Are they for real?"

From the perspective of mindfulness, our lives as we ordinarily live them seem profoundly out of touch with what is real. Few people appear to live in accord with what seem to be some sobering truths—that death will overtake us all, that the world is in constant change, that suffering is pervasive. Racing about in hot pursuit of trivial successes, possessions, and pleasures; working and amusing ourselves to death; filling our minds with useless junk—that's what seems to me to be an escape from reality.

Just as meditation has sometimes been criticized as escapist, it has also been charged with being self-centered. The expression "navel-gazing" has entered the English language as a term to refer to both meditation and egotism. In the view of some, both are forms of self-absorption.

Apparently, they regard the meditating practitioner as someone only interested in attaining a state of bliss while the rest of the world goes to hell in a hand-basket. I can only assume that such a criticism must be based on the most superficial of understandings.

While the practice of mindfulness meditation no doubt begins with turning inward toward one's own experience, the sharp distinction between self and world gradually begins to fade. A mindfulness practice reveals the intricate ways our lives are intertwined with one another. As a consequence, meditation begins to awaken our empathy and helps develop our natural sense of compassion. In the Buddhist tradition, compassion and wisdom are twin virtues: Both are cultivated by the practice of meditation. It is not possible to have true wisdom without genuine compassion, and vice versa. To be wise is to see things clearly, without delusion. Wisdom thus means to recognize the interdependence of our lives with the lives of others. Seeing our interdependence with others evokes our compassion. Knowing that your life is intrinsically connected to mine makes your well-being a matter for my concern. By the same token, when I act compassionately and generously toward others, I alleviate the egotism that obstructs my clear insight into reality. When my life is self-absorbed, I'm unable to perceive the world as it is. The world is merely a reflection of my own needs and desires, assumptions and beliefs. Letting go of the ego that distorts my vision clears the way for the insight that leads to wisdom.

This dialectical relationship between compassion and wisdom may not yet be completely lucid to you, but as we proceed through the course it should become so. For now, it is only necessary to affirm that a meditation practice that produces only self-satisfaction is not a genuine mindfulness practice. You can certainly begin to meditate because you want to be blissfully absorbed in your own little world, but along the way, that goal is just another thing that will have to be relinquished.

Finally, your conventional ideas of success and failure may also need to be abandoned when you take up meditation. Soon, we'll discuss the specific instructions involved in meditation. I'll tell what you need to do with your body, how to focus your attention, and what to do with your mind.

You'll probably discover, however, that you have a hard time doing these things—or at least some of them. When you're unable to follow the instructions exactly, you may be tempted to judge your effort as a failure. But that would be a mistake. In meditation practice, you fail only when you do not pay attention. But even failing to pay attention is not a failure if you realize you're not paying attention. Eventually, you'll see that you cannot fail at meditation, if you just do it. By the same token, you'll see that you cannot succeed at it either.

I hope by means of this true paradox, that you'll understand that meditation practice is an activity that is best approached with an openness of mind and sincerity of heart. But if you can't muster openness and sincerity, that's all right. Meditation can teach you that as well.

Preparation—Taking Moral Inventory
Lecture 4

C onduct a moral inventory in the spirit of five moral aspirations: harming others, stealing, sexual misconduct, lying, and intoxication. Consider whether any of your behaviors in these five areas might in some way impede your attentiveness to your experience and jeopardize your happiness. You'll find this exercise more meaningful if you write down your reflections. If your reflections reveal that your conduct falls short of what you think it should be, consider taking these five vows—or whichever ones you find relevant.

Mindfulness and Morality

- The religious and philosophical traditions that promote mindfulness foreground the significance of the connection between personal conduct and the practice of mindfulness in the discipline. Many of the psychological and medical approaches to mindfulness, though, tend to downplay it.

- However, to some extent, all mindfulness perspectives recognize that meditation must be practiced within the wider context of one's life, and that context necessarily involves the dimension of human experience we call ethical. The religious and philosophical traditions insist that this larger context must be in place before one attempts to delve deeper into mindfulness meditation.

- It is not possible to compartmentalize the various aspects of our lives. Our physical, mental, ethical, and spiritual dimensions are interrelated; we are holistic beings. A disordered ethical life will disrupt our efforts to practice meditation.

- The mindfulness approach to matters of personal ethics differs from moral perspectives that are governed by rules. Unlike ethical systems based on obedience to specific regulations, the practices governing ethical conduct in the mindfulness tradition are centrally concerned with shaping personal character.

- The precepts associated with mindfulness practice are put forth as tools for refining the personal qualities that enable us to become wiser and more compassionate—the principal virtues in this tradition. Observing these precepts is considered essential to sharpening the skills of mindfulness and, hence, to eliminating suffering and fostering happiness.

- The particular formulation of these principles that we'll use for this course comes from the teachings of the Buddha, but the principles are not uniquely Buddhist. In fact, most of them are included in almost all ethical perspectives—religious and secular.

- What distinguishes the Buddhist articulation is the way they are presented as aspirations rather than as commands or laws. Each of these precepts is formulated as a promise that one makes to try to behave in a specific way.

- If one falls short of the promise, he or she simply takes note of the shortcoming and vows to do better on the next occasion—without the feeling of moral guilt. Gradually, the skill to follow the precepts becomes increasingly stronger, to the point where acting otherwise becomes unthinkable.

- This particular way of approaching ethical conduct invites individuals to act morally—not to avoid punishment, but for the more positive purpose of refining one's character and promoting the well-being of the world. Attending to one's actions for this reason helps one recognize how wholesome actions condition a wholesome mind, promoting a sense of greater responsibility for the quality of our personality.

- When we fall short of our aspirations, we simply relinquish our mistake and try again. This pattern of observing and letting go is the basic dynamic of mindfulness. Thus, in attending to our conduct, we aren't only cultivating an appropriate context for mindfulness; we're actually practicing mindfulness as we do so.

The Five Ethical Aspirations

- The Buddha taught a great number of ethical aspirations to his followers, but we need only concern ourselves with five, the foundational precepts of them all. These promises are all related to the principle of not harming—a notion that resounds throughout the world's philosophical and ethical traditions.

I will endeavor not to harm sentient beings.

- From a metaphysical perspective, one might argue that harming sentient beings—beings that can feel pain and pleasure—is a violation of our innate nature or that it defies the dignity and inherent worth of others. More pragmatically, not harming others minimizes the chances that we ourselves will be harmed because people have a tendency to retaliate against those who hurt them.

- From a mindfulness perspective, striving not to cause harm helps us to be more mindful. Deliberately hurting others has a profound effect on our state of mind. Causing harm to others thus causes harm to us.

- Generally, the intention to harm arises from anger, hatred, or fear. When we act on that intention, we reinforce the emotion that underlies it, thus increasing the likelihood that the emotion will arise again.

- When our minds are flooded with anger, hatred, and fear, we lose our capacity to view things clearly, and we often make poor choices. By refusing to inflict injury when such negative emotions occur, we are given an opportunity to seek more constructive and skillful ways to respond to them.

- Not all harm we cause, however, is intentional; we often hurt others simply by being thoughtless. To vow not to harm is a promise to be more aware of our words and actions and their effect on others. It is an intention to be more mindful and to refuse to revert to the mindless state where selfishness rules.

- When we consider the unintended harm we may cause, fulfilling the first mindfulness precept seems impossible. The value of the precept, however, lies not in performing it perfectly, which we may never do, but in the objective to become more fully aware of ourselves.

I will endeavor not to steal.

- The promise not to steal follows a universal moral principle. No ethical system condones stealing, except in the rarest of cases. Proscribing stealing is an absolute necessity for the sustainability of any society.

- Whereas the intention to harm arises out of anger, hatred, and fear, stealing is usually motivated by greed and envy. Like anger, hatred, and fear, greed and envy are disruptive to the mental serenity that mindfulness needs and intends to develop.

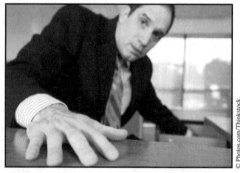

- Stealing, however, need not be prompted by greed or envy. Lurking behind so much of what we do is a self

Although some people might pilfer a few office supplies from work, most don't steal cars or televisions.

that wants godlike powers: to be at the center of the universe, to exert control over reality, to feel unconstrained by anything. The problem is that for finite beings like us, these desires are not only unrealistic—they lead to behaviors that thwart our happiness and cause misery to others.

- Stealing need not be defined merely as the taking of material things. The more insidious forms of theft are of the abstract variety, such things as taking credit for another person's ideas or illegally downloading music from the Internet. Because we live in a materialistic culture, these types of stealing often seem less real or less severe than stealing tangible objects.

- From the mindfulness perspective, there is little difference between the kinds of things one steals—the effect is the same. Taking what does not belong to us strengthens a sense of self that is unwholesome and obstructs the clarity that mindfulness practice seeks to develop.

- The promise not to steal signals our intention to restrain greed and envy and commits us to a practice of honesty, especially when we think we have the opportunity to escape without penalty. In mindfulness practice, every act leaves its mark on our character, and the small things we do, or do not do, add up.

I will endeavor not to misuse sexuality.

- Like stealing, the principle of not misusing sexuality is a near-universal ethical standard—and with good reason. The abuse of sexuality causes tremendous destruction to individual lives and threatens the stability of human social life.

- Although the proscription of abusing sexuality is a near-universal principle, the concrete meaning of that principle often varies from culture to culture. The vagueness of the mindfulness precept is deliberate and, perhaps, constructive.

- Simply vowing not to misuse sexuality, rather than promising to act on more specific rules, ultimately implies that we must take responsibility for our own sexual ethic. Because we're ultimately responsible in these situations, we must remain keenly attentive to our thoughts, words, and deeds and act in a manner that refrains from harming others and ourselves.

- The misuse of sexuality can be an especially powerful threat to mindfulness. As our own culture amply shows, sexuality can easily become an obsession that renders us mindless. Even more serious are all the things a sexually obsessed individual might be willing to do to satisfy his or her lust.

- Deeper still is the effect of a disordered sexuality on the mind. We spend so much of our lives looking for something that will make us happy—only to find that nothing provides it. The desire for happiness is wholesome, but our quest is misguided because of our distorted ideas about what will give us the satisfaction we crave.

I will endeavor not to use false speech.

- False speech is lying, gossiping and slander, cursing and harsh language, and idle chatter—frivolous talk with no constructive purpose. Try to go an entire day avoiding these forms of false speech and being attentive to the times you slip.

- The real challenge of observing this precept is to be aware of when we use false speech. We are so conditioned to this kind of behavior that we're usually oblivious when our tongues go astray until after the fact, and even then, some of us remain totally unaware of the effects of our language.

- In view of the damage caused by our mindless words and the attentiveness required to keep them in check, the significance of the promise to watch our language for mindfulness practice ought to be apparent.

I will endeavor not to consume toxins.

- Historically, the precept to refrain from consuming toxins referred specifically to the use of alcohol, but the intent of this principle was simply to diminish the destructive effects of drunkenness and to foster the clarity of mind necessary for practicing mindfulness.

- The use of alcohol can obviously affect the ability to be attentive and think clearly, but alcohol isn't the only substance that stupefies the mind. Adhering to the spirit of this precept would necessarily mean becoming aware of any substance that could impair our mental and bodily functions, such as tobacco and mind-altering drugs.

- In short, promising to observe this precept means nothing less than trying to stay as physically healthy and as mentally sharp as possible by keeping a close eye on the things we allow into our bodies and into our minds.

- Today, guarding our minds from intoxication would necessarily include being mindful about the kinds of information we take in. Surely, the amount and quality of data we permit into our heads shapes the character of our minds. And, like other stupefying substances, we can become addicted to media stimulation.

- Try to spend a day fasting from the media—that is, going 24 hours without reading a paper or magazine, listening to music, watching television, going to a movie, playing video games, or using the Internet or cell phones (except in an emergency). Those who find the fast refreshing and those who find it irritating both attest to the way heavy reliance on media stimulation can detract from mindfulness.

1. What is the relationship between moral conduct and mindfulness?

2. Dedicate a weekday to observing how well you follow each of the five precepts. For example, on Monday, watch your capacity to refrain from harming; on Tuesday, see how well you refrain from stealing, and so on.

Preparation—Taking Moral Inventory
Lecture 4—Transcript

At first blush, this talk may seem out of sequence. For the last three sessions, we've been discussing mindfulness and meditation.

In this lecture, however, we're turning—rather precipitously it might seem—to the subject of moral behavior. Yet, the turn to morality is not as odd as it might appear at first. There is an essential and intrinsic relationship between personal conduct and the practice of mindfulness.

The religious and philosophical traditions that promote mindfulness are fully aware of this connection and foreground its significance in the discipline. Many of the psychological and medical approaches to mindfulness, though, tend to downplay it. However, to some extent, all mindfulness perspectives recognize that meditation must be practiced within the wider context of one's life, and that context necessarily involves the dimension of human experience we call ethical. The religious and philosophical traditions insist that this larger context must be set in order before one attempts to delve deeper into mindfulness meditation.

The reasoning is simple: It is not possible to compartmentalize the various aspects of our lives. Our physical, mental, ethical, and spiritual dimensions are interrelated; we are holistic beings. A disordered ethical life will disrupt our efforts to practice meditation. How can one attain tranquility and clarity of mind if one's behavior weighs heavily on the conscience? This does not mean, however, that you must be a morally perfect individual before you can start to meditate. Since all aspects of our lives are interconnected, mindfulness practice will enable us to be morally better persons. Yet it is important that certain kinds of behavior be curtailed, if necessary, before one attempts the more demanding practice of meditation.

The mindfulness approach to matters of personal ethics differs from moral perspectives that are governed by rules. Unlike ethical systems based on obedience to specific regulations, such as the Ten Commandments, the practices governing ethical conduct in the mindfulness tradition are centrally concerned with shaping personal character. The precepts associated with mindfulness practice are put forth as tools for refining the personal qualities that enable us to become wiser and more compassionate, the principal virtues in this tradition. These precepts are not regarded as rules sent down from on high; no one is threatened with divine punishment for failing to observe them. Instead, they are presented as practices that are in our nature and best interest to follow. Observing these precepts is considered essential to sharpening the skills of mindfulness, and hence to eliminating suffering and fostering happiness.

The particular formulation of these principles that we'll use for this course comes from the teachings of the Buddha, but the principles are not uniquely Buddhist. In fact, most of them are included in almost all ethical perspectives, religious and secular. What distinguishes the Buddhist articulation is the way they are presented as aspirations rather than as commands or laws. Each of these precepts is formulated as a promise that one makes to behave in a specific way. If one fails to fulfill that promise, he or she simply takes note of the shortcoming and vows to do better on the next occasion. No moral guilt is incurred for falling short of the promise, although one will inevitably have to face any personal or legal consequences of so doing. Gradually, by resolving to start afresh each time one falls short, the skill to follow the precepts becomes increasingly stronger, to the point where acting otherwise becomes unthinkable.

This particular way of approaching ethical conduct is especially valuable for promoting mindfulness. It invites individuals to act morally, not to avoid punishment but for the more positive purpose of refining one's character and promoting the well-being of the world. Attending to one's actions for this reason helps one recognize how wholesome actions condition a wholesome mind, promoting a greater sense of responsibility for the quality of our personality.

When we fall short of our aspirations, we don't need to carry around a sense of guilt that serves no good purpose. We simply relinquish our mistake and try again. This pattern of observing and letting go is the basic dynamic of mindfulness. Thus, in attending to our conduct, we aren't only cultivating an appropriate context for mindfulness, we're actually practicing mindfulness as we do so.

The Buddha taught a great number of ethical aspirations to his followers, but we need only concern ourselves with five, the foundational precepts of them all. In the manner in which they are most frequently stated, the five aspirations are these: I will endeavor not to harm sentient beings; I will endeavor not to steal; I will endeavor not to misuse sexuality; I will endeavor not to use false speech; I will endeavor not to consume toxins.

These promises are all related to the principle of not harming, a notion that resounds throughout the world's philosophical and ethical traditions. We'll discuss each of these five precepts in turn to examine how they are connected to the practice of harmlessness as well as to the practice of mindfulness.

There are many good reasons to refrain from harming sentient beings, that is, beings that can feel pain and pleasure. From a metaphysical perspective, one might argue that doing harm is a violation of our own innate nature or that it defies the dignity and inherent worth of others. To hurt others, therefore, goes against the grain of who we truly are. More pragmatically, one could say that not harming others minimizes the chances that we ourselves will be harmed, since people have a tendency to retaliate against those who hurt them. These are excellent—and perhaps sufficient—reasons to cultivate a practice of harmlessness. The mindfulness practice, however, offers additional incentives.

Striving not to cause harm helps us to be more mindful. Deliberately hurting others has a profound effect on our state of mind. Generally, the intention to harm arises from anger, hatred, or fear. When we act on that intention, we reinforce the emotion that underlies it, thus increasing the likelihood that the emotion will arise again. When our minds are flooded with anger, hatred, and fear, we lose our capacity to see things clearly, and we often make poor choices. Causing harm to others thus causes harm to us. By refusing to inflict injury when such negative emotions occur, we are given an opportunity to seek other, more constructive and skillful ways to respond to them. Later in the series, we'll discuss specific techniques for handling these situations without resorting to the conditioned impulse to hurt others or ourselves.

Not all harm we cause, however, is intentional. We often hurt others simply by being thoughtless. Sometimes we say things without regard for how our words might affect another. Consider how many car accidents occur because people simply do not pay sufficient attention to their driving. Think about how many bugs you squash just walking across the sidewalk, or reflect on the size of your carbon footprint. To vow not to harm is a promise to be more aware of our actions and words and their effect on others. It is an intention to be more mindful and to refuse to revert to the mindless state where selfishness rules.

When we consider the unintended harm we may cause, fulfilling the first mindfulness precept seems well-nigh impossible. It is certainly difficult to go through life without hurting someone or something. The value of the precept, however, lies not in performing it perfectly, which we may never do, but in the objective to become more fully aware of ourselves and to create a peaceful mind that minimizes the damage we cause and promotes a clearer perception of reality and our place in it. It awakens within us what Albert Schweitzer called a "reverence for life," an awe and respect for all living things and for life itself.

The promise not to steal follows what is a universal moral principle. I can think of no ethical system that condones stealing, except in the rarest of cases. Proscribing stealing is an absolute necessity for the sustainability of any society. Like the precept of non-harming, the principle of non-stealing can be justified in any number of ways, but it has special meaning for those who wish to become more mindful. Whereas the intention to harm arises out of anger, hatred, and fear, stealing is usually motivated by greed and envy. Acting on these negative states tends to reinforce them, conditioning the mind in such a way that greed and envy crop up at the slightest provocation. Like anger, hatred, and fear, greed and envy are disruptive to the mental serenity that mindfulness needs and intends to develop.

Stealing, however, need not be prompted by greed or envy. In the *Confessions*, Saint Augustine relates a fascinating story from his childhood in which he and a bunch of youthful companions stole pears from a neighbor's orchard. Augustine himself was initially perplexed about what inspired this theft. He wasn't hungry and didn't need or even want the pears. In fact, he had better pears at home. He wasn't even intending to cause harm to the owner of the orchard. After reflection, Augustine concluded that the primary drive behind the act was the pure thrill of doing wrong; he did it for the hell of it. His profound insight displays the great complexity and subtlety of the mind. So often, the motives underlying our deeds are simply unknown to us.

But Augustine's depth of understanding allowed him to recognize that beneath this puzzling act was his own ego, a sense of self craving to feel the pleasure of a power that Augustine believed only belonged to God. One need not subscribe to Augustine's theism to appreciate his insight. Lurking behind so much of what we do is a self that wants godlike powers: to be at the center of the universe, to exert control over reality, to feel unconstrained by anything. The problem is that for finite beings like us, these desires are not only unrealistic, they lead to behaviors that thwart our happiness and cause misery to others. The vow to try not to steal thus serves to recondition the impulses that ultimately cause us great harm.

Stealing, of course, need not be defined merely as the taking of material things like pears. Probably most of us don't steal cars or television sets, although we might pilfer a few office supplies from work or sample the occasional strawberry in the grocery store. If we do take material goods, they're probably of the minor sort that allows us to rationalize the act with comparative ease. The more insidious forms of theft, however, are of the abstract variety—the kinds of things that are less tangible—such things as taking credit for another person's ideas, illegally downloading music or software from the Internet, or failing to speak up when the checkout cashier makes an error in our favor. Because we live in a materialistic culture, these types of stealing often seem less real or less severe than stealing tangible objects. We might not consider them stealing at all.

From the perspective of mindfulness, there is little difference between the kinds of things one steals; the effect is the same. Taking what does not belong to us strengthens a sense of self that is unwholesome and obstructs the clarity that mindfulness practice seeks to develop. On the other hand, the promise not to steal signals our intention to restrain greed and envy and commits us to a practice of honesty, especially when we think we have the opportunity to get away scot-free. In mindfulness practice, however, there is no getting away scot-free. Every act leaves its mark on our character, and the small things we do, or do not do, add up.

The Buddha admonished his followers: "Do not think lightly of evil, saying 'It will not come to me,' for drop by drop a water jar is filled. The fool fills himself with evil, soaking it up little by little."

But the same is true with the cultivation of a good character. The Buddha also said: "Do not think lightly of goodness, saying 'It will not come to me,' for drop by drop a water jar is filled. The sage fills himself with goodness, soaking it up little by little."

Like stealing, the principle of not misusing sexuality is a near-universal ethical standard—and with good reason. The abuse of sexuality causes tremendous destruction to individual lives and threatens the stability of human social life. The point is so patent that it requires no further commentary from me.

What does bear analysis, however, is the significance of this precept in mindfulness practice. Let's begin with what is meant by the expression "misuse of sexuality." Although, the proscription of abusing sexuality is a universal, or near-universal, principle, the concrete meaning of that principle often varies from culture to culture. In some communities, premarital sex is wrong; in others, it is acceptable and even expected. The vagueness of the mindfulness precept is deliberate and, I think, constructive. Simply vowing not to misuse sexuality, rather than promising to act on specific rules, ultimately implies that we must take responsibility for our own sexual ethic. What constitutes misuse may vary from situation to situation, and it's up to us to determine what that may mean concretely. Because we're ultimately responsible in these situations, we must remain keenly attentive to our thoughts, words, and deeds, and act in a manner that refrains from harming others and ourselves, the principal guideline we must use.

The misuse of sexuality can be an especially powerful threat to mindfulness. As our own culture amply shows, sexuality can easily become an obsession that renders us mindless. In fact, much of Western commerce counts on the mindlessness of sexual obsession to persuade us to buy products and services that we don't really need. Even more serious are all the things a sexually obsessed individual might be willing to do to satisfy his or her lust.

The list includes the violation of every conceivable ethical principle—lying, stealing, cheating, and even murder.

Deeper still is the effect of a disordered sexuality on the mind. Once again, my favorite Christian saint—Augustine—provides a compelling example. Augustine has been called the most famous sex addict in history. If you've read his *Confessions*, you'll understand why. Like his theft of the pears, Augustine sought to understand his sexual debauchery as a young man. Again, his insight was profound. According to the later, celibate Augustine, his youthful lust was love gone awry. What really motivated Augustine's sexual exploits, he concluded, was the thoroughly wholesome desire to love and be loved. Yet, because he was unable to see that clearly—because, we might say, he was mindless—Augustine came to believe that copious sex would satisfy this deeper longing, a yearning he really didn't understand. We can say that Augustine was, in the words of the immortal country and western song, "lookin' for love in all the wrong places." Through years of agony, Augustine eventually discovered what he was really seeking could only be found in God. Again, you don't need to accept Augustine's theology to appreciate his insight into the human condition: We spend so much of our lives looking for something that will make us happy, only to find that nothing provides it. The desire for happiness is wholesome, but our quest is misguided because of our distorted ideas about what will give us the satisfaction we crave. The promise not to misuse sexuality, then, can be understood as a principle for keeping us on the right track. There is no happiness in disordered sexual behavior.

In some of my courses, I assign students a simple task to acquaint them with the practice of abstaining from false speech. False speech is lying, gossiping, and slander, cursing and harsh language, and idle chatter, or frivolous talk with no constructive purpose. I ask my students to go an entire day trying to avoid these forms of false speech and to be attentive to the times they slip. The assignment is made, along some other ascetical practices, but students usually find this one the hardest. I understand why; it's also the hardest for me. The author of the book of James in the New Testament tells us, "Every species of beast and bird, of reptile and sea creature, can be tamed and has been tamed by the human species, but no one can tame the tongue—a restless evil, full of deadly poison." A bit of poetic hyperbole, perhaps, but who can deny the power of our words to cause tremendous harm and the difficulty of keeping our words under control?

The real challenge of observing this precept is to be aware of when we use false speech. As my students discover, we are so conditioned to this kind of behavior that we're usually oblivious when our tongues go astray until after the fact, and even then, some of us remain totally unaware of the effects of our language. In view of the damage caused by our mindless words and the attentiveness required to keep them in check, the significance of the promise to watch our language for mindfulness practice ought to be apparent. Its importance is so great, in fact, that we will devote an entire discussion later in the course to the practice of mindful speech. In the meantime, I invite you to make a deliberate effort to watch the patterns of your words for a single day.

Historically, the precept to refrain from consuming toxins referred specifically to the use of alcohol, or "stupefying drink," as it was then called. The intent of this principle was simply to diminish the destructive effects of drunkenness and to foster the clarity of mind necessary for practicing mindfulness. The use of alcohol can obviously affect the ability to be attentive and think clearly. But alcohol isn't the only substance that stupefies the mind, of course. Adhering to the spirit of this precept would necessarily mean becoming aware of any substance that could impair our mental and bodily functions, such as tobacco and mind-altering drugs. In short, promising to observe this precept means nothing less than trying to stay as physically healthy and as mentally sharp as possible by keeping a close eye on the things we allow into our bodies and into our minds.

Today, guarding our minds from intoxication would necessarily include being mindful about the kinds of information we take in. Since he did not live in the age of Twitter, Facebook, and cable TV, the Buddha did not anticipate the potentially deleterious effects of being exposed to as much information as we moderns are. Yet surely, the amount and quality of data that we permit into our heads shapes the character of our minds. Feeding our minds a steady of diet of pointless and trivial information can dull the mind as much as other intoxicants. And, like stupefying substances, we can become addicted to media stimulation.

In the same assignment I give my students for refraining from false speech, I ask them to spend another day fasting from media—that is, going 24 hours without reading a paper or magazine, listening to music, watching TV, going to a movie, playing video games, or using the Internet or cell phones except in an emergency. Their responses to the assignment are quite revealing. Many of them find the experiment to be refreshing. They discover how much time they usually waste in meaningless activities and how more aware they are of their world and inner experience when their minds are not cluttered with inessential information. They find that they have more time in the day than they realized. Others find the media fast to be very difficult to endure. They report irritability and a sense of aimlessness, the kinds of things one might experience trying to quit an addiction cold turkey. Those who find the fast refreshing and those who find it irritating both attest to the way heavy reliance on media stimulation can detract from mindfulness.

There is a great deal more that can be said about these five precepts and their importance in the practice of mindfulness. As we proceed through the course, we'll have more opportunities to discuss them. At this point, though, I merely want to invite you to conduct a moral inventory in the spirit of these five aspirations. Set aside some time and honestly look at the way you conduct your life. Consider whether any of these behaviors in these five areas— harming others, stealing, sexual misconduct, lying, and intoxication—might in some way impede your attentiveness to your experience and jeopardize your happiness. You'll find this exercise more meaningful if you write down your reflections. To help with this inventory, consider taking a media fast and practicing a day of refraining from false speech. These exercises will assist in bringing these aspects of your life into greater awareness. If your reflections reveal that your conduct falls short of what you think it ought be, consider taking these five vows—or whichever ones you find relevant. If you choose to do so, you will find them easier to observe if you recite them each day.

In our next session, we'll begin to discuss the practice of sitting meditation. See you then.

Position—Where to Be for Meditation

Lecture 5

Establishing a suitable setting for practicing mindfulness is not complicated or difficult, but it requires some forethought and perhaps a bit of imagination and experimentation. The basic physical preparations for beginning a practice to cultivate the mind include putting the body in a safe, pleasant environment and taking up a posture that will allow it to remain still and feel stable for a longer-than-usual period. With these external factors in place, the mind will start to follow and will find it easier to become calm and focused.

Establishing a Suitable Setting

- Because our minds have been conditioned to become easily distracted, it is essential to set aside a special place and time to minimize those distractions and allow the mind to concentrate on learning to concentrate. As the mind is reconditioned in more skillful ways, it will become easier to move beyond the special practice setting to everyday life.

- This is not to say, however, that you should strictly confine your practice to special times and places until you've mastered mindfulness. Exercising mindfulness in a special context is intended only to support the development of moment-to-moment awareness throughout the rest of our lives.

Three Key Elements

Determining the Most Appropriate Time for Your Practice

- Deciding on the best time to practice meditation is probably the most individual of all the decisions you'll make concerning the external factors of this discipline. You alone are able to determine the best time to practice, and you may have to try different times to figure out your answer.

- Because you'll ultimately want to set aside about 20–45 minutes for your daily meditation, it is important to decide when you can carve out that much time to be free from interruptions or other distractions.

- You'll also want to take into consideration the times your body and mind are most conducive to practice. You might even dabble with times that seem counterintuitive.

- Less important than the time of day is the regularity with which you practice; it matters greatly that you make an effort on a daily basis. At first, it will probably be difficult to devote 20–45 minutes a day to the practice, so 5 minutes is fine as long as you commit to a regular schedule.

- As the benefits of the discipline become more apparent, you'll find it easier to make time to practice, and you'll probably begin to protect those times with great zeal. However, do not expect this at first; the benefits of mindfulness practice are gradual and cumulative.

- Finally, you should have access to a timer of some sort. The timer allows you to determine before you start how long you intend to practice, and it will help keep you committed to fulfilling that intention.

Creating the Most Congenial Location for Your Practice

- Your physical environment needs to be conducive to the facilitation of moment-to-moment awareness. Accordingly, the place you choose to meditate needs to be as quiet as possible and free from distractions and interruption.

- Whether you create a special space or just use a chair in the dining room, you may find it helpful to use the same place each time you practice. Returning to the same location helps your mind and body readily prepare for meditation and obviates the need to become familiar with a new setting.

- Ideally, your practice space should be relatively free of visual as well as other distractions—especially noise. It is very important that your practice space be pleasant; it should be inviting and calming in whatever way you see fit.

- If you're a traditionalist, you may find the time-honored forest setting to your liking. In the ancient days, when the techniques of yoga and mindfulness were being refined and practiced by great numbers of people in South Asia, it was customary to meditate out of doors.

- Most importantly, the Hindu **Upanishads**, some of the earliest documents to record instructions in contemplative practice, urge the aspirant to find a quiet, safe, uncluttered, and agreeable place to practice.

Learning to Put the Body in a Proper Position for Meditation

- Like time and place, the bodily posture for meditation practice is governed by the aim of crafting a calm and alert mind. To create these conditions, it is helpful, at least initially, to bring the body into a still and stable position.

- The classic position for meditating, of course, is sitting. Seasoned meditators, in fact, often refer to the discipline simply as "sitting" or "sitting practice." Just as one can be mindful anywhere, one can cultivate mindfulness skills in any physical position—including standing, lying down, and walking.

- With practice, the unaccustomed body can be trained to sit directly on the ground in, for example, the classic **lotus position**. In this traditional pose, one sits on the bare floor or a thin cushion and places the right foot on top of the left thigh and the left foot on top of the right thigh.

- While it is relatively easy to get into the full lotus position, maintaining it can be quite difficult and painful for the novice. Using a cushion or chair works just as well in the beginning, and the urgency of getting to mindfulness practice outweighs the need to learn the traditional position.

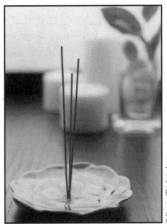

- If you choose to use a cushion, find one that will elevate your body at least five to six inches from the floor—maybe more if you are tall. This elevation allows you to cross your legs comfortably without tiring too quickly and permits necessary circulation throughout the body.

Your meditation practice space should be pleasant; some people prefer to scent it with incense.

- You will also find it very helpful to wear loose-fitting, comfortable clothes for your practice. In addition, you should remove your shoes because shoes can restrict the flow of circulation—just as tight-fitting clothes can.

- What is wonderful about sitting on a cushion is that you don't have to entangle your legs in the compact way required by the lotus position. You may simply cross your legs at the ankles without having to place your feet on opposite thighs—a position known as the **Burmese style**.

- A posture called *seiza* involves sitting on your calves with your knees, shins, and feet resting on the ground. This manner of sitting is very common throughout Japan, even among those who do not practice meditation.

- Using a chair for mindfulness practice is almost the same as using it for ordinary sitting—but with a few important exceptions. First, you should keep both feet flat on the floor without crossing them. This position promotes a feeling of stability and prevents cramping or other painful sensations.

- Second, you should not use the back of the chair for support. Sit away from the back of the chair to avoid leaning on it. Although it feels more comfortable initially, you will soon be tired and will find yourself moving your body to find a more comfortable position. Remember, we are seeking a posture that will enable us to avoid unnecessary movement.

- All forms of sitting—on the ground, on a cushion, on a bench, and in a chair—are designed to prevent the back from resting against an external object. The purpose of this design is to encourage the back to remain in a position conducive to mental alertness and the smooth flow of breathing.

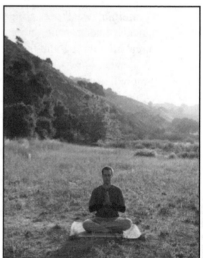

The Position of the Back

- Wherever you choose to sit, the position of the back will be ultimately the same. Keep your back straight but not rigid. There should be a slight curvature following the natural contours of the spine. To achieve this

The place you choose to meditate needs to be quiet and free from distractions and interruptions.

© Valueline/Thinkstock.

position, you may find it helpful to roll your hips forward a bit as you elongate your back.

- Regardless of what you sit on, it may be useful to imagine a string attached to the crown of your skull that is pulling it upward toward the ceiling. This visualization helps lengthen the backbone while drawing down the shoulders and keeping the head in its proper position for practice.

- At first, remaining in this position may be uncomfortable because we are not accustomed to using the lower back muscles in this way. Over time, though, those muscles will strengthen and maintaining this posture will not be difficult at all.

- Now that you have found a steady place for your legs, focus your attention on the back. Allow it to elongate and follow its natural curvature. Permit your shoulders to relax by coaxing them down toward the floor and drawing them toward the spine.

Other Physical Preparations

- With legs and back in place, we can now attend to the hands and arms. Traditionally, the upper extremities find their place in two locations. First, you may put the hands in your lap, one on top of the other. A second approach is to place the hands on the knees— either palms down or up.

- You will probably need to experiment with your arms and hands to decide which position is right for you. Your criteria for making this determination are comfort and stability: Choose the posture that allows you to remain still for the longest period.

- With the chin essentially level with the floor, we now consider what to do with the various elements of the head. Because a great deal of muscular tension accrues in this region of the body, try to relax those muscles systematically. Move your jaw around and allow it to hang slightly from the rest of the head. Keep your lips lightly closed or slightly parted. Let your tongue relax in your mouth.

- Next, you must decide what to do with your eyes. You can meditate with the eyes open or shut; both approaches have their advantages. Keeping the eyes closed helps eliminate external visual distractions, but closed eyes permit a range of rather amazing internal distractions.

- Open-eye practice, though, promotes alertness. You may find that keeping your eyes closed for an extended time makes you drowsy, but keeping the eyes open works against that. If you choose to practice with open eyes, you should direct your vision to a point on the ground in front of you about six feet away from your body.

- You may wish to try both open and closed eyes to determine which approach is most helpful. If you have never practiced meditative disciplines before, you might want to begin with closed eyes simply to assist in removing visual distraction and promoting concentration. Later, you can try to practice with eyes open and see how that style suits you.

Important Terms

Burmese style: In this position, one sits on a cushion, crossing the legs at the ankles without having to place the feet on opposite thighs—as when sitting on the floor.

lotus position: In this traditional pose, one sits on the bare floor or a thin cushion and places the right foot on top of the left thigh and the left foot on top of the right thigh.

seiza: A posture that involves sitting on one's calves with the knees, shins, and feet resting on the ground. This manner of sitting is very common throughout Japan, even among those who do not practice meditation.

Upanishad: One of the earliest Hindu documents in which instructions in contemplative practice were recorded.

Questions to Consider

1. Why is it important to set aside a specific place and time for practicing mindfulness?

2. If you have chosen a time and place for your sitting practice, how does the environment make you feel? Relaxed, anxious, happy, or uncomfortable? Is there anything you can do to make the setting more conducive to meditating?

Position—Where to Be for Meditation
Lecture 5—Transcript

In our last conversation, we discussed the importance of providing a suitable context for cultivating mindfulness. We talked about that context in a broad sense as the way we act and comport ourselves throughout our lives.

We noted that committing ourselves to following certain ethical precepts helps provide a congenial environment in which mindfulness can flourish. Today, we'll narrow that context considerably as we turn to the more specific circumstances for practicing meditation, the fundamental instrument for strengthening our mindfulness skills.

Since our minds have been conditioned to become easily distracted, it is essential to set aside a specific place and time to minimize those distractions and allow the mind to concentrate on learning to concentrate. As the mind is reconditioned in more skillful ways, it will become easier to move beyond the special practice setting to everyday life. This is not to say, however, that you should strictly confine your practice to special times and places until you've mastered mindfulness. Exercising mindfulness in a special context is intended only to support the development of moment-to-moment awareness throughout the rest of our lives.

Establishing a suitable setting for practicing is not difficult or complicated, but it requires some forethought and perhaps a bit of imagination and experimentation to make it work. We'll discuss three key elements you'll need to take into consideration. The first is determining the most appropriate time for your practice. The second is environment—creating the most congenial location for your practice. And the third is posture—learning to put the body in a proper position to facilitate the goals of mindful development. Today, we will talk about each of these in turn.

Deciding the best time to practice meditation is probably the most individual of all decisions you'll make concerning the external factors of this discipline. You alone are able to determine the best time to practice, and you may have to try different times to figure out your answer. Your decision will depend in part on what works best for your schedule and in part on the condition of your body and mind at various times of the day. Since you'll ultimately want to set aside about 20 to 45 minutes for your daily meditation, it is important to decide when you can carve out that much time to be free from interruptions or other distractions. If you're a busy parent, for example, you may have to wake up well before your children arise or wait until they have gone to bed. You'll also want to take into consideration the times your body and mind are most conducive to practice. If you're a morning person, that may be the best time for you. If your mind is more alert and your body more relaxed late at night, you may decide that is your time. You might even dabble with times that seem counterintuitive.

Several years ago, I began to practice my meditation immediately after coming home from work in the evening. I was physically and mentally tired and had gotten into the habit of crashing on the sofa and watching TV for an hour or so until I felt refreshed. I discovered that I could more readily and more assuredly regain my energy by meditating instead of wasting time being passively entertained. Whatever time you choose, you'll find it best to practice when your stomach is relatively empty. Trying to meditate on a full stomach is difficult.

Less important than the time of day is the regularity with which you practice. It matters little if you meditate at 9:00 in the morning or 9:00 at night, but it matters greatly that you make an effort on a daily basis. At first, it will probably be difficult to devote 20 to 45 minutes a day to the practice. Perhaps you can only manage 5 minutes. That is fine. It is better to practice for five minutes for 6 days than 30 minutes for only 1 day in 6. The benefits of mindfulness practice are gradual and cumulative, and regularity is key to the process. As the benefits of the discipline become more apparent, you'll find it easier to make time to practice, and you'll probably begin to protect those times with great zeal. You'll discover a pleasantness about your practice that draws you to it. But don't expect that at first. You may find the initial days or weeks of meditating to be rather difficult. But as with any skill, the difficulties and awkwardness of the initial phase will soon give way to more agreeable sensations as the practice develops.

One final note about time: You should have access to a timer of some sort. An ordinary kitchen timer will do nicely. So will a cell phone. Most cell phones today have a timer application that can be used for this purpose. Some phones or portable media players can be installed with software that simulates the sounding of a gong or bell to signal the end of the practice in traditional settings. The timer allows you to determine before you start how long you intend to practice, and it will help you stay committed to fulfilling that intention. As your practice proceeds, you will discover yourself developing a most fascinating love-hate relationship with your timer.

The criteria for establishing an appropriate place to practice are essentially the same as those for determining a suitable time. Your physical environment needs to be conducive to the facilitation of moment-to-moment awareness. Accordingly, the place you choose to meditate needs to be as quiet as possible and free from distractions and interruption.

You may not have the luxury of being able to dedicate a particular space in your home exclusively to the practice of mindfulness. Sitting quietly on a chair in the living room or bedroom will serve just as well. If you are able to afford a special location, such as the corner of room or an entire room itself, having a dedicated space may symbolize the seriousness of your dedication to your discipline and may provide an inducement to staying committed to it. But whether you create a special space or just use a chair in the dining room, you may find it helpful to use the same place each time you practice, although it is not essential. Returning to the same location helps your mind and body readily prepare for meditation and obviates the need to become familiar with a new setting.

Ideally, your practice space should be relatively free of visual as well as other distractions, especially noise. If you find it inspiring to display a Buddha image or hang an icon of Jesus or a picture of Gandhi, that is fine. But it isn't necessary. I personally prefer an empty space devoid of images that might take attention away from concentrating on mental cultivation. But it is very important that your practice space be pleasant. It should be inviting and calming in whatever way you see fit. If that means decorating it with flowers or candles or scenting it with a few sticks of incense as you practice, by all means do so. But fussing too much with one's setting can easily become a substitute for actually practicing mindfulness. During meditation, I've sometimes found myself daydreaming about how I can better decorate my practice space! It is very easy to get caught up in attending to the externalities of the discipline rather than engaging in the practice itself. For that reason, it is best to keep the decoration of your space as nice but as uncomplicated as possible.

If you're a real hard-core traditionalist, you may find the time-honored forest setting to your liking. In the ancient days, when the techniques of yoga and mindfulness were being refined and practiced by great numbers of people in South Asia, it was customary to meditate out of doors. This was the setting of the Buddha on the night his awakening. The Hindu *Upanishads*, some of the earliest documents to record instructions in contemplative practice, urge the aspirant to "find a quiet retreat for the practice of meditation, sheltered from the wind, level and clean, free from rubbish, smoldering fires, and ugliness, and where the sound of waters and the beauty of the place help thought and contemplation." Once these conditions have been met, the ancient sages suggest laying out a deer or tiger skin over a bed of fragrant *kusha* grass under the shade of a large tree. But if you find it difficult to get your hands on a tiger skin or *kusha* grass, the basic principles of space remain the same, whether you're practicing in the forest or within your own home. Make sure your place is quiet, safe, uncluttered, and agreeable.

As I prepared these lectures, I had the great luxury of using a small room at an Eastern Orthodox church near where I work in Memphis. This place was really little more than a big closet that had been used for storage for many years. When I mentioned to the pastor my desire for a quiet place where I could work free of distractions, he kindly made this space available to me. Not only was this space beneficial for my work, it did wonders for my spirit. I noticed that simply by going to this little room, located above the church's main sanctuary, and sitting there for a few hours, my entire disposition would become serene. Mind you, I wasn't even meditating or deliberately attempting a mindfulness practice. Just being in this simple room, where it was so quiet, with soft, gentle light filtered through the yellow stained glass windows and the remnants of liturgical incense wafting throughout, my entire being would settle into tranquility. My experience pointedly reminded me of the profound effect that space has on our lives, a fact to which we often fail to give sufficient attention in our daily lives.

Like time and place, the bodily posture for meditation practice is governed by the aim of creating a calm and alert mind. To create these conditions, it is helpful, at least initially, to bring the body into a still and stable position. Later, we will discuss the practice of mindfulness as the body moves, but in the training stages it is most useful to develop the fundamental skills while keeping the body as free from movement as possible. The classic position for meditating, of course, is sitting. Seasoned meditators, in fact, often refer to the discipline simply as "sitting" or "sitting practice."

But just as one can be mindful anywhere, one can cultivate mindfulness skills in any physical position, including standing, lying down, and walking. Sitting, however, has remained the favored posture for millennia—and with that we will begin.

Most of us living in the West require a chair or at least a cushion in order to sit. That is not the case in Asia, where people learn to sit comfortably on the floor or the ground from a very early age. But Westerners may need some assistance to avoid what can be an initially painful experience. With practice, the unaccustomed body can be trained to sit directly on the ground in, say, the classic lotus position. Many meditation instructors insist on the lotus posture for sitting practice. In this traditional pose, one sits on the bare floor or a thin cushion and places the right foot on top of the left thigh and the left foot on top of the right thigh. While it is relatively easy to get into the full lotus position, maintaining it can be quite difficult and painful for the novice.

Using a cushion or chair works just as well, and I think the urgency of getting to mindfulness practice outweighs the need to learn the traditional position. For that reason, I strongly suggest you at least begin with a cushion or chair. If you choose to use a cushion, I recommend that you find one that will elevate your body at least five to six inches from the floor, maybe more if you are tall. This elevation allows you to cross your legs comfortably without tiring too quickly and permits necessary circulation throughout the body.

You will also find it very helpful to wear loose-fitting and comfortable clothes for your practice. I learned that lesson the hard way by wearing tight blue jeans to my first meditation session. It wasn't long before I was in sheer agony because of the restriction of my circulation. You should remove your shoes, as well, since shoes can restrict the flow of circulation. Comfortable clothing and bare feet will serve you well, whether you're sitting on a cushion or adopting some other posture.

There are two basic types of cushions made especially for the purpose of sitting meditation. One is called a zafu, and the other is known as a gomden. The zafu is a Japanese cushion originally designed for Zen practice. It is a round pillow, about a foot in diameter and 6–8 inches thick, and stuffed with fibers such as kapok or with buckwheat hulls, to provide a firm support as you sit. You may also find the zafu designed in a crescent shape.

The gomden is a Tibetan cushion. It is rectangular, about 18 by 12 inches, and 6 inches high. It is made of hard foam, which I like because it provides firmer support than a zafu. Both types of cushions are readily available from several meditation supply companies around the country. You can easily find one simply by Googling "meditation cushion." The only sure way to decide which cushion is right for you is to try them both. I own both types and find them equally comfortable, although I usually favor the gomden because of my size.

If you want to try sitting on the floor, I recommend that you first get a zabuton. A zabuton is a large rectangular cushion, roughly 3 feet by 2 feet, on which your sitting cushion rests. If you do not have access to a zabuton, you can simply use a sofa or bed pillow or place the sitting cushion on a high pile carpet. The zabuton can be used with any sort of sitting cushion. But whether gomden or zafu, you will sit on them in essentially the same way. This particular position is known as the Burmese style. The zabuton allows your feet and ankles to rest softly rather than press against the hard floor or ground, which over time can prove painful.

One final way to sit on the floor involves a posture called seiza. Seiza is sitting on your calves, with your knees, shins, and feet resting on the ground. This manner of sitting is very common throughout Japan, even among those who do not practice meditation.

Some meditators use what is called a seiza bench—like the one I have here. This apparatus alleviates the weight placed on the calves and makes it much easier to hold this posture for a long period. The bench is placed over the calves as one kneels on the ground and then sits back on the bench's seat. Unfortunately for me, my knees are too weak for me to sustain the seiza position for a significant length of time. You, however, may find this position to your liking.

Finally, let us consider the good old chair. Using a chair for mindfulness practice is almost the same as using it for ordinary sitting, but with a few important exceptions. First, you should keep both feet flat on the floor without crossing them. This position promotes a feeling of stability and prevents cramping and other painful sensations. Second, you should not use the back of the chair for support. Sit away from the back of the chair to avoid leaning on it. Although it feels more comfortable initially, reclining against the back of the chair will soon cause you to tire, and you will find yourself moving your body to find a more comfortable position. Remember, we are seeking a posture that will enable us to avoid unnecessary movement.

All forms of sitting—on the ground, on the cushion, on a bench, and in the chair—are designed to prevent the back from resting against an external object. The purpose of this design is to encourage the back to remain in a position conducive to mental alertness and the smooth flow of breathing. Whether you choose the floor, the cushion, the bench, or the chair, the position of the back will ultimately be the same. Keep your back straight but not rigid. There should be a slight curvature following the natural contours of the spine. To achieve this position, you may find it helpful to roll your hips forward a bit as you elongate your back. One of the virtues of the seiza bench is that it is designed to put your pelvis in just the right position for the proper spinal alignment.

Regardless of what you sit on, it may be useful to imagine a string attached to the crown of your skull pulling it upwards to the top of the ceiling. This visualization helps lengthen the backbone while drawing down the shoulders and keeping the head in its proper position for practice. Remaining in this position may be uncomfortable at first, because we are not accustomed to using the lower back muscles in this way. Over time, though, those muscles will strengthen and maintaining this posture will not be difficult at all.

Let's briefly review before adding the final elements for posture. If you are on the ground or on a cushion, sit down and cross your legs in the way you find most comfortable and stable. If you are on a chair, sit slightly away from the backrest with feet flat on the floor. Now that you have found a steady place for your legs, focus your attention on the back. Allow it to elongate and follow its natural curvature. Permit your shoulders to relax by coaxing them down toward the ground and drawing them toward the spine.

With legs and back in place, we can now attend to the hands and arms. Traditionally, the upper extremities find their place in two locations. First, you may put the hands in your lap, one top of the other. Some practitioners like to allow the thumbs to touch lightly. Allow the arms to relax and let the inner thighs bear the weight of the hands. The second approach is to place the hands on the knees. You can either rest the hands on the knees with palms down or allow them to rest palms up, usually with some of the fingers touching. You will probably need to experiment with your arms and hands to decide which position is right for you. Your criteria for making this determination are comfort and stability: Choose the posture that allows you to remain still for the longest period.

With the chin essentially level with the floor, we will now consider what to do with the various elements of the head. Since a great deal of muscular tension accrues in this region of the body, it is good to try to relax those muscles systematically. Move your jaw around a little and allow it to hang slightly from the rest of the head. Do not clench it. Keep your lips lightly closed or slightly parted. Let your tongue relax in your mouth.

The next thing is deciding what to do with your eyes. You can meditate with the eyes open or shut. Both approaches have their advantages. As you would expect, keeping the eyes closed helps eliminate external visual distractions. But you may also discover that closed eyes permit a range of rather amazing internal distractions. If you gaze at the insides of your eyelids for a while, you'll see what I mean. Still, closed eyes are helpful for permitting the mind to settle down by not becoming too stimulated by events outside the body. What recommends the opened-eye practice, though, is the fact that it promotes alertness. You may find that keeping your eyes closed for an extended time makes you drowsy. Keeping the eyes open, on the other hand, works against that. If you choose to practice with open eyes, you should direct your vision to a point on the ground in front of you about six feet away from the body. You may wish to try both opened and closed eyes to determine which approach is most helpful. If you have never practiced meditative disciplines before, let me recommend that you begin with closed eyes simply to assist in removing visual distraction and promoting concentration. Later, you can try to practice with eyes open and see how that style suits you. I practice both styles at different times.

We have now completed the basic physical preparations for beginning a practice to cultivate the mind. The body is located in a safe, pleasant environment, and it has taken up a posture that will allow it to remain still and feel stable for a longer than usual period.

With these external factors in place, the mind will start to follow and will find it easier to become calm and focused. When we return in our next talk, we will pick up from here and begin to discuss the methods for allowing the mind to return to its fundamental tranquility and alertness.

Breathing—Finding a Focus for Attention
Lecture 6

Y ou can imagine the mind in its usual state as a bottle of muddy water. Your thoughts are swirling and chaotic; it's not easy to think clearly in this situation. However, if you simply set the jar down and refrain from stirring it up, the dirt will settle and the water will become clear as the sediment simply falls to the bottom. When the mind is given a chance, it will naturally settle and become clear and serene—just like muddy water.

Preparing the Mind and Body

- To allow our mind to settle, we need a focus, or an anchor—a fixed place to direct our attention while the mind calms itself. This anchor serves the same purpose as setting down a jar of muddy water. It simply helps keep us from stirring things up.

- As we continue with instructions for beginning to meditate, try to read while sitting in one of the meditative postures described earlier. This will help condition your body to the proper position, and you'll be prepared to follow instructions as they are presented. When your body is properly positioned, take a few deep breaths to help you settle in.

- As your sitting meditation proceeds, you may discover that some part of your body requires readjustment. If you find yourself needing to shift your body a bit, it is perfectly fine to do so. You goal is not to remain absolutely still but to attain some reasonable stability that allows you to focus on developing your awareness.

- As you meditate, it's a good idea to occasionally check each of the items mentioned for posture to ensure that your body is in the best position possible. The only rule is that if you make adjustments during your practice, do so with complete mindfulness.

Attending to the Mind

- Once the body is where it needs to be, we turn our attention to the mind. We take a brief moment to acknowledge our intention to practice mindfulness. As we deepen our practice, we will discover how critical it is to set proper intentions; when we are sincere and determined about our purposes, they have an amazing capacity to be realized.

- Now, we are ready to begin the meditation. Our initial task is to establish a focal point, or anchor. What we wish to do is to let the mind settle down, like a jar of muddy water, allowing its mindless hyperactivity to subside gradually.

- All forms of meditation use such an anchor, although the particular focal point varies from tradition to tradition. Some practitioners use a **mantra**, which is usually a short saying or set of syllables that the meditator repeats to him- or herself. Virtually anything—an object, a sound, a thought, or a bodily sensation—can become the focus of meditative practice.

Attending to the Breath

- In the basic mindfulness exercises taught here, we use the breath as the anchor for our attention. Although we will not focus solely on the breath, at the beginning of our training, it is a good place to start.

- For one thing, the breath is always present. Because of this, the breath is something to which we can return—no matter where we are—when our mind begins to wander, as it inevitably will. That fact is essential to strengthening our powers of concentration.

- Second, simply attending to the rhythms of breathing as we inhale and exhale brings profound calmness to the body. Watching the breath serves two important purposes: to calm us and to focus our awareness. Observing the breath can also teach us many things about the world and about ourselves, as we will see when we start to meditate.

- There are several ways you can observe the breath, and you'll need to experiment a bit to see which technique works best for you. First, you can watch your breath by focusing attention on the sensations of the air flowing through your nostrils. Simply pay attention to where the sensation feels most prominent and direct your awareness to that area. Take a few moments to try this technique.

- A second way to observe breathing is by attending to the abdomen or the chest as either expands and contracts with each breath. You may prefer directing your concentration to one of these locations if the sensation at the nostrils seems too subtle or too faint to hold your attention. Again, take a moment to try this method. Simply guide your awareness to the place where you most prominently sense the rhythms of your inhalation and exhalation.

- As you advance in your practice, you may discover other places to attend to your breathing, which is fine. The important thing is to choose a site and stay with it, at least in the initial training stages. The breath functions as a focal point for awareness, so that point needs to remain constant.

- Once you have determined where you will observe your breath, then sit there and watch yourself breathe. Now, stay there for a few moments and pay attention to your breath. Let your breathing be as effortless as possible. Just let it be what it will be.

- Your task is merely to watch what happens. If you can do this, you are being mindful. Pay attention to the minute qualities of this process, but refrain from making judgments or evaluating your experience.

- Try to notice the things you usually ignore. Observe the start of your inhalation; observe when the inhaled breath has come to an end. Then, watch as you begin to exhale, and watch as the exhalation comes to an end. As you focus on your breathing, try to remain merely observant, and stay attentive to your breath for as long as you can.

Breathing and Mindfulness

- No matter how hard we try, it's very difficult at the beginning of this discipline to stay concentrated. After only a short time, attention usually begins to wander elsewhere, and a torrent of thoughts and judgments flood the brain.

- When you notice that your mind has wandered away from its focal point, simply observe the fact that it has strayed and then—ever-so gently—return your attention to the breath. Occasionally, what distracts the mind isn't a thought but a sensation or a sound. Try not to make judgments about what has happened; simply observe and move on.

- What we've just described is the fundamental practice of developing concentration. Concentration is the capacity to stay attentive to a single thing. Hindu yogis call this ability *ekgrata*, or one-pointedness.

- To train the mind to attain one-pointedness, we must learn to become aware of when the mind wanders from its anchor and then bring it back to its focal point. In learning to concentrate, we'll repeat this process over and over: The mind strays, and we return it to the breath.

- In doing so, we are doing more than simply learning to concentrate; we are also sharpening our awareness. The real challenge in the process of learning one-pointedness is to be attentive to the mind when it drifts. Because we are conditioned to be mindless, we're usually not aware of when we have lost our focus.

- When you notice your attention has gone astray—even if it takes 15 minutes before you realize it—just return your awareness to the breath. Don't criticize yourself. Being self-critical merely agitates the mind and thwarts the very serenity you're trying to realize.

- The important thing at this stage of the practice is not to prevent the mind from wandering away from its anchor, but simply to be aware of when it does. In other words, the real goal of this practice is awareness—not one-pointedness. Being able to concentrate our attention on one thing is simply a means for helping to attain greater consciousness of our experiences as they occur.

The Problem of Boredom

- As modern people, we have become accustomed to being constantly stimulated. Our minds crave novelty and excitement, and the ubiquity of technology has only exacerbated that hunger. When faced with the idea of paying attention to our breath for 15— or even 5—minutes, many of us recoil in horror. In fact, we expend a great deal of money and time trying to avoid being bored.

- Most of us think boredom is caused by our circumstances. We think the situation we find ourselves in is simply not interesting. The mindfulness traditions, on the other hand, regard boredom as the product of inattention. We get bored, in other words, when we withdraw our full awareness from whatever it is we are experiencing at the moment.

- Boredom isn't caused by our external circumstances but by our own mind. The antidote to boredom is paying complete attention. Rather than paying attention, though, most of us are inclined continually to seek out new mental stimulants to keep our minds occupied with trivialities.

- The practice of mindfulness encourages us to relinquish the craving for stimulation and simply be attentive to what is. Boredom itself can be interesting if you simply observe it patiently without judgment.

Complete Focus on the Breath

- When you can relinquish your fear of being bored and direct your full, receptive attention to your breath, you might be amazed at what you'll discover. You might notice what a pleasant sensation relaxed breathing brings. When you can be wholly engaged with the simple pleasure of breathing, you'll find yourself with a refined sense of completeness in that moment.

- Observing the breath might also teach you about our interconnectedness with the world. As we breathe, we are exchanging substances with the rest of reality. We take in the fresh oxygen produced by plant life and offer them the carbon dioxide they need. We depend on each other. Breathing also reminds us of our connectedness to our fellow human beings.

- Attending to the breath, we become acutely conscious of the passage of time. We can see that each breath is a fleeting event. This is something we know, of course, but careful observation reveals this fact in a vivid and profound way. You'll see that each breath is remarkably unique, just as each moment that contains it is unique.

- Focusing attention on the breath and returning to it when the mind strays constitutes the basic mindfulness practice. Before you proceed to the next lecture, you should practice this exercise. Everything else in this course is based on the simple discipline of attending to the breath, so it is important that you learn this practice and become as proficient as possible.

- Whether you decide to spend a few weeks—or even a few months—on the basic practice or choose to spend only a few minutes with it, try to incorporate sitting into your daily routine. Determine in advance how long you'd like to sit. Forty-five minutes is considered to be an optimal length of practice time, but like everything in this discipline, we take things in increments.

ekgrata: The term that Hindu yogis use for concentration, or one-pointedness.

mantra: A short saying or set of syllables that a meditator repeats to him- or herself.

1. What is the purpose of finding a focal point in the cultivation of mindfulness?

2. What makes the breath a particularly useful anchor?

Breathing—Finding a Focus for Attention
Lecture 6—Transcript

You can imagine the mind in its usual state as a bottle of muddy water. Your thoughts are swirling and chaotic. It's not easy to think clearly in this situation. But if you simply set the jar down and refrain from stirring it up, the dirt will settle, and the water will become clear as the sediment simply falls to the bottom.

When given a chance, the mind will naturally become clear and serene, just like muddy water. To allow our mind to settle, we need a focus or an anchor, a fixed place to direct our attention while the mind calms itself. This anchor serves the same purpose as setting down a jar of muddy water. It simply helps us from stirring things up. Today, the focus of our conversation will be finding such a stable point for the mind.

When we met last, we discussed the spatial and temporal requisites for mindfulness practice. As we continue with instructions for beginning to meditate, I suggest that you try to listen while sitting in one of the meditative postures we described earlier. This will help condition your body to the proper position, and you'll be prepared to follow instructions as I offer them. If you're not able to take up a meditating posture—if, for example, you're hearing me as you're driving—then just listen for now, and you can begin the practice when conditions are better suited to it.

Let me start by reviewing the key steps in preparing for sitting meditation. First, make sure your physical environment is quiet, safe, and conducive to mental alertness. Choose your sitting style and make sure you have the necessary items at hand—your cushion, your chair, your bench, or your tiger skin. Then take your place on your item of choice and systematically check and adjust the following parts of your body to ensure they are properly positioned. First, observe your legs. Make sure they are in the right place for your particular style: crossed if on a cushion or the floor or tucked under the thighs for a seiza bench. If you're in a chair, sit normally with your feet flat on the ground.

Then consider your hands and arms. Your hands should be resting comfortably on your knees or in your lap and your arms should be relaxed.

Draw your shoulders down towards the floor and allow your shoulder blades to move a bit toward each other, slightly opening your chest. Next, take stock of your back. The spine should not be reclining against the back of a chair or a wall but should remain erect without any external support. Imagine a string attached to the top of your skull gently pulling your head and spine upwards, allowing the back to elongate. Roll your pelvis forward slightly to ensure a slight curvature in the small of your back. Now, close your eyes or, if you choose, allow them to remain open and focused on a point about six feet away from your body. Let your jaw relax and let your tongue rest lightly in your mouth. When your body is properly positioned, take a few deep breaths to help you settle in.

As your sitting meditation proceeds, you may discover that some part of your body requires readjustment. Your foot might go to sleep or you might get an itch or your back gradually begins to slouch. If you find yourself needing to shift your body a bit, it is perfectly fine to do so. Mindfulness practice should not become a trial for enduring pain. Your goal is not to remain absolutely still, but to attain some reasonable stability that allows you to focus on developing your awareness. If your back is in great pain, it may cause too great a distraction for you to attend to your mind. So use common sense. As you meditate, it's a good idea to occasionally check each of the items we've mentioned for posture to ensure that your body is in the best position possible. The only rule is that if you make adjustments during your practice, do so with complete mindfulness.

When the body is where it needs to be, we turn our attention to the mind. We take a brief moment to acknowledge our intention to practice mindfulness. Silently, we may say to ourselves something like, "For the next few moments, I will try to devote myself wholeheartedly to being aware of my experience, whatever it may be." As we deepen our practice, we will discover how critical it is to set proper intentions. When we are sincere and determined about our purposes, they have an amazing capacity to be realized.

Now, we are ready to begin the meditation. Our initial task is to establish the focal point that we mentioned earlier. What we wish to do is to let the mind settle down, like a jar of muddy water, allowing its mindless hyperactivity to gradually subside.

All forms of meditation use such an anchor, although the particular focal point varies from tradition to tradition. Some practitioners use a mantra, which is usually a short saying or set of syllables that the meditator repeats to him or herself. Contemplatives in the Eastern Orthodox tradition of Christianity recite the "Jesus Prayer": "Lord Jesus Christ, son of God, have mercy upon me, a sinner." These words are repeated—often tens of thousands of times a day—to keep the straying mind attentive and focused on the theological meaning of this statement. Some Hindu yogis recite a sacred syllable like Om or the name of God. Other practitioners focus attention on a mental image. In the Tibetan Buddhist tradition, meditators often visualize an enlightened being or a teacher whose qualities they wish to emulate. Virtually anything—any kind of object, a sound, a thought, or a bodily sensation—can become the focus of meditative practice.

In the basic mindfulness exercises that I teach, we use the breath as the anchor for our attention. Although we will not focus solely on the breath, at the beginning of our training, it is a good place to start. For one thing, the breath is always present. As long as you are alive, you have breath. Our very existence depends on this evanescent and almost unnoticeable process. We can live for 40 days without food or four days without water, but we can't go four minutes without breathing. Because it is ever-present, the breath is something to which we can return, over and over again, no matter where we are. That fact, as we'll see, is essential to strengthening our powers of concentration. We need some place or thing to come back to when our mind begins to wander, as it inevitably will.

Second, simply attending to the rhythms of breathing as we inhale and exhale brings profound calmness to the body. You're probably already familiar with the technique of taking several deep breaths when you're feeling angry or anxious. Just a little attention to the breath can soothe an agitated spirit. So watching the breath serves these two important purposes: 1) to calm us, and 2) to focus our awareness. But observing the breath can also teach us many things about the world and ourselves, as we'll see when we start to meditate.

There are several ways you can observe the breath, and you'll need to experiment a bit to see which technique works best for you. As I describe them, and if you're able, try out each method. First, you can watch your breath by focusing attention on the sensations of the air flowing through your nostrils. Simply pay attention to where the sensation feels most prominent and direct your awareness to that area. At first, the sensation will probably seem very subtle, but that is perfectly fine—in fact, it's even desirable. Take a few moments to try this technique.

A second way to observe breathing is by attending to the abdomen or to the chest, as they expand and contract with each breath. You may prefer directing your concentration to one of these locations if the sensation at the nostrils seems too subtle or too faint to hold your attention. Again, take a moment to try this method. Simply guide your awareness to the place where you most prominently sense the rhythms of your inhalation and exhalation.

As you advance in your practice, you may discover other places to attend to your breathing. That's fine. The important thing is to choose a site and stay with it, at least in the initial training stages. The breath functions as a focal point for awareness, so that point needs to remain constant.

Once you have determined where you will observe your breath, then, as they say, just do it: Sit there and watch yourself breathe. That's it: Now you're meditating. It's simple! It's easy! It's the most natural thing in the world! Now, stay there for a few moments and pay attention to your breath. Let your breathing be as effortless as possible. There's no need to exert any control over it. There's no need to make the breath deep or shallow. Just let it be what it will be. Your task is merely to watch what happens, as if you were a disinterested observer. If you can do this, you are being mindful.

Pay attention to the minute qualities of this process, but refrain from making judgments or evaluating your experience. Try to notice the things you usually ignore. Observe the start of your inhalation; observe when the in-breath has come to an end. Then watch as you begin to exhale, and watch as the exhalation comes to an end. Is the breathing easy or difficult? Are you controlling your breath or do you allow it to proceed on its own? Is the sound of your breath quiet or not-so-quiet? Can you feel the flow of air through your nose and into your lungs? Notice if the sensation is warm or cool. Or, are you unable to tell? As you focus on your breathing, try to remain merely observant; refrain from engaging in thinking about what you observe. Stay attentive to your breath for as long as you can. If it possible for you to do so, I suggest that you turn off the sound of my voice for just a few minutes and practice the exercise I've just described. You will find it easier to attend to your breath without having my instructions as a potential distraction. When you've had a chance to practice for a brief while, return to the lecture.

Now that you've had an opportunity to practice observing your breath, let's discuss your experience. How long were you able to stay focused on your breathing, merely observing the sensations? If you're like most of us, you probably noticed that you weren't able to keep your attention on your breath for very long.

After only a short time, the attention usually begins to wander elsewhere and a torrent of thoughts and judgments flood the brain: Am I doing this correctly? My back is starting to hurt. How boring is this? I wonder what's for lunch. No matter how hard we try, it's very difficult at the beginning of this discipline to stay concentrated. The good news is that's OK. We begin with the mind in its conditioned mindless state and train it to stay attentive.

When you notice that your mind has wandered away from its focal point, simply observe the fact that it has strayed and then, ever-so gently, return your attention to the breath. You might find it helpful at first to note this fact to yourself by silently saying "thinking" and then, without further ado, return your awareness to the breathing process. Occasionally, what distracts the mind isn't a thought but a sensation or a sound. To make note of these distractions, just silently say "feeling" or "hearing" or "hurting." If you choose to make note of the times your mind wanders from its focus, don't get involved in more thought. Try not to make judgments about what has happened. Simply observe and move on. After some practice, you'll find that you will not even need to make these silent notes. You can just notice that the mind has gotten involved in thinking or some other process and then nudge the attention back to the breath.

What we've just described is the fundamental practice of developing concentration. Concentration is the capacity to stay attentive to a single thing. Hindu yogis call this ability *ekāgratā*, or one-pointedness. To train the mind to attain one-pointedness, we must learn to become aware of when the mind wanders from its anchor and then bring it back to its focal point. In learning to concentrate, we'll repeat this process over and over. The mind strays, and we return it to the breath. But we are doing more than simply learning to concentrate; we are also sharpening our awareness. The real challenge in the process of learning one-pointedness is to be attentive to the mind when it drifts. Because we are conditioned to be mindless, we're usually not aware of when we have lost our focus.

You can be seated on your chair or cushion for 5 or 10 or 15 minutes, totally lost in your thoughts, oblivious to the fact that you're even thinking. One moment you're intently observing your breath, and then you wake up ten minutes later realizing that you're planning your summer vacation in Orlando. Furthermore, it's an absolutely mystery how you got from the cushion in your bedroom to the Shamu show at Sea World. Be prepared for the mind to wander off like this. Once again, the good news is this is OK. When you notice your attention has gone astray—even if it takes 15 minutes before you realize it—just return your awareness to the breath. Avoid commentary and judgment. Don't criticize yourself for your quarter hour of mindlessness. Being self-critical merely agitates the mind and thwarts the very serenity you're trying to realize. But if you do find yourself being self-critical, don't start criticizing yourself for being self-critical!

The important thing at this stage of the practice is not to prevent the mind from wandering away from its anchor, but simply to be aware of when it does. Let me repeat that point: The real goal of this practice is awareness, not one-pointedness. Being able to concentrate our attention on one thing is simply a means for helping to attain greater consciousness of our experiences as they occur.

Gradually, the process of observing the way the attention strays and gently returning it to the breath will strengthen both the skill of concentration and the skill of mindfulness. Meditation teacher Jack Kornfield calls this technique "training the puppy" because it is like housebreaking a young dog.

You put the puppy down and say "Stay!" But the puppy won't listen. It gets up and wanders where it will. Then you simply pick up the puppy again, put it down on the old newspapers, and say "Stay!" The puppy jumps up again and runs somewhere else, perhaps creating a mess on your new carpet. It does no good to treat the puppy harshly. Every time it runs away, you firmly but kindly pick it up and set it down again. You do it over and over and over, until, one day—voilà—the puppy stays. Likewise, firmly but kindly returning the awareness to the breath sharpens your attentiveness to what the mind is doing and accustoms it to staying put.

Now, training your mental puppy may seem to be, for many, a rather boring prospect. As modern people, we have become accustomed to being constantly stimulated. Our minds crave novelty and excitement—and the ubiquity of technology has only exacerbated that hunger. When faced with the idea of paying attention to our breath for 15—or even 5—minutes, many of us recoil in horror. In fact, we expend a great deal of money and time trying to avoid being bored, as if boredom were tantamount to death. We even use expressions like "bored to death" and "bored stiff." Consider the vast expanse of amusements, entertainments, and diversions that we create and indulge just to keep from feeling bored.

Yet the problem of boredom is not new. Ages ago, there was a Zen novice who complained to his master that he didn't enjoy meditation because he found focusing on the breath boring. "Oh, you don't find breathing interesting, huh?" asked the teacher. "Well, come with me." The student accompanied the master to a stream outside the temple. At the water's edge, the master told his student to gaze closely at his reflection in the water. As soon as the novice bent over to look, the master thrust his head deep into the water and forcibly held it there as the poor student struggled not to drown. "So," said the master, "do you still find breathing boring?"

Most of us think boredom is caused by our circumstances. We think the situation we find ourselves in is simply not interesting. The mindfulness traditions, on the other hand, regard boredom as the product of inattention. We get bored, in other words, when we withdraw our full awareness from whatever it is we are experiencing at the moment. Boredom isn't caused by our external circumstances but by our own mind. The antidote to boredom is paying complete attention. Rather than paying attention, though, most of us are inclined continually to seek out new mental stimulants to keep our minds occupied with trivialities. The practice of mindfulness encourages us to relinquish the craving for stimulation and simply be attentive to what is. This discipline can take something that appears to be boring and make it into something positively interesting, just as a submerged head can become fascinated with the breath. Boredom itself can become interesting if you simply observe it patiently without judgment. Hence, if you're concerned about being bored while you meditate, don't worry about it. It's only boredom, a fleeting experience like everything else.

When you can relinquish your fear of being bored and direct your full, receptive attention to your breath, you might be amazed at what you'll discover. You might notice what a pleasant sensation relaxed breathing brings. It's very mild and hardly perceptible, but it's there. When you can be wholly engaged with the simple pleasure of breathing, you'll find yourself with a refined sense of completeness in that moment. You know that the joy of breath is all you need. You know that just this moment is enough. You want nothing else.

Observing the breath might also teach you about our interconnectedness with the world. As we breathe, we are exchanging substances with the rest of reality. We take in the fresh oxygen produced by plant life and offer them the carbon dioxide they need. We depend on each other. Breathing also reminds us of our connectedness to our fellow human beings.

Enrico Fermi, the great 20th-century physicist, mathematically demonstrated that with each breath, we inhale at least one molecule breathed by virtually every human being—indeed every living being, human or not—who has ever lived. Thus, our breathing reveals our interdependence with all life, and with the past and the future.

Attending to the breath, we become acutely conscious of the passage of time. We can see that each breath is a fleeting event. This is something we know, of course, but careful observation reveals this fact in a vivid and profound way. You'll see that each breath is remarkably unique, just as each moment that contains it is unique.

When you start feeling bored, try to observe the source of the breath. Who is breathing? Are you breathing or are you being breathed? If you take the time, you'll discover there is a lot to learn from the breath.

In this lecture, we have covered the fundamental elements of sitting meditation. Focusing attention on the breath and returning to it when the mind strays constitutes the basic mindfulness practice. Before you proceed to the next lecture in this series, I recommend that you become further acquainted with this exercise by practicing it. Everything else we'll discuss in this course is based on the simple discipline of attending to the breath, so to move forward it is important that you learn this practice and become as proficient as possible.

Many meditation instructors, in fact, ask their students to practice attention to the breath exclusively for weeks or months to ensure that they have mastered the basic technique. When I was first learning sitting practice, learning to be attentive to the breath was all I did for at least a year. There are, of course, other valuable techniques in the mindfulness tradition, and we will discuss them, later in the series. You may choose to work only with the simple mindfulness practice we discussed today for a while before taking up the other topics. Or you may go ahead and learn about the other mindfulness techniques, knowing that you can always return to the basic practice. After over 25 years of practicing meditation, I often return to the fundamental exercise of simply watching the breath. In this sense, meditation is a matter of always beginning again.

Whether you decide to spend a few weeks—or even a few months—on the basic practice or choose to spend only a few minutes with it, try to incorporate sitting into your daily routine. Determine in advance how long you'd like to sit. Be modest at first. Many people will find it a challenge to meditate for only five minutes. Gradually, you can lengthen your sitting period. Forty-five minutes is considered to be an optimal length of practice time. But like everything in this discipline, we take things in increments.

When you feel you've had sufficient experience at practicing this basic technique, you can move on to the next lecture. The next talk will be most meaningful once you've had some meditation experience. So, set your timer and begin.

Problems—Stepping-Stones to Mindfulness
Lecture 7

P roblems are inevitable with this discipline; they should be expected. The problems you will necessarily face on this path are precisely the means that will help you progress along the way. Facing these difficulties in meditation will give us practice in confronting problems in the rest of our lives. In time, you'll see that what you thought were problems turn out to be stepping-stones to greater mindfulness. Remember that the most important aspect of any mediation practice is persistence. Never give up, and you will never fail.

Facing Difficulties with Courage

- Meditation is a microcosm of the rest of our life. Just as our lives are fraught with difficulties, so too is our meditation practice. Perhaps it is even more so, for in meditating we bring the manifold problems of our lives to sit with us while we face the special challenges that come with meditation itself.

- However, we should do more than just expect difficulties; we should welcome them. The real key to dealing with the problems we face in meditation is the attitude we take toward them. Often, our approach to life's difficulties is avoidance rather than confrontation.

- Only the complete acceptance of suffering leads to its end. To accept suffering, rather than flee from it, requires **courage**—the determination to look at difficulty straight in the eye. Courage is the fundamental attitude for facing problems.

- Although we sometimes equate courage and fearlessness, courage is not the absence of fear. Fear, in fact, is an essential component of courage. You cannot truly be courageous unless you can feel your fear fully. If you're able to stand your ground rather than averting your gaze or taking flight, that's courage.

- The very posture we assume as we meditate symbolizes the courage to which we aspire. When we determine to be still for 30 minutes, we're declaring our intention to look bravely at whatever our mind churns up without implementing our usual exit strategy.

- Facing difficulties is made easier by viewing them as opportunities to grow in awareness—to deepen our self-knowledge and our skills of compassion. We progress further by courageously meeting our difficulties than by not having them at all.

- As you reflect on the history of your life, you can see that the things that have contributed most to your personal development have been the trials you've faced and passed through.

- As we consider our difficulties in prospect, rather than in retrospect, the fears begin to well up in us. Perhaps we fear them because we think they'll overwhelm us, but the vast majority of our fears never materialize.

- Consider thinking of difficulties as merely things that require attention. Many times, there is nothing to do and nothing to solve—only something to watch, embrace, and learn from.

The Difficulties of Meditation

- There are certain difficulties associated with the discipline of meditation that are qualitatively no different than similar issues that arise when we're not meditating, but the specific aspects of meditation practice make them seem more prominent and more urgent.

- Pain may be the most common of these problems. Almost everyone has to adjust somehow to the physical discomfort that comes with meditation: Backs begin to ache, knees start to hurt, or legs go to sleep. Some of these discomforts will subside after continued practice, but some discomforts never go away.

- When you begin to experience pain, do what you can to eliminate it. If your clothes are too restrictive, change them. If you find sitting on a cushion too painful, try a chair. There is enough pain in life without adding more of it to mindfulness practice.

- There are certain discomforts that cannot be removed by altering our circumstances. However, meditation practice shows us that many of those discomforts can be mitigated by mindfulness.

Pain versus Suffering

- The mindfulness tradition understands pain as an unpleasant sensation. Because we comprise physical bodies, pain is inevitable. Suffering, however, is not the same as pain, although most of us equate the two.

- Suffering, as it's understood in mindfulness practice, is a mental and emotional response. It may or may not be associated with the sensation of pain. It's possible to suffer without pain, just as it's possible to feel pain without suffering.

- When the sensation of pain arises, we usually respond immediately with resistance, which is why pain and suffering are so closely associated in our minds. The slightest discomfort might cause us to wince and groan.

- Our minds may begin to go through any number of conditioned reactions: We feel a sense of unfairness, lodge a protest, and then fear sets in. Sometimes, fear turns to panic.

- Underlying all of these forms of resistance is the same belief: Pain shouldn't happen to us. That belief is a great source of our suffering. It can condition anger, fear, panic, and disillusionment.

- One way to reduce our suffering, then, is to align our minds with reality. Believing that pain shouldn't happen to us is delusional; it is inconsistent with the nature of the world. Rather than resist, we can be open to pain—to respond to it with compassionate mindfulness.

- It is possible, with sufficient training, to become an observer of our pain. Refining this technique can lessen one's suffering and may, in fact, lessen one's pain.

Dealing with Pain

- If physical discomfort appears as you meditate, allow the pain to become the object of your attention. Simply let the sensation itself provide the anchor for your awareness and become mindful of the pain as you would be of your breath. Watch the pain as you would watch your own inhalation and exhalation.

- Try to relax any tension or contraction of muscles surrounding the painful sensation. Observe the sensation with curiosity. Try to narrow your focus on the pain. Watch the pain change and move. If your focus is sharp enough, you can perceive the impermanent nature of pain. If you cannot stay focused on the sensation itself, direct your attention to how you're reacting to it.

- As you study your pain, you may find your resistance to it diminishing. It may continue to hurt, but you may suffer less because you are no longer struggling against it. With enough practice, you may find yourself simply watching pain as nothing more than a sensation, like any other.

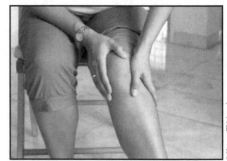

- In the early stages of practice, it is unrealistic to expect that this technique of

Most people have to adjust to the physical discomfort that comes with meditation, including backaches and knee pain.

observation will substantially lessen the suffering associated with severe pain, such as migraines. However, even that kind of pain can be ameliorated with mindfulness over time.

- Begin your work with pain on a minor discomfort, such as an itch. With itching, as with most sorts of discomforts, we reflexively try to stop it. The next time you get an itch as you're meditating, don't scratch. Instead, observe. Draw your attention to the itch and investigate it. Notice its qualities and its impermanence.

- After a few minutes of mindfulness, you may be able to watch the itch dissolve. If it doesn't, it's okay to scratch. When you scratch, however, just make sure you do so with complete awareness.

- As you continue working with little sensations, you will eventually become skilled enough to use these methods with more intense expressions of pain. People who endure chronic pain, in particular, have found the mindfulness approach to be helpful in ameliorating the sorts of pain that medicines are unable to treat.

Dealing with Strange Sensations

- As you meditate, you may feel a wide variety of strange things. These weird sensations probably occur all the time, but it's often only in meditation that we become sharply conscious of them. These sensations may be unpleasant, but they can just as well be pleasant or neutral. Such feelings are totally normal for meditation.

- Some of the commonly reported odd sensations include tingling in the arms, hands, legs, and feet; feeling the entire body becoming lighter, even to the extent of floating; and feeling the body—or parts of it, such as the hands—becoming larger.

- Unusual feelings can also involve vision and sound. If you meditate with your eyes closed, you may become distracted by the displays of lights on the insides of your eyelids. If you keep your eyes open, you might see odd patterns on the floor. If it is extremely quiet, you may find the silence deafening.

- If one of these strange sensations arises as you meditate, you should treat it like anything else: You should observe it and watch your reaction to it. If it is unpleasant, view it without aversion; if it is a pleasant sensation, view it without desire or attachment.

Dealing with Concentration

- Difficulty concentrating is hardly a problem unique to meditation, but it can be particularly vexing in this practice because so much in meditation concerns this skill.

- Focusing attention on the breath and returning to it when the mind wanders is the fundamental exercise for developing concentration and refining mindfulness. Over time, diligence with this practice can dramatically improve our ability to attain one-pointedness.

- If you're finding it hard to stay focused, first consider whether this difficulty might derive from experiences apart from meditation. For example, drowsiness is a potential threat to concentration that can often be dealt with before meditation begins by getting more sleep or eating less.

- While we can eliminate certain external circumstances that disrupt concentration, it is not always possible to do so. If it were, perhaps we wouldn't need to meditate at all.

- Just the ups and downs of a typical day can take their toll on the mind's capacity to remain attentive. If you cannot settle those disrupting influences before sit down to meditate, sit down anyway.

- There are several exercises you may use to regain and strengthen your concentration. First, simply try to take deeper breaths, inhaling and exhaling more forcibly than usual. This will heighten the sensation of breathing, giving your attention a more prominent object of focus. You can continue this exercise until you are able to stay more attentive to the breath.

- Another concentrative practice involves counting. There are a number of variations of this technique. When your attention is able to remain with the breath for longer periods, you can drop the counting. Counting itself can become a distraction, so use it only as a prop and then let it go.

Dealing with Discouragement

- Discouragement often comes when we meet with little success in coping with physical discomfort, weird sensations, and the inability to concentrate. Discouragement leads us to want to quit the practice altogether.

- There are some good ways to face discouragement in meditation— and they happen to be good ways to deal with it in the rest of our lives. The first way is to remind ourselves that the only way to fail at meditation is not to do it. The struggles we face and the ostensible "failures" we have are part of the process.

- The second thing you can do is to examine your experience of being disheartened. Look at it dispassionately. See where it comes from. Watch it come and go. Discouragement is just an emotion like any other. It will pass away.

- Sometimes the greatest problem we face in meditation is just sitting down. Regardless of how you feel about meditation at a particular moment, you should just do it anyway—no argument, no excuses. If that strategy fails, try to remind yourself of the many benefits to be gained by developing your mindfulness.

- Usually, any aversive feelings toward the practice evaporate after a few minutes once you sit down. Once you settle into your meditation, you can begin to explore the source of your aversion. You'll probably discover some sort of fear lurking underneath your resistance, which you can meet with courage.

Important Term

courage: The ability to accept suffering rather than flee from it; the determination to look at difficulty straight in the eye.

Questions to Consider

1. How do you define courage? Why is courage important in living a full life? What aspects of your life could most benefit from the application of the virtue of courage?

2. What role does fear play in your life? What fears restrict your life the most?

Problems—Stepping-Stones to Mindfulness
Lecture 7—Transcript

By now, you should have sufficient experience with meditation to have encountered some problems. That's good. Problems are inevitable with this discipline; they should be expected.

Meditation is a microcosm of the rest of our life. Just as our lives off the cushion are fraught with difficulties, so too is our meditation practice. Perhaps it is even more so, for in meditating we bring the manifold problems of our lives to sit with us while we face the special challenges that come with meditation itself.

But we should do more than just expect difficulties; we should welcome them. The problems you will face on this path are precisely the means that will help you progress along the way. Facing these difficulties in meditation will give us practice in confronting the problems in the rest of our lives. In time, you'll see that what you thought were problems turn out to be stepping-stones to greater mindfulness.

The real key to dealing with the problems we face in meditation is the attitude we take toward them. Often, our approach to life's difficulties is avoidance. Rather than confront the deeper fears of our lives, we often attempt to mask or evade them. Our constant search for momentary pleasures is one of our strategies for hiding from our inner conflicts. It's much easier—so we think—to keep ourselves amused or intoxicated than to gaze deeply within. Ironically, the very motivation of this strategy—the desire to escape suffering—drives us right into it. Now juxtapose this irony to another: Only the complete acceptance of suffering leads to its end.

To accept suffering, rather than flee from it, requires courage—the determination to look at difficulty straight in the eye. Courage is the fundamental attitude for facing problems, both on and off the cushion. Although we sometimes equate courage and fearlessness, courage is not the absence of fear. In fact, fear is an essential component of courage. You cannot truly be courageous unless you can feel your fear fully. You could be trembling in terror and still be courageous. If you're able to stand your ground rather than averting your gaze or taking flight, that's courage. The very posture we assume as we meditate symbolizes the courage to which we aspire. When we take the cushion or chair and determine to be still for 30 minutes, we're declaring our intention to look bravely at whatever our mind churns up, without implementing our usual exit strategy. What helps me keep my place when difficulties arise is knowing that running away will ultimately cause me more suffering than staying put. Fleeing problems and facing them can both be fearful, but experience has made me more afraid of the consequences of evasion. To me, courage has become a matter of choosing the thing I fear less.

Facing difficulties is made easier by viewing them as opportunities to grow in awareness, to deepen our self-knowledge and our skills of compassion. We progress farther by courageously meeting our difficulties than by not having them at all. You already know this. As you reflect on the history of your life, you can see that the things that have contributed most to your personal development have been the trials you've faced and passed through. Yet as we consider our difficulties in prospect, rather than in retrospect, the fears begin to well up in us. Perhaps we fear them because we think they'll overwhelm us. But we usually exaggerate their power. The vast majority of our fears never materialize. As Mark Twain put it, "Some of the worst things in my life never happened."

Consider thinking of difficulties as merely things that require attention. Many times, there is nothing to do, nothing to solve, only something to watch, embrace, and learn from. Rainer Maria Rilke said it well when he suggested that "Perhaps everything that frightens us is, in its deepest essence, something helpless that wants our love." Like a crying child, the thing we fear may only need our notice and comfort.

As you've probably discovered in your meditation, there are certain difficulties associated with the discipline. These difficulties are qualitatively no different than similar issues that arise when we're not meditating, but the specific aspects of meditation practice make them seem more prominent and more urgent. Let's discuss the most common problems.

Pain may be the most common of these common problems. Almost everyone has to adjust somehow to the physical discomfort that comes with meditation. This is especially true as one is learning the rudimentary components of meditating. Most of us simply aren't used to sitting still for very long. Soon our backs begin to ache, our knees start to hurt, or our legs go to sleep. Some of these discomforts will subside after continued practice. Aching backs often get relief when the muscles we use to sit upright without support have gotten stronger. Some discomforts, though, never go away. After over 25 years of meditating, my legs still go to sleep.

When you begin to experience pain, use the common sense approach first: Do what you can to eliminate it. If your clothes are too restrictive, change them. If you find sitting on a cushion too painful, try a chair. If you're too cold, wrap yourself in a blanket or turn up the heat. There is enough pain in life without adding more of it to mindfulness practice.

Not all pain, of course, is easily dispatched with a change of clothes or a blanket. There are certain discomforts that cannot be removed by altering our circumstances. Yet meditation practice shows us that many of those discomforts can be mitigated by mindfulness.

This technique of amelioration is based on a crucial distinction between pain and suffering. The mindfulness tradition understands pain as an unpleasant sensation. Because we comprise physical bodies, pain is inevitable. We all experience pain; there's just no way around it. Suffering, however, is not the same as pain, although most of us equate the two. Suffering, as it's understood in mindfulness practice, is a mental and emotional response. It may or may not be associated with the sensation of pain. It's possible to suffer without pain, just as it's possible to feel pain without suffering. Suffering can be defined in many ways, of course, but I think of it simply as sustained resistance to reality or as a mental and emotional struggle against the way things are.

When the sensation of pain arises, we usually respond immediately with resistance, which is why pain and suffering are so closely associated in our minds. The slightest discomfort might cause us to wince or groan. Our muscles may contract around the area of pain. Our minds may begin to go through any number of conditioned reactions. Our first thought is often, This shouldn't be happening to me! We feel a sense of unfairness. This is unjust! This isn't right! I don't deserve this! In other words, we lodge a protest. Then, fear sets in. What does this mean? Is it cancer? What's causing this? What if it continues? Sometimes, fear turns to panic. I've got to stop this immediately! What can I take?

My dear mother, bless her heart, always responds to any report of my discomfort or illness with the same refrain: "Have you taken anything?"—as if for every unpleasant sensation there is a corresponding little pill to take it away. As a society, we've come to expect medical science to remove our pains, and when it doesn't, we experience profound disappointment and even anger.

Underlying all of these forms of resistance is the same belief: Pain shouldn't happen to us. That belief is a great source of our suffering. It can condition anger, fear, panic, and disillusionment. One way to reduce our suffering, then, is to align our minds with reality. Believing that pain shouldn't happen to us is delusional; it is inconsistent with the nature of the world. When pain makes its appearance, it does us no good to protest or panic. We're better served by simply accepting its advent. That's not to say we can't wish for it to leave, but to complain about its arrival or to cringe in fear only makes matters worse. Indeed, it's likely to intensify the pain itself. Rather than resist, we can be open to pain, to respond to it with compassionate mindfulness.

It is possible, with sufficient training, to become an observer of our pain. Refining this technique can lessen one's suffering and may in fact lessen one's pain. Later in the series, we'll spend an entire lecture discussing the role of mindfulness in working with pain, but for now I'll only outline some of the basic steps to assist with the minor to moderate pains that may arise in meditation practice.

If physical discomfort appears as you meditate, allow the pain to become the object of your attention. Simply let the sensation itself provide the anchor for your awareness and become mindful of the pain as you would be of your breath. Watch the pain as you would watch your own inhalation and exhalation. Try to relax any tension or contraction of the muscles surrounding the painful sensation. Observe the sensation with curiosity. What kind of pain is it? Would you characterize it as sharp or dull, throbbing, or continuous? Is it deep or shallow, intense or mild? Try to narrow your focus on the pain, as if you were pinpointing it with a laser. Does it have a shape? Watch the pain change and move. If your focus is sharp enough, you can perceive the impermanent nature of pain. If you cannot stay focused on the sensation itself, direct your attention to how you're reacting to it. Do you notice resistance or aversion? If you study your pain, you may find your resistance to it diminishing. It may continue to hurt, but you may suffer less because you are no longer struggling against it. With enough practice, you may find yourself simply watching pain as nothing more than a sensation, like any other.

In the early stages of practice, it is unrealistic to expect that this technique of observation will substantially lessen the suffering associated with severe pain, such as migraines. But with time, even that kind of pain can be ameliorated with mindfulness. Like everything else in meditation, we progress gradually.

Begin your work with pain on a minor discomfort, such as an itch. Almost every practitioner has to deal with itches, and they can be absolutely wonderful to watch. With itching, as with most sorts of discomforts, we reflexively try to stop it. You may start to itch and begin to scratch without an ounce of awareness. Let me suggest that the next time you get an itch as you're meditating, don't scratch. Instead, observe. Draw your attention to the itch and investigate it. Treat it in the same way I just suggested for any kind of pain. Become a bystander. Notice its qualities and its impermanence. Believe it or not, the common itch can be fascinating. After a few minutes of mindfulness, you may be able to watch the itch dissolve. But if doesn't, it's OK to scratch. Remember, meditation is difficult, but it shouldn't become an ordeal. When you scratch, however, just make sure you do so with complete awareness.

Working with little irritations like itching will give you practice in working with other manifestations of pain. You can apply these techniques to other forms of unpleasant sensation, such as your legs falling asleep. As you continue working with these sensations, you will eventually become skilled enough to use these methods with more intense expressions of pain. Persons who endure chronic pain, in particular, have found the mindfulness approach to be helpful in ameliorating the sorts of pain that medicines are unable to treat. We'll return to this topic later in the course when you've had more experience with meditation practice.

Not exactly in the category of pain is another set of bodily sensations that I can only classify as "weird." As you meditate, you may feel a wide variety of strange things. These weird sensations probably occur all the time, but it's often only in meditation that we become sharply conscious of them. These sensations may be unpleasant—mainly because they're unusual and we're unaccustomed to them—but they can just as well be pleasant or neutral. The main thing you should know is that such feelings are totally normal for meditation.

Some of the commonly reported odd sensations include tingling in the arms, hands, legs, and feet; feeling the entire body becoming lighter, even to the extent of floating; and feeling the body—or parts of it, such as the hands—becoming larger. You can expand so much that you feel one with the universe. Unusual feelings can also involve vision and sound. If you meditate with your eyes closed, you may become distracted by the displays of lights on the insides of your eyelids. You might see reflections of what ophthalmologists call "floaters," those unusually shaped images that seem to float slowly before your eyes. If you keep your eyes open, you might see odd patterns on the floor. You may begin to recognize faces or other shapes as you do when you watch clouds. The floor may even appear to move. The light in the room may seem to get darker or brighter. If it is extremely quiet, you may find the silence deafening.

What should you do if one of these strange sensations arises as you meditate? Treat it like anything else. You observe and watch it come and go. You watch your reaction to it. If it is unpleasant, you view it without aversion; if it is a pleasant sensation, you view it without desire or attachment. Like pain, these are just sensations. They arise and fall away. They're nothing special. Even if you feel the rapture of being one with everything, let it go.

Difficulty concentrating is hardly a problem unique to meditation, but it can be particularly vexing in this practice since so much in meditation concerns this skill. Focusing attention on the breath and returning to it when the mind wanders is the fundamental exercise for developing concentration and refining mindfulness. Over time, diligence with this practice can dramatically improve our ability to attain one-pointedness. Yet even with this practice, some meditators find it difficult to concentrate. If you're finding it hard to stay focused, first consider whether this difficulty might derive from experiences apart from meditation. I once got in the habit of watching the evening news just before beginning my sitting practice. I was perplexed as to why I was finding it hard to concentrate during these sessions until I realized that unsettling images and commentary from these newscasts were disrupting my concentration. It was almost impossible to stay attentive to my breathing as hurricanes and suicide bombers swept across my imagination.

Once identified, however, the solution was clear: I stopped watching the news before meditation. Drowsiness is another potential threat to concentration that can often be dealt with before meditation begins. Drowsiness, of course, can be induced by a large meal, insufficient sleep, or a hard day at work. These contributing factors can be easily managed by eating less, sleeping more, and scheduling your practice at optimal times.

While we can eliminate certain external circumstances that disrupt concentration, it is not always possible to do so. If it were, perhaps we wouldn't need to meditate at all. Just the ups and downs of a typical day can take their toll on the mind's capacity to remain attentive. How often do your thoughts drift back to a conversation you had earlier in the day as you're chopping carrots for supper? By the way, reflecting on the day while slicing vegetables can be particularly hazardous. If there's ever a time you need your concentration, it's while a sharp knife is in motion near your fingers. Fortunately, meditation does not involve sharp instruments, but as you meditate you may still find that the recollection of the day's events will interrupt your attentiveness.

If you can't settle those disrupting influences before sitting down to meditate, sit down anyway. There are several exercises you may use to regain and strengthen your concentration. First, simply try to take deeper breaths, inhaling and exhaling more forcibly than usual. This will heighten the sensation of breathing, giving your attention a more prominent object of focus. You can continue this exercise until you are able to stay more attentive to the breath.

Another concentrative practice involves counting. There are a number of variations to this technique. Here's one: As you inhale, silently count from 1 to 5 or 1 to 10, depending on the length of your in-breath. As you exhale, count backwards, from 5 to 1 or 10 to 1. Breathing in, it's 1, 2, 3, 4, 5. Breathing out, it's 5, 4, 3, 2, 1.

Or try this one: As you inhale, count to 10; then exhale. It's not necessary to count on the exhalation. On the next in-breath, count to 9 and then exhale. The next time make it 8, then 7, and so on until you reach 1. Then, count to 10 again and start the process over until the mind can stay better focused on the breath.

Or consider this technique: Count 1 on the inhalation and 2 on the exhalation; 3 on the inhalation and 4 on the exhalation; and so on to 10. Then start back at 1, then 2, 3, then 4.

There are a great number of ways you can vary the counting technique. I suggest you try the ones I've recommended and then invent some of your own. There is nothing sacrosanct about any particular form of this practice. Just find what works for you and use it. When your attention is able to remain with the breath for longer periods, you can drop the counting. Counting itself can become a distraction, so use it only as a prop and then let it go.

Another common problem in meditation practice is discouragement. Discouragement often comes when we meet with little success in coping with physical discomfort, weird sensations, and the inability to concentrate. Discouragement leads us to want to quit the practice altogether.

There are some good ways to face discouragement in meditation—and they happen to be good ways to deal with it in the rest of our lives. The first thing is to remind ourselves about failure and success. We usually get discouraged because we're not "succeeding" as we think we should. As I indicated in an earlier talk, the only way to fail at meditation is not to do it. The struggles we face, the ostensible "failures" we have, are part of the process. Even discouragement is part of the practice! Meditation has everything to do with so-called "failing" and starting over. Try to relinquish your conventional ideas about success. They do not apply in meditation. The second thing you can do is to examine your experience of being disheartened. Look at it dispassionately. See where it comes from. Watch it come and watch it go. Discouragement is just an emotion like any other. It will pass away.

Sometimes the greatest problem we face in meditation is just sitting down. Even though we may know that meditating is one of the best things we can do, we often find it hard to muster the desire to do it. Sometimes, it seems like an odious chore, and we begin to think of better things to do. "Tomorrow, I'll do it tomorrow," we say. "Today, though, I absolutely must wash my hair." You can easily come up with a hundred reasons not to meditate. My suggestion is to do it anyway, regardless of how you feel about it. Don't allow the issue to become a matter of debate or struggle. Don't wait for inspiration. Plan a time, put it on your calendar, and do it. That's it. No argument, no excuses.

If that strategy fails, then by all means try to reason with yourself. Remind yourself of the many benefits to be gained by developing your mindfulness. Think of how much happier you'll be. Think of how much happier those you love will be when they see how much happier you are. Think of the good you're doing for the world by becoming less of a grouch. Think of how disappointed I'll be if you don't do it.

Usually, any aversive feelings toward the practice evaporate after a few minutes once you sit down. You will discover that the resistance to meditating happens mainly in anticipation of doing it. Once you settle into your meditation you can begin to explore the source of your aversion. Sometimes, you'll probably discover some sort of fear lurking underneath your resistance. If so, you'll simply need to summon some of that courage that we talked about earlier and see what's down there.

The most important aspect of any mediation practice is persistence. Never, never give up, and you will never fail. But if you ever give up, just know that you can always start again—and again, and again, and again, and again.

Body—Attending to Our Physical Natures
Lecture 8

You can consider the body scan as one element in the practice of self-compassion. By carefully watching the various components of your body with curiosity and openness, you are extending to your own physical nature the same compassionate attentiveness you might offer to a good friend. Sometimes we find it harder to be kind to ourselves than we do to others. That difficulty reflects an estrangement within us. By giving compassionate attention to our bodies, we come closer to healing that alienation.

The Body Scan

- Mindfulness of the breath is not the only form of meditation in this tradition. Another kind of practice that builds upon the basics is known as a body scan. Because this technique uses some of the same skills as meditation that is focused on breathing, it can serve as a way to augment and support it.

- Some instructors, in fact, use the body scan as the foundational practice for teaching mindfulness. In becoming proficient with both techniques, you may find that you prefer one to the other, or you might discover them equally helpful in fostering moment-to-moment awareness.

- In the body scan, we'll take the same skill of directing attention that is used in the practice of attending to the breath and use it to focus our awareness on various aspects of our body. This operation gives us the opportunity to build up the skill of concentration by systematically surveying the body using focused attention.

- This process is similar to the way we can shine a flashlight to help illumine an object in the dark. The light brings the object of our choosing into relief while what surrounds it remains darkened. If we wish, we can move the light to other areas to bring them into view. This is the way focused attention operates.

- This practice does more than simply strengthen our concentrative abilities; it also helps acquaint us with our own bodies. Just as we are strangers to the operation of our own minds, we're often strangers to our physical entities. The body scan fosters awareness of our bodies by allowing us to feel its sensations on a part-by-part basis.

- The body scan also has the great benefit of promoting relaxation—perhaps even to a greater extent than sitting meditation. In fact, you can become so relaxed using this technique that you may fall asleep, which is fine. However, to gain the greatest benefit from this exercise, you should be well rested before you begin.

- Like meditation on breathing, the body scan can be practiced alone, but to learn this particular form of meditation, it is especially helpful to be guided through it in a step-by-step format. Once you have been led through a body scan, you can conduct it on your own at any time.

- You will need to allocate about 20 minutes for the entire body scan meditation exercise that follows, and you will need to have access to a quiet place free from distractions and interruptions.

- The body scan can be practiced in either a sitting or lying position, and you should try both postures at some point to see which best suits you. For our introduction to this exercise, however, we will use the lying position because many people find this posture easier. If you're a practitioner of hatha yoga, you may recognize the position as *shavasana*, the corpse pose.

- Before we begin, you'll need to be wearing comfortable, loose-fitting clothes, and you'll need some sort of padding to provide a little cushioning if you'll be lying on the bare floor. A lightly padded but firm surface is best. You might also want to use a thin pillow to cushion your head.

The Body Scan in Practice

- When you're prepared, lie down on your back in a supine position—with your face upward. If you want to relieve some of the tension in your back, place a pillow or blanket under your knees to elevate them slightly.

- Allow your shoulders, middle back, lower back, and hips to settle into the surface on which you're lying. Try to move your shoulder blades together slightly to allow your arm sockets to move toward the ground. Gently coax your shoulders toward your feet. Allow your hands to be open, palms up. Let your feet fall open, away from each other. Allow your head to feel heavy against the ground. Take a few deep breaths and become attentive to the inhalation and exhalation as the breath returns to its natural rhythm. Focus your attention on the sensation of breathing at the nostrils or with the rising and falling of the abdomen.

- If your mind begins to drift and dwell on thoughts or sounds, lightly return it to the sensation of breathing. Concentrate your efforts on being fully present to your experience. With each exhalation, feel your body become heavier and more relaxed.

- Now, direct your attention to your feet: Let go of any tension you may feel, and allow your feet to relax as you breathe out. Pay attention to your legs. Release any tension you may feel in this area of your body, and let your legs relax as you breathe out. Be aware of your arms and hands. If you feel any tension, let it go; allow your arms and hands to relax as you breathe out.

- Direct your awareness to your abdomen, chest, and back. Let go of any tension you may feel, and relax this area as you breathe out. Bring your attention to your neck, shoulders, and head. Allow any tightness you may feel to dissolve, and relax these parts of your body as you breathe out.

- Now that you have settled into position, allow yourself to feel your whole body as a single organism; continue to breathe naturally, letting yourself become deeply relaxed as you do.

- Now, focus your awareness on your scalp and the area on the top of your head. Allow your attention to move systematically throughout this area. Be open and inquisitive. Try to feel the sensation in that area of your body as it is. Be aware of the quality of the sensation. You may feel tightness, tingling, pressure, stiffness, or nothing in particular. If there is no sensation, just notice. Whatever the sensation, just permit it to be what it is, without judgment. Now, let go of those sensations in this part of the body and continue to breathe naturally.

- Now, bring your attention to your face: For a few moments, focus on your forehead and temples and become aware of any sensation in this area. Allow your attention to survey this part of your body with openness, simply accepting what is there. Note the quality of those sensations and relinquish them.

- Direct your awareness to your eyes and the area surrounding your eyes, and continue to note and accept the sensations you feel. If your mind has begun to wander from its attentiveness to the body, gently return it to where it should be.

- Now, allow your attention to move to other parts of your face, focusing on the nose, cheeks, and mouth. Then, become mindful of your chin, jaw, and ears—all the while observing and accepting the sensations in these areas as they are.

- Move your awareness now to the back of your head and to the top of your neck. Notice if there is tension, tingling, stiffness, or no sensation at all. Just take note of whatever you feel and let that be sufficient. Be aware and open to whatever you sense. Allow your attention to move down your neck and throat and to the top of your shoulders. Feel every aspect of these areas.

- Now, bring your awareness to your arms. Feel the inside and outside of your upper arms—noticing any sensations—as you move your attention down to the elbows, forearms, wrists, and then hands. Survey each of your fingers. Carefully try to feel every sensation, every bit of tension or pressure, tingling or lightness. Examine if the area feels warm or cool—or has no sensation at all. Don't struggle with what you feel; simply have a caring interest in what is happening. Try to be fully attentive to your experience.

- Now, relinquish your attention to your arms and hands, and direct it to the top of the chest, noticing any sensation as you move along. From the chest, follow the ribs to the upper back and to the shoulder blades. The sensation may be pleasurable, unpleasant, or simply absent. Accept whatever is there with gentleness and compassion.

- Next, let your attention move down the spine to your lower back, and then bring your awareness to the abdomen. Take a moment to feel yourself breathe, as your belly and lower back expand and contract with each inhalation and exhalation. Feel the subtle movements of the breath, noticing the slight pressure of your clothing as you breathe. In this area of your body, you may feel sensations in your internal organs as they function to keep you alive.

- Allow your awareness to move to your hips and groin. If your mind has begun to drift, gently refocus your attention on this part of the body. Sense the physical impressions in this area and note their qualities. Accept each sensation as it is; just observe and move on.

- Bring your attention to your upper legs. First, observe the way the muscles and skin of your inner thighs feel, and then do the same for the muscles and skin of your outer thighs. Slowly scan downward to your knees. Feel each and every sensation. Be aware of everything, and continue to breathe. If your mind has wandered, escort it back to where you want it to be.

- Continue to move your awareness down your legs, shifting attention to your shins and then your calves, noticing any tension or tingling—any pleasant or unpleasant feelings. Be mindful as you give attention to your ankles and heels, to the tops and soles of your feet, and finally to your toes. Try to bring your awareness to each of your toes, feeling whatever sensation might be perceptible.

- Now, allow your awareness to encompass your entire body as a whole. Take time to feel the sensation of being alive in this moment. You may feel deeply relaxed and suffused with a sense of well-being and peacefulness. You can return to this peacefulness at any time.

- When you are ready to end the meditation, slowly move your fingers and toes—and then your arms and legs. Open your eyes and gently move the other parts of your body. Then, very carefully, roll over to one side and use your arms and hands to bring yourself to a sitting position.

Variations on the Body Scan

- Now that you have become acquainted with the basic features of the body scan, feel free to vary the practice in ways you find most beneficial. As mentioned, the body scan can be performed in the sitting posture or in a standing pose. You can conduct the practice at a faster or slower pace, or you can scan your body from toes to head or right to left or left to right. The variations are many, and you should determine for yourself which possibilities you find most valuable in promoting awareness and relaxation.

Important Term

shavasana: This position is known as the corpse pose and is practiced in hatha yoga.

1. How do you imagine the relationship between the body and mind?

2. In what ways does the body scan augment the practice of sitting meditation?

Body—Attending to Our Physical Natures
Lecture 8—Transcript

In an earlier lecture, I introduced the fundamental technique of attending to the breath to cultivate mindfulness. This simple exercise constitutes the basic practice of sitting meditation. But as I indicated then, mindfulness of the breath is not the only form of meditation in this mindfulness tradition.

Today, I'll introduce another kind of practice that builds upon the basics we've discussed earlier. This technique is known as a body scan. Because this technique uses some of the same skills we discussed earlier, it can serve as a way to augment and support meditation that is focused on breathing.

Some instructors, in fact, use the body scan as the foundational practice for teaching mindfulness. I invite you to become proficient with both techniques; you may find that you prefer one to the other, or you might discover them equally helpful in fostering moment-to-moment awareness.

Our practice of attending to the breath is based on our capacity to direct attention to whatever dimension of our experience we choose. As we begin the breathing practice, our intention is to focus awareness on the breath. Initially, we're able to concentrate on breathing for only a brief while before the mind starts to wander and drift into thought or attend to a sensation. Our goal is to become aware of the mind's waywardness and gently escort the attention back to the breath. As we continue to practice this technique, we become more adept at being attentive to our experience and directing our awareness to the aspects of experience that we choose. In so doing, we gain greater control of our attention, and our mind begins to give up its nomadic ways.

In the body scan, we'll take this same skill of directing attention and use it to focus our awareness on various aspects of the body. You might liken this process to the way we can shine a flashlight—or torch, as we say in my household—to help illumine an object in the dark. The light brings the object of our choosing into relief, but what surrounds it remains darkened. If we wish, we can move the light to other areas to bring them into view. This is the way focused attention operates. Using this operation on the body gives us the opportunity to build up the skill of concentration. In the body scan, we systematically survey the body using focused attention.

Yet the practice does more than simply strengthen our concentrative abilities; it also helps acquaint us with our own bodies. Just as we are strangers to the operation of our own minds, we're often strangers to the physical entities that we are. The body scan fosters awareness of our bodies by allowing us to feel its sensations part-by-part. In later discussions, we'll see how directing awareness to different areas of the body helps us to cope with pain and the body's mortality. The body scan also has the great benefit of promoting relaxation, perhaps even to a greater extent than sitting meditation. In fact, you can become so relaxed using this technique that you may fall asleep. If that occurs, it's fine. Most Westerners are terribly sleep-deprived, and a bit of extra sleep will probably do you some good. However, to gain the greatest benefit from this exercise, you should be well-rested before you begin, since the chief purpose of this practice is strengthening awareness.

Like meditation on breathing, the body scan can be practiced alone, without any assistance from another. But to learn this particular form of meditation, it is especially helpful to be guided through it step-by-step. Once you have been led through a body scan, you can conduct it on your own at any time.

Or you may find it beneficial to be guided through the process each time you practice it. One of the great advantages of having these recorded lectures is the opportunity to play them over and over. You might find that you'd like to listen to my instructions each time you practice the body scan.

Now, for the remainder of this session, I will lead you through an entire body scan meditation. I invite you to participate if you can. You will need to allocate about 20 minutes for this exercise and have access to a quiet place free from distractions and interruptions. The place you use for sitting meditation will work fine. The body scan can be practiced in either a sitting or lying position, and I recommend that you try both postures at some point to see which best suits you. For our introduction to this exercise, however, we will use the lying position since many people find this posture easier to use. If you're a practitioner of hatha yoga, you may recognize the position we'll take as *shavasana*, the corpse pose. And if you're not a yogi or yogini, don't be alarmed by the name. Remember that in many traditions, rebirth is always preceded by death.

Before we begin, you'll need to be wearing comfortable, loose-fitting clothes, as for sitting meditation. You'll also need some sort of padding to provide a little cushioning if you'll be lying on the bare floor. A yoga mat or a folded blanket or quilt would work well. If your floor is carpeted, you may not require additional cushioning. You can even use a sofa or the bed, but these may actually be too comfortable and may induce sleep. As I said, sleep is fine, but the real benefits from this practice are gained by staying alert. A lightly padded but firm surface is best. If you have back problems, you may want to place a pillow or rolled up blanket under your knees to relieve some of the stress on your back muscles. You might also want to use a thin pillow to cushion your head. If you need to make preparations, you can turn off your media player at this point and turn it back on when you're ready.

When you're prepared, lie down on your back in a supine position and follow my instructions. If you want to relieve some of the tension in your back, place a pillow or rolled blanket under your knees to elevate them slightly. Close your eyes. Now allow your shoulders, middle back, lower back, and hips to settle into the surface on which you're lying. Try to move your shoulder blades together slightly to allow your arm sockets to move toward the ground. Gently coax your shoulders toward your feet. Allow your hands to be open, palms up. Let your feet fall open, away from each other. Allow your head to feel heavy against the ground. Take a few deep breaths and become attentive to the inhalation and exhalation as the breath returns to its natural rhythm. Focus your attention on the sensation of breathing at the nostrils or with the rising and falling of the abdomen. If your mind begins to drift and dwell on thoughts or sounds, lightly return it to this sensation. Concentrate your efforts on being fully present to your experience. With each exhalation, feel your body become heavier and more relaxed.

Now direct your attention to your feet; let go of any tension you may feel; and allow your feet to relax as you breathe out. Pay attention to your legs; release any tension you may feel in this area of your body; and let your legs relax as you breathe out. Be aware of your arms and hands; if you feel any tension, let it go; and allow your arms and hands to relax as you breathe out.

Direct your awareness to your abdomen, chest, and back; let go of any tension you may feel; and relax this area as you breathe out. Bring your attention to your neck, shoulders and head; allow any tightness you may feel to dissolve; and relax these parts of your body as you breathe out. Now that you have settled into position, allow yourself to feel your whole body as a single organism; continue to breathe naturally, letting yourself become deeply relaxed as you do.

Now focus your awareness on your scalp and the area on the top of your head. Allow your attention to move systematically throughout this area. Be open and inquisitive. Try to feel the sensation in that area of your body as it is. Be aware of the quality of the sensation. You may feel tightness, tingling, pressure, stiffness, or nothing in particular. If there is no sensation, just notice. Whatever the sensation, just permit it to be what it is, without judgment. Now, let go of those sensations in this part of the body and continue to breathe naturally.

Now bring your attention to your face: For a few moments, focus on your forehead and temples and become aware of any sensations in this area. Allow your attention to survey this part of your body with openness, simply accepting what is there. Note the quality of those sensations and relinquish them.

Direct your awareness to your eyes and the area surrounding your eyes, and continue to note and accept the sensations you feel. If your mind has begun to wander from its attentiveness to the body, gently return it to where it should be. Now allow your attention to move to other parts of your face, focusing on the nose, cheeks, and mouth. Then become mindful of your chin, your jaw, and ears, all the while observing and accepting the sensations in these areas as they are.

Move your awareness now to the back of your head and the top of your neck. Notice if there is tension, tingling, stiffness, or no sensation at all. Just take note of what you feel and let that be sufficient. Be aware and open to whatever you sense. Allow your attention to move down your neck and throat and to the top of your shoulders. Feel every aspect of these areas.

Now, bring your awareness to your arms. Feel the inside and outside of your upper arms, noticing any sensations, as you move your attention down to the elbows, to your forearms, your wrists, and then your hands. Survey each of your fingers. Carefully try to feel every sensation, every bit of tension or pressure, tingling or lightness. Examine if the area feels warm or cool or has no sensation at all. Don't struggle with what you feel; simply have a caring interest in what is happening. Try to be fully attentive to your experience.

Now relinquish your attention to your arms and hands, and direct it to the top of your chest, noticing any sensation as you move along. From the chest, follow the ribs to the upper back and to the shoulder blades. The sensation may be pleasurable, unpleasant, or simply absent. Accept whatever is there with gentleness and compassion.

Next, let your attention move down the spine to your lower back, and then bring your awareness to the abdomen. Take a moment to feel yourself breathe, as your belly and lower back expand and contract with each inhalation and exhalation. Feel the subtle movements of the breath, noticing the slight pressure of your clothing as you breathe. In this area of your body you may feel sensations in your internal organs as they function to keep you alive.

Allow your awareness to move to your hips and groin. If your mind has begun to drift, gently refocus your attention on this part of the body. Sense the physical impressions in this area and note their qualities. Accept each sensation as it is. Just observe and move on.

Bring your attention to your upper legs. First observe the way the muscles and skin of your inner thighs feel, and then do the same for the muscles and skin of your outer thighs. Slowly scan downward to your knees. Feel each and every sensation. Be aware of everything, and continue to breathe. If your mind has wandered, escort it back to where you want it to be.

Continue to move your awareness down your legs, shifting attention to your shins and then your calves, noticing any tension or tingling, any pleasant or unpleasant feelings. Be mindful as you give attention to your ankles and heels, to the tops and soles of your feet, and finally to your toes. Try to bring your awareness to each of your toes one-by-one, feeling whatever sensation might be perceptible.

Now, allow your awareness to encompass your entire body. Take time to feel the sensation of being alive in this moment. You may feel deeply relaxed and suffused with a sense of well-being and peacefulness. You can return to this peacefulness at any time.

When you are ready to end the meditation, slowly move your fingers and toes, and then your arms and legs. Open your eyes and gently move the other parts of your body. Then very carefully, roll over to one side and use your arms and hands to bring yourself to a sitting position.

Now that you have become acquainted with the basic features of the body scan, you should feel free to vary the practice in ways you find most beneficial. As I mentioned, the body scan can be performed in the sitting posture, or in a standing pose for that matter. You can conduct the practice at a faster or slower pace, as you find helpful or convenient. You can scan your body from toes to head or right to left or left to right. The variations are many, and you should determine for yourself which possibilities you find most valuable in promoting awareness and relaxation.

In a conversation later in the series, we'll talk about the importance of treating ourselves with compassion. Anticipating that discussion, let me say now that you can consider the body scan as one element in the practice of self-compassion. By carefully watching the various components of your body with curiosity and openness, you are extending to your own physical nature the same compassionate attentiveness you might offer to a good friend. Sometimes we find it harder to be kind to ourselves than we do to others. That difficulty reflects an estrangement within us. By giving our bodies compassionate attention, we come closer to healing that alienation.

Mind—Working with Thoughts
Lecture 9

W e may not be able to control particular thoughts, but we can influence the conditioned mind that gives rise to particular thoughts. We can prepare a fertile mental soil that increases the likelihood of germinating wholesome, skillful ideas and decreases the likelihood of growing distracting ones—but such a mind must be tended with a watchful eye. Unwholesome thoughts grow fast and wild and leech vital nutrients from the thoughts that are conducive to our freedom and happiness.

The Tamed Mind

- The mind is a double-edged sword: It is capable of doing us great benefit as well as great injury. Naturally, we want to cultivate our mental processes in such a way that we maximize the mind's capacity for doing good and minimize its tendencies for causing suffering. The skills we refine as we develop moment-to-moment awareness in sitting meditation are the same used in shaping the mind to function in more wholesome ways.

- As we've observed both casually and in formal meditation, the untamed mind tends to operate in a rather haphazard way, bounding from thought to thought with little or no apparent prompting or direction. The mind seems to have a mind of its own. Thus, it might appear that our thoughts are thoroughly beyond our control—that we have no choice about the kinds of things that drift across our minds.

- Although thoughts may seem to come out of the blue, they are, in fact, conditioned by previous patterns of thought. The thoughts that our mind produces now have been shaped by its history of thinking.

- Recent neuroscientific research has shown that routine patterns of thought make incremental but substantial changes in the way the brain is structured and the way the mind functions. These structural alterations make the brain more effective at doing what it is asked to do.

- If we habitually think in certain ways, the mind becomes more adept at those patterns of thought. Thus, as the concept of conditioning suggests, wholesome thoughts create a propensity for more wholesome thoughts, and unwholesome thoughts predispose the mind to produce more unwholesome thoughts.

- Fortunately, we can use this dynamic principle to our advantage. While we may not be in conscious control of each and every thought, meditation practice shows us that we can choose which thoughts to entertain and develop and which to observe and release. In this manner, we can influence the kinds of thoughts we are likely to produce in the future.

- In the meditation practices we've discussed so far, our practice of releasing thoughts has been indiscriminate. We've been training the mind to drop any thought as soon as we become aware of it, without regard to its content or quality. The purpose of this particular practice is to reinforce our ability to focus and be attentive.

- When we have become sufficiently proficient at using these techniques, we can add another component to the practice that will enable us to manage our thinking more consciously. In this new method, we will endeavor not only to become aware of thoughts as they arise, but also to identify the kind of thoughts we are having. Once identified, we can make conscious choices about how we will handle them.

The Unskilled Mind

- Because of our conditioning, the great majority of our thoughts are not conducive to our well-being. In the mindless state, our thoughts can be highly critical of others—and of ourselves. When you attend carefully to the quality of your thoughts, you might easily conclude that most of them serve little constructive purpose in our lives.

- Because of the mind's overproduction of unwholesome thoughts, it redounds to our benefit to be able to respond appropriately and immediately when such thoughts arise. Doing this, of course, requires sharp attention and the capacity to discern wholesome from unwholesome thoughts.

- Unfortunately, the unskilled mind finds this difficult to do. Just as the untrained mind has difficulty even knowing when it is absorbed in thought, it finds it hard to know when a thought is edifying or corrosive. Often, the undisciplined mind even fails to appreciate the importance of this distinction.

- The mindfulness tradition offers very specific ways of identifying harmful thoughts and enables us to see why they are problematic. According to this tradition, an unwholesome thought is one that is not conducive to freedom and happiness but, rather, promotes suffering. Conversely, wholesome thoughts diminish suffering and foster happiness and freedom.

Unwholesome Thoughts

- Unwholesome thoughts may be recognized by certain telltale traits. Specifically, unwholesome thoughts—which we can also call unskillful thoughts—are connected to selfish desire, hatred, or delusion.

- Thoughts associated with selfish desire are predicated on our voracious appetite for pleasure. An unwholesome thought of this sort may prompt us to act or speak in a way that provides us with momentary gratification.

- Whereas thoughts based on selfish desire draw us toward an act that we believe will give us pleasure, thoughts associated with hatred repel us from people or situations we think will cause us pain or make us feel uncomfortable.

- Deluded thoughts are at odds with reality and result from our failure to see ourselves and the world as they really are. On the basis of delusion, we can generate grandiose thoughts about our own importance or our own worthlessness, or we can somehow come to believe that we are immune to the vicissitudes to which everyone else is subject.

- It requires skill, of course, to recognize these unskillful thoughts, and ultimately, it takes knowing ourselves very well—the kind of self-knowledge that comes only with ruthless honesty and dispassionate observation.

- To give you some practice at identifying unskillful thoughts, try this simple exercise the next time you meditate or sit in the park. Whenever you catch your mind drifting in its usual haphazard way, take a moment to examine the character of the thought that has captured your attention.

- The great danger of entertaining any thought that arises from selfish desire, hatred, and delusion is its eventual effects on the shape of our minds. Even the thoughts that remain confined to the interior of our skulls can proliferate, generating habits of thought that form our personality and character.

Attending to Unwholesome Thoughts

- The mindfulness tradition offers a variety of very practical ways to assist us in disempowering unwholesome thoughts and relaxing their corrosive effects on the mind. They're all forms of relinquishment, and they're all dependent on our ability to recognize an unwholesome thought when it arises.

Replacement

- In some ways, replacement is the simplest and most effective method of disarming a harmful thought. When an unwholesome thought arises, we immediately supplant it with a wholesome one. The

Buddha likened this method to the way a woodworker might knock out a coarse peg with a fine one.

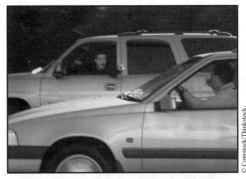
© Comstock/Thinkstock.

Initially, the practice of replacing unwholesome thoughts with wholesome ones may seem artificial in situations such as road rage.

- This approach is most effective when the unskillful thought is replaced by a skillful one that directly counteracts it. Thoughts based on selfish desire, for example, can be substituted by thoughts about the impermanence of the object of desire. Thoughts grounded in hatred can be replaced with notions of friendliness and compassion. Finally, thoughts founded on delusion can be overcome by thoughts based in reality.

- Initially, the technique of replacing thoughts may seem awkward and artificial, but if you act in a certain way over time—even when it doesn't feel authentic—those actions will eventually begin to feel and be real and genuine.

Reflecting on Results

- We can also contemplate the consequences of the unwholesome thought by reflecting on the results. When unwholesome thoughts arise, we think about the effects of holding these unwise notions. Consider the kind of person you become when you entertain and foster a particular unwholesome thought. If mind shapes our experience, then our thoughts have ineluctable consequences.

- Follow the trajectory of an unwholesome thought. It's not even necessary to reflect on the consequences of acting on these thoughts; you can simply think about having your mind packed with such ideas.

- The Buddha compares the unwholesome thought to a snake or animal carcass around the neck of a well-dressed person. Such a thought, he argues, is unbecoming to a wise and compassionate human being. When the unskillful thought appears, don't denounce it; just let it go, reminding yourself that it is not reflection of who you truly are.

Redirecting

- Redirecting is simply diverting attention away from the unwholesome thought to something more beneficial. The Buddha compared this technique to averting one's gaze to avoid staring at certain objects.

- In sitting meditation, when the mind has been distracted by thought, we simply escort the attention back to the breath. Thus, our practice of meditation strengthens our ability to employ this technique.

- Redirecting attention relies on the impermanence of reality to work. We're all aware that everything in the world will change and pass away. That thought usually occasions within us a feeling of sadness or melancholy. However, the impermanence of reality can be a source of comfort and happiness when we accept it, and we have to be constantly reminded to accept it.

- Redirecting attention helps us to accept the impermanence of the world and to use that fact to our benefit. Thoughts, like everything else, pass away. To maintain a thought, we have to renew it, which is why we have to be reminded of life's transience. Of course, if we renew the unwholesome thought, it will arise again, at which point we escort our attention elsewhere. Eventually, by redirecting attention, the unwholesome thought will lose its power and fade.

- Redirecting attention need not use the breath as its anchor; any wholesome thought or activity can suffice. Far better to keep oneself diligently engaged with wholesome activity lest the straying mind comes to dwell in greed, aversion, and delusion.

Reconstructing

- Reconstructing involves analyzing the formation of the unskillful thought. In reflecting on results, we contemplate the forward trajectory of an unwholesome thought, considering its consequences for the future. With reconstructing, on the other hand, we examine the antecedents that have given rise to the unwholesome notion.

- Through the process of reconstructing, we can begin to examine the assumptions supporting a particular belief. This allows us to see how unwholesome thoughts can be rooted in untenable assumptions that we make about the things that will make us happy, and it allows us to examine those assumptions more rationally.

- When we've analyzed the root causes of envy enough times, we come to recognize a peculiar pattern of unskillful thinking that most of us routinely practice. It's a manner of thought strongly encouraged by our competitive culture.

- The mindfulness tradition calls restructuring "comparing mind," which is the insidious habit of seeing how we measure up to other people. Our culture is obsessed with it and, in a sense, thrives on it.

- The foremost disadvantage of comparing mind is the unnecessary suffering it causes: We not only feel bad about ourselves, but we often begin to wish ill upon the person we envy—sometimes to the point where we take steps to realize those wishes.

- Whether we judge ourselves favorably or unfavorably, the practice of comparing mind is unwholesome. It causes us harm, expends our precious mental energy, and erodes our relationships with others.

- Although it is generally unskillful, there are times when comparing mind can be used skillfully, but doing so is an advanced practice that requires great wisdom. For most of us, however, certainly in the early stages of mindfulness practice, it is a habit that is best acknowledged and then relinquished.

Questions to Consider

1. As you meditate, try to identify patterns of unwholesome, or unskillful, thinking. What kinds of negative thoughts seem to dominate your thinking life?

2. Which techniques to deal with unwholesome thoughts work best for you?

Mind—Working with Thoughts
Lecture 9—Transcript

The mind is a two-edged sword. It is capable of doing us great benefit as well as great injury.

Naturally, we want to cultivate our mental processes in such a way that we maximize the mind's capacity for doing good and minimize its tendencies for causing suffering. The skills we refine as we develop moment-to-moment awareness in sitting meditation are the same used in shaping the mind to function in more wholesome ways. Today, we'll discuss how to take those skills in meditation practice and use them to nurture a mind that will bring us greater happiness.

As we've observed both casually and in formal meditation, the untamed mind tends to operate in a rather haphazard way, bounding from thought to thought with little or no apparent prompting or direction. The mind seems to have a mind of its own. Thus, it might appear that our thoughts are thoroughly beyond our control, that we have no choice about the kinds of things that drift across our minds.

Although thoughts may seem to come out of the blue, they are, in fact, conditioned by previous patterns of thought. The thoughts that our mind produces now have been shaped by its history of thinking. Recent neuro-scientific research has shown that routine patterns of thought make incremental but substantial changes in the way the brain is structured and the way the mind functions. These structural alterations make the brain more effective at doing what it is asked to do. If we habitually think in certain ways, the mind becomes more adept at those patterns of thought. Thus, as the concept of conditioning suggests, wholesome thoughts create a propensity for more wholesome thoughts; unwholesome thoughts predispose the mind to produce more unwholesome thoughts.

Fortunately, we can use this dynamic principle to our advantage. While we may not be in conscious control of each and every thought, meditation practice shows us that we can choose which thoughts to entertain and develop and which to observe and release. In this manner, we can influence the kinds of thoughts we are likely to produce in the future. The power to select and then foster or relinquish thoughts is a tool we can use to cultivate a skillful mind that will serve us well.

In the meditation practices we've discussed so far, we have exercised our capacities to concentrate and be attentive to our experience. In sitting meditation, we've learned to focus our awareness on our breath and try to be attentive to moments when the mind strays, mindlessly getting lost in thought. In the body scan, we've seen how to develop the same skills of focusing awareness and gently returning attention to the body when the mind wanders. Both practices help strengthen our skill at observing thoughts as they appear and then relinquishing them.

Now up to this point, our practice of releasing thoughts has been indiscriminate. We've been training the mind to drop any thought as soon as we become aware of it, without regard to its content or quality. The purpose of this particular practice is to reinforce our ability to focus and be attentive. When we have become sufficiently proficient at using these techniques, we can add another component to the practice that will enable us to manage our thinking more consciously. In this new method, we endeavor not only to become aware of thoughts as they arise but also to identify the kinds of thoughts we are having. Once identified, we can make conscious choices about how we will handle them.

Because of our conditioning, the great majority of our thoughts are not conducive to our well-being. In the mindless state, our thoughts can be highly critical of others—and of ourselves. They can dwell on pointless and trivial matters of little real significance. They may lead us to eat when we're not hungry and to say things we immediately regret. They can anxiously focus on the future, anticipating things that have little likelihood of being realized, or sorrowfully focus on the past, regretting things that cannot be changed. When you attend carefully to the quality of your thoughts, you might easily conclude that most of them serve little constructive purpose in our lives.

Because of the mind's overproduction of unwholesome thoughts, it redounds to our benefit to be able to respond appropriately and immediately when such thoughts arise. Doing this, of course, requires sharp attention and the capacity to discern wholesome from unwholesome thoughts.

Unfortunately, the unskilled mind finds this difficult to do. Just as the untrained mind has difficulty even knowing when it is absorbed in thought, it finds it hard to know when a thought is edifying or corrosive. Often, the undisciplined mind even fails to appreciate the importance of this distinction. An apocryphal anecdote from the life of Sigmund Freud puts this difficulty in an amusing light. Freud supposedly asked one his patients if she were ever troubled by lustful thoughts. "No," she replied, "I rather enjoy them."

The mindfulness tradition offers very specific ways of identifying harmful thoughts and enables us to see why they are problematic. According to this tradition, an unwholesome thought is one that is not conducive to freedom and happiness, but rather, promotes suffering. Conversely, wholesome thoughts diminish suffering and foster happiness and freedom. Unwholesome thoughts may be recognized by certain telltale traits. Specifically, unwholesome thoughts—which we can also call unskillful thoughts—are connected to selfish desire, hatred, or delusion.

Thoughts associated with selfish desire are predicated on our voracious appetite for pleasure. An unwholesome thought of this sort may prompt us to act or speak in a way that provides us with momentary gratification. A thought might arise suggesting that we make a witty remark at the expense of a friend to make us appear clever and funny. Thoughts of hatred arise out of feelings of aversion or our desire to avoid unpleasant experiences. Whereas thoughts based on selfish desire draw us toward an act that we believe will give us pleasure, thoughts associated with hatred repel us from people or situations we think will cause us pain or make us feel uncomfortable.

My fear of others different from me might generate thoughts that exaggerate another's faults or lead me to accept misleading stereotypes about another's character. Deluded thoughts are at odds with reality and result from our failure to see ourselves and the world as they really are. On the basis of delusion, we can generate grandiose thoughts about our own importance or about our own worthlessness; or we can somehow come to believe that we are immune to the vicissitudes to which everyone else is subject, such as getting old and dying. It requires skill, of course, to recognize these unskillful thoughts, and ultimately, it takes knowing ourselves very well, the kind of self-knowledge that comes only with ruthless honesty and dispassionate observation.

To give you some practice at identifying unskillful thoughts, try this simple exercise the next time you meditate or sit in the park. You can also turn off your media player and do it now. Whenever you catch your mind drifting in its usual haphazard way, take a moment to examine the character of the thought that has captured your attention. Look carefully to see if it is a thought that is rooted in selfish wanting or aversion or in unrealistic beliefs about the nature of the world. With patience and practice, you can become quite skilled at recognizing your unskillful thoughts.

The great danger of entertaining any thought that arises from selfish desire, hatred, and delusion is its eventual effects on the shape of our minds. True, the biting comment that comes to mind in conversation seems relatively harmless if we keep our mouths shut and resist saying aloud what's running through our heads. Yet, even the thoughts that remain confined to the interior of our skulls, not immediately coming to expression as word or deed, can proliferate, generating habits of thought that form our personality and character. Inevitably, the shape of our mind determines the person we become.

Unwholesome thoughts, therefore, need attention. The mindfulness tradition offers a variety of very practical ways to assist us in disempowering these thoughts and relaxing their corrosive effects on the mind. Somehow, I've been able to come up with names for these techniques that all begin with the letter "R," which ought to make them a little easier to remember. They're all forms of that other R-word we've been brandishing about: relinquishment. And they're all dependent on our ability to recognize an unwholesome thought when it arises.

I call the first technique "replacement." In some ways, it is the simplest and most effective method of disarming a harmful thought. When an unwholesome thought arises, we immediately supplant it with a wholesome one. The Buddha likened this method to the way a woodworker might knock out a coarse peg with fine one. This approach is most effective when the unskillful thought is replaced by a skillful one that directly counteracts it.

Thoughts based on selfish desire, for example, can be substituted by thoughts about the impermanence of the object of desire. As your mind is salivating over the latest electronic gadget to hit the market, you might remind yourself that within a few months the device you think you must have right now will be obsolete and within a few years will be a useless heap of plastic and silicon.

Thoughts grounded in hatred can be replaced with notions of friendliness and compassion. When you feel animosity towards the lunatic who cuts you off in traffic, immediately wish him well. You might think flipping him off will make you feel better, but it really only builds hostility. Is that the kind of person you really want to be? Finally, thoughts founded on delusion can be overcome by thoughts based in reality. The unskilled mind, of course, mistakes delusional thoughts for reality, but meditation helps the practitioner to see the difference. One is deluded, for example, by thinking she can escape growing old and remain youthful-looking. What a relief it is simply to replace that fantasy with the realistic acceptance of aging.

Initially, the technique of replacing thoughts may seem awkward and artificial. Wishing godspeed to the speed demon in the car next to you might seem forced and stilted at first, and it might even seem insincere. That's all right. I'm a believer in the power of "faking it till you make it," which is the idea that if you act in a certain way over time—even when it doesn't feel authentic—those actions will eventually begin to feel and be real and genuine. You don't feel compassionate? Just act compassionately and the feeling will follow.

If replacing unskillful thoughts with skillful thoughts proves unsuccessful, the mindfulness tradition offers a second practice: We can contemplate the consequences of the unwholesome thought. To keep with my alliterative scheme, I call this "reflecting on results." When unwholesome thoughts arise, we think about the effects of holding these unwise notions. Consider the kind of person you become when you entertain and foster a particular unwholesome thought. If mind shapes our experience—if as we think, so we become—then our thoughts have ineluctable consequences, not unlike the way high-caloric foods have consequences for our physical health.

Just as I might reflect on my clogged arteries as I contemplate eating a slice of cheesecake—as pleasurable as that might be—so I follow the trajectory of an unwholesome thought. I envision where a diet of such thoughts might lead. Do I really want to become the kind of person whose life has been shaped by thoughts of greed and hatred? It's not even necessary to reflect on the consequences of acting on these thoughts; you can simply think about having your mind packed with such ideas. Do you really want to live with a mind that routinely churns up thoughts rooted in selfishness and condemnation? The Buddha compares the unwholesome thought to a snake or animal carcass around the neck of a well-dressed person. Such a thought, he argues, is unbecoming to a wise and compassionate human being. When the unskillful thought appears, don't denounce it; just let it go, reminding yourself that it is not a reflection of who you truly are.

The third method is "redirecting." Redirecting is simply diverting attention away from the unwholesome thought to something more beneficial. The Buddha compared this technique to averting one's gaze to avoid staring at certain objects. This practice should seem familiar, since it is one of the fundamental skills of sitting meditation. When the mind has been distracted by thought, we simply escort the attention back to the breath. Thus, our practice of meditation strengthens our ability to employ this technique, because we do it over and over again.

Redirecting attention relies on the impermanence of reality to work. We're all aware that everything in the world will change and pass away. That thought usually occasions within us a feeling of sadness or melancholy. But it need not do so; in fact, the selfsame thought can generate hope and happiness. You may be familiar with the old tale, claimed by both the Sufi and Jewish traditions, of an ancient king who asked his wise men to construct a single sentence that would sober him when he was happy and would cheer him when he was sad. The expression they offered him has become well-known: "This, too, shall pass." The monarch was so moved that he had the saying inscribed on a ring, so he could see it all the time. The phrase has become a cliché, of course, but it is true nonetheless. The fable tells us two important things: One, the impermanence of reality can be a source of comfort and happiness when we accept it; and two, we have to be constantly reminded to accept it.

Redirecting attention helps us to accept the impermanence of the world and to use that fact to our benefit. Thoughts, like everything else, pass away. Of their own accord, they dissolve. To maintain a thought, we have to renew it, which is why we have to be reminded of life's transience. If we simply divert attention to more wholesome objects or activities, the unskillful thought will vanish. All things that rise must fall. Of course, if we renew the unwholesome thought, it will arise again, and once again, we escort our attention elsewhere. Eventually, by redirecting attention, the unwholesome thought will lose its power and fade. I've found this method especially useful for dealing with obsessive thoughts, those annoying ideas or images that seem to persist in the mind.

This technique can be easily practiced in meditation, of course, but it can also work well off the cushion. Redirecting attention need not use the breath as its anchor. Any wholesome thought or activity can suffice. That wonderful and now almost extinct Christian community, the Shakers, has an old expression that nicely reflects the wisdom of redirecting attention. Their motto is "Hands to work and hearts to God." This admonishment recognizes the importance of continually redirecting attention to wholesome activity and thoughts. For the Shakers, hard manual labor and reflection on the divine helps keep the mind constructively occupied. Undisciplined attention becomes the workshop of the devil. Far better to keep one's self diligently engaged with wholesome activity lest the straying mind comes to dwell in greed, aversion, and delusion.

The fourth technique I call reconstructing, by which I mean analyzing the formation of the unskillful thought. In reflecting on results, we contemplate the forward trajectory of an unwholesome thought, considering its consequences for the future. With reconstructing, on the other hand, we move in the opposite direction, to examine the antecedents that have given rise to the unwholesome notion in the first place. Since the mind is a conditioned phenomenon, distracting thoughts are predicated on previous thoughts. It is possible, then, carefully to explore the deeper roots of unskillful thinking.

Let's say I am having unkind thoughts about another person. I recognize these thoughts as unwholesome. With a bit of honest reflection, I am able to acknowledge that those unkind thoughts emerge out of strong feelings of envy. Pursuing this insight further, I notice that my envy derives from a barely perceptible sense of personal inadequacy, which has led me to crave something that the person I envy has. I might want her intelligence, success, good looks, or fancy sports car because I believe that I, too, should have those things. Now, having gotten to this point in our reconstruction, we can begin to examine the assumptions supporting this belief. What's the great benefit in owning a sports car? Will it really make me happier? Or is it possible that a sports car might actually bring me unhappiness? Or why do I want an intelligence like hers? What do I believe that I'm lacking that would lead me to want something other than what I have? Is there a way to improve my intelligence without developing an envy that leads to unkind thoughts about this person whom I otherwise like? Is it possible for me simply to appreciate her intelligence, knowing that I have other, equally valuable gifts? Taking our reconstruction of negative thinking down to this level allows us to see how unwholesome thoughts can be rooted in untenable assumptions that we make about the things that will make us happy, and it allows us to examine those assumptions more rationally. Such a process is often effective in rendering the thought totally harmless.

When we've analyzed the root causes of envy enough times, we come to recognize a particular pattern of unskillful thinking that most of us routinely practice. It's a manner of thought strongly encouraged by our competitive culture.

The mindfulness tradition calls it "comparing mind." Comparing mind is that insidious habit of seeing how we measure up to other people. You know what I'm talking about; we expend a lot of mental energy engaged with it. Our culture is obsessed with it and, in a sense, thrives on it. Comparing mind carries with it a host of negative side effects. Its foremost disadvantage is the unnecessary suffering it causes. Envy is a nasty emotion; it makes us feel just plain yucky. I have no better word for it. The English philosopher and mathematician Bertrand Russell called envy one of the most powerful causes of human unhappiness. Furthermore, we not only feel bad about ourselves, we often begin to wish ill upon the person we envy, sometimes to the point where we take steps to realize those wishes.

You may remember the stepmother of a girl called Snow White. Even if we stop short of reaching for the poisoned apples, the mind puts itself through mental gymnastics to rid itself of all that yuck. "She may be prettier than me, but my children are smarter than hers." "I could be as successful as she is, if I were willing to compromise my integrity." Or, to cite my own personal trump card, "At least I have a Harvard Ph.D. So there!"

Whether we judge ourselves favorably or unfavorably, the practice of comparing mind is unwholesome. It causes us harm, expends our precious mental energy, and erodes our relationships with others. Although it is generally unskillful, there are times when comparing mind can be used skillfully, but doing so is an advanced practice and requires great wisdom. For most of us, however, certainly in the early stages of mindfulness practice, it is a habit that is best acknowledged and then relinquished.

We may not be able to control particular thoughts, but we can influence the conditioned mind that gives rise to particular thoughts. We can prepare a fertile mental soil that increases the likelihood of germinating wholesome, skillful ideas and decreases the likelihood of growing distracting ones. But such a mind must be tended with a watchful eye. A seasoned gardener once gave me this advice: "When you see a weed, pluck it." In other words, it's in the nature of weeds to grow fast and wild; don't wait until the garden is overrun with unwanted foliage before you remedy the situation. Unwholesome thoughts are the same. They grow fast and wild and leech vital nutrients from the thoughts that are conducive to our freedom and happiness.

We've spent our time today discussing the methods of working with unwholesome thinking. There's another aspect to this practice that we have yet to consider: cultivating wholesome thoughts. That discussion will come later in the series when we take up the subjects of compassion and generosity.

Walking—Mindfulness While Moving
Lecture 10

W e often overlook the tremendous potential of the simplest things in our lives. Consider walking. It's something virtually all of us do every day of our lives, yet how much attention do we even give to this basic aspect of our existence? The vast majority of our walking is spent in mindlessness, eager to get from one place to another with nary a thought about how we're getting there. It's quite a metaphor for the way we live our lives.

Walking Meditation

- Although most of us give little consideration to the activity of walking, some of the most thoughtful among us have been keenly aware of its importance. Walking need not be just a way to move our brains around; walking can help improve the way those brains work.

- Being physically calm, as we have observed, helps foster the mental tranquility necessary for moment-to-moment awareness. However, bodily stillness is not essential to mindfulness; it merely helps promote it, especially for those who are in the initial stages of learning the practice.

- Walking meditation shares the same goal as all practices in this tradition—that of gaining deeper awareness—but it approaches that objective in a different and complementary way from the techniques that involve physical stillness. In this way, walking meditation provides a balance to the other practices.

- Many practitioners have come to prefer walking mindfulness to the motionless forms of meditation because walking practice can be more versatile than sitting: It doesn't require a particular setting or equipment, such as a chair or cushion.

- Before you try this form of meditation during a stroll in the park or on the way from the car to the office, it's a good idea to get some experience in a special setting that is free from distractions and hazards so that you can master the basic technique.

- Like sitting meditation, walking has a number of variations that you can explore to help you design the practice that is most effective for you. Experiment with these variations to determine which techniques best sharpen your awareness.

Preparing for Walking Meditation

- To begin the practice of walking meditation, you must first find a suitable location. You can walk within the privacy of your own home, your own backyard, or any other space free from dangers and distractions. The fresh air of the outdoors, of course, has much to recommend it.

- The space for walking doesn't need to be large, but you will be walking back and forth on this space. You'll start at one end, walk to the other end, turn around, and walk the other way—repeating this many times.

- The space doesn't need to be demarcated in any way; you can simply set the boundaries in your imagination. The surface of the walkway only needs to be level and stable. If you walk barefoot—which is a very pleasant thing to do—just make sure the walking surface will not endanger your feet.

- Like sitting meditation, there is no single best time for practicing walking meditation. If you are able to do so, however, walking just before or just after sitting meditation is beneficial; walking and sitting alternately has a synergistic effect on mindfulness. Whereas sitting meditation after a meal can lead to drowsiness, research suggests that a gentle walk after eating can be healthy and invigorating.

- Before you begin, make sure you're wearing comfortable clothing, appropriate to your environment. Divest yourself of needless sources of distraction or discomfort, such as cell phones or music players. You may want to stretch a bit to loosen and relax your muscles. Do whatever is necessary to maximize your sense of freedom.

Walking Meditation in Practice

- When you're ready to start your mediation, take your place at one end of your walkway. Stand tall with your spine upright and your shoulders relaxed, letting your arms hang naturally by your sides. Keep your chin level with the ground. Relax your jaw and smile slightly. Take a few slow, deep breaths.

- Using a body scan, briefly survey the different areas of your body from the feet to the top of your head, releasing any tension as you do. For a few moments, simply stand there and observe the sensations of your body. Take a moment to appreciate your surroundings and the feel and fragrance of the air.

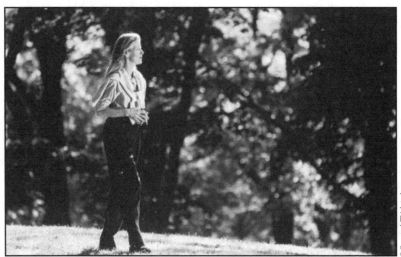

It may be beneficial to engage in basic walking practice outdoors with fresh air.

- Pay special attention to the sensations at the bottom of your feet. If you're barefoot, allow yourself to completely feel the qualities of your walking surface. Wiggle your toes a bit to let them sense the textures under your feet.

- As you prepare to walk, remind yourself of your intention to be mindful during this exercise, just as you do at the beginning of sitting meditation. Now, focus your vision on the ground about five or six feet in front of you, but don't gaze at anything in particular. You'll keep your eyes open during the entire meditation.

- You can place your hands in front of you or behind. If you hold them in front, you may put one hand in the other, as in sitting meditation. If you put them behind you, let one hand clasp the other and allow them to rest against the back. You can also allow the arms to remain at your sides and swing slightly as you move.

- Now, begin to walk, using small, careful steps. Mindfully, lift your right foot, move it forward, and place it on the ground a few inches beyond the toes of your left foot. Then, allow your weight to shift onto your right leg, and mindfully lift your left foot. Then, move it and place it on the ground a few inches beyond the toes of your right foot. Shift the weight of your body forward onto your left leg. Repeat.

- It's basic walking, of course, except with greater attention to the experience. At first, walking with attentiveness may feel awkward. Beginning practitioners sometimes even lose their balance because they're trying to be conscious of what is ordinarily an unconscious process. The awkwardness will dissipate as you become accustomed to the pace and deliberate style of the practice.

- As you move, be sure to retain an upright posture. Many people walk improperly, allowing their head and upper torso to lead their body. To maintain a correct carriage as you walk, imagine the rest of your body being led forward by the belly rather than by the head and chest.

- Initially, you may find it helpful to coordinate your movements with your breath. On the inhalation, you can lift and move the foot, and as you exhale, you can place the foot and shift your weight. You'll probably discover, however, that your breath and bodily movements will fall into a natural, synchronized rhythm after a while.

- This natural rhythm will allow your mind and body to relax. When you sense this harmony, you can withdraw your attention from the breath. Unlike sitting, in walking practice, we allow the breath to fade into the background and place our attention on other bodily sensations.

Focusing Awareness

- There are several places where you may focus your awareness. Some instructors recommend attending to the legs and feet while silently labeling the three parts of each step—lifting, moving, and placing. You may find this technique helpful for your practice, but only use it in the initial stages of learning.

- An alternative method involves focusing your awareness on the sensations of your feet as they make contact with the ground. This technique is most effective when you're walking barefoot. Due to a high concentration of nerve endings, the bottoms of the feet are among the most sensitive areas of the body. Consequently, they provide an excellent anchor for the attention.

- If you find yourself distracted by a thought or an emotion, you can gently return attention to the soles of the feet. If you find it helpful, you can pause to refocus your awareness and then resume your walk. As in other forms of meditation, allow your mind to be relaxed and focused.

- A third technique is to direct your awareness to the sensation of your body as a whole. Rather than concentrate on a particular part, try to gain a sense of the body as a single organism. Be open and attentive to whatever experiences come your way. This method is especially useful when you want to practice walking mindfully at a faster pace.

- Regardless of the technique you choose, your objective is to keep your attention on each moment, as time moves from one instant to the next. If at any moment you wish to stop and enjoy your environment—to watch the leaves fall or to listen to a sparrow's chirp—you should feel free to do so.

Completing the Walk

- When you reach the end of your path, come to a complete stop. Stand still and observe your whole body. If you wish, you can do a brief body scan or simply take a few moments to enjoy the sensation of being alive. You can walk for as long or as short a period as you like, but 30 minutes is a good time for beginners and experienced practitioners.

- When you are ready, begin slowly and mindfully to turn around 180 degrees. Stop your turn when you're facing the other end of the walkway. Once again, set your intention to be mindful during the next segment and begin again.

- Once you've become accustomed to the basic skills of mindful walking, you're free to vary the practice in ways that you find meaningful. As you walk, you might recite a *gatha*, a short verse from the Buddhist tradition that focuses the mind on a wholesome thought.

- Walking practice can also be modified to emphasize our full attentiveness in the present moment. One way to use walking for this purpose is to stop at each step and bring your complete attention to that moment before taking another step. By so doing, you're reminding yourself that life is a series of present moments.

- Walking can also be a way of imagining letting go. With each pace, you can envision leaving your anxieties and worries behind and taking a fresh step into a new moment. It's important to remember that although you're walking, you're not going anywhere. Walking meditation has no destination but awareness.

Being Mindful Anywhere

- Anytime you walk, you can be mindful. Your pace will probably be more brisk than the formal practice, and you'll probably find it most helpful to stay aware of your entire body as it moves, rather than focusing on the feet. Rather than thinking about your destination, stay focused on the act of walking.

- Anytime is a good time to walk mindfully, but this practice is especially helpful when you get angry. The next time you're taken with anger, try to walk mindfully. You'll discover that it cools the fires of rage.

- Another variation on the practice involves using a contemplative tool that has regained popularity among many Christians in recent years. **Labyrinths** are intricate structures or patterns that define a pathway; they have been found in a wide range of cultures throughout history and assume a variety of different shapes.

- A labyrinth should not be confused with a **maze**, which is a kind of puzzle with many pathway options. You can get lost in a maze, and the goal is to find a way out. A labyrinth, however, has only a single route. It has twists and turns like a maze—but no branches offering alternative paths.

Important Terms

gatha: A short verse from the Buddhist tradition that focuses the mind on a wholesome thought.

labyrinth: Intricate structures or patterns that define a pathway; it has twists and turns but only a single route.

maze: A kind of puzzle with many pathway options; one can get lost in a maze, and the goal is to find a way out.

1. Why do you think philosophers such as Nietzsche, Kant, and Thoreau considered walking essential to their creativity?

2. Do sitting and walking meditation affect your mind differently? What are the differences? Which style do you prefer and why?

Walking—Mindfulness While Moving
Lecture 10—Transcript

We often overlook the tremendous potential of the simplest things in our lives. Consider walking. It's something virtually all of us do every day of our lives, yet how much attention do we even give to this basic aspect of our existence? The vast majority of our walking is spent in mindlessness, eager to get from one place to another with nary a thought about how we're getting there. It's quite a metaphor for the way we live our lives.

Walking need not be just a way to move our brains around. Walking can help improve the way those brains work. No less a thinker than Friedrich Nietzsche once remarked, "All truly great thoughts are conceived by walking."

Nearly a century earlier, Nietzsche's fellow philosopher, Immanuel Kant, had become well-known in his hometown for his daily afternoon strolls, which were so consistent, it was said, that the citizens of Königsberg set their clocks by them. Neither Nietzsche nor Kant could hardly be described as a poster boy for the practice of mindfulness, yet they were each aware of the intellectual and spiritual benefits of walking. Closer to the spirit of mindfulness was Henry David Thoreau. In a little-known essay entitled *Walking*, Thoreau wrote: "I think that I cannot preserve my health and spirits unless I spend four hours a day at least—and it is commonly more than that—sauntering through the woods and over the hills and fields absolutely free from all worldly engagements."

Although most of us give little consideration to the activity of walking, some of the most thoughtful among us have been keenly aware of its importance. Today, we'll join these illustrious strolling thinkers by giving the act of walking some well-deserved attention.

Up to this point in the course, we've emphasized the importance of stillness as a component in the practice of mindfulness. Being physically calm, we observed, helps foster the mental tranquility necessary for moment-to-moment awareness. But bodily stillness is not essential to mindfulness; it merely helps promote it, especially for those who are in the initial stages of learning the practice. After gaining acquaintance with sitting meditation and body scans, it's desirable to learn the skills of walking meditation, another fundamental practice of the mindfulness tradition. Walking meditation shares the same goal as all practices in this tradition—that of gaining deeper awareness—but it approaches that objective in a completely different and complementary way from the techniques that involve physical stillness. In this way, walking meditation provides a balance to the other practices.

During longer periods of meditation such as retreats, meditators usually alternate between sitting and walking practices. They might sit for 45 minutes and then walk for 45, followed by more sitting and then more walking, all throughout the day. Alternating these disciplines in this manner helps break the routine of simply sitting and gives the body some much needed exercise to revitalize it for sustained mindfulness. Although it serves this vital purpose, walking meditation is a valuable instrument in its own right, and many practitioners come to prefer it to the motionless forms of meditation. Because it doesn't require a particular setting, or equipment like a chair or a cushion, walking practice can be more versatile than sitting. With walking meditation, you can practice mindfulness wherever and whenever you go.

But before you try this form of meditation during a stroll in the park or on the way from the car to the office, it's a good idea to get some experience in a special setting, free from distractions and hazards, so you can master the basic technique. So, just as we did for sitting meditation, let's discuss some of the basic conditions for engaging this practice. Like sitting meditation, walking has a number of variations that you can explore to help you design the practice that is most effective for you. Experiment with these variations to determine which techniques best sharpen your awareness.

First, find a suitable location. You can walk within the privacy of your own home, your own backyard, or any other space free from dangers and distractions. The fresh air of the out-of-doors, of course, has much to recommend it. Basic walking practice may look a little strange to those unfamiliar with it, so if you're concerned about what the neighbors will think, you may want to stay out of public view.

The space for walking doesn't need to be large. A walkway 10 to 12 feet in length and 3 feet wide will suffice. It can also be longer if you wish. You'll be walking back and forth on this space. You'll start at one end, walk to the other end, turn around and walk the other way, and repeat that many times. The space doesn't need to be demarcated in any way; you can simply set the boundaries in your imagination. There are no requirements about the surface of the walkway; it can be carpeted, a bare floor, concrete, or grass. It only needs to be level and stable. If you walk barefoot—which is a very pleasant thing to do—just make sure the walking surface will not endanger your feet.

Like sitting meditation, there is no single best time for practicing walking. Anytime that suits your schedule is a good time. If you are able to do so, however, walking just before or just after sitting meditation is beneficial; walking and sitting alternately has a synergistic effect on mindfulness. Whereas sitting meditation after a meal can lead to drowsiness, walking doesn't have that drawback. In fact, research suggests that a gentle walk after eating can be healthy and invigorating. If you find drowsiness to be particularly troubling during sitting meditation, try walking instead.

Before you begin, make sure you're wearing comfortable clothing, appropriate to your environment. Divest yourself of needless sources of distraction or discomfort, such as cell phones, music players, or cumbersome articles in your pockets. If possible, avoid purses or bags. You may want to stretch a bit to loosen and relax your muscles. Do whatever is necessary to maximize your sense of freedom.

When you're ready to start your mediation, take your place at one end of your walkway. Stand tall with your spine upright and your shoulders relaxed, letting your arms hang naturally by your sides. Keep your chin level to the ground. Relax your jaw and smile slightly. Take a few slow, deep breaths. Using a body scan, briefly survey the different areas of your body from the feet to the top of your head, releasing any tension as you do. For a few moments, simply stand there and observe the sensations of your body. Take a moment to appreciate your surroundings and the feel and fragrance of the air. Pay special attention to the sensations at the bottom of your feet. If you're barefoot, allow yourself to completely feel the qualities of your walking surface. Wiggle your toes a bit to let them sense the textures under your feet. Take your time. You're in no rush. Although you'll be walking, you're not going anywhere. Walking meditation has no destination but awareness.

As you prepare to walk, remind yourself of your intention to be mindful during this exercise, just as you do at the beginning of sitting meditation. Now, focus your vision on the ground about 5 or 6 feet in front of you, but don't gaze at anything in particular. You'll keep your eyes open during the entire meditation. You can place your hands in front of you. You may put one hand in the other, as in sitting meditation. Or behind, let one hand clasp the other and allow them to rest against the back. You can also allow the arms to remain at your sides and swing slightly as you move.

Now begin to walk, using small, careful steps. Mindfully, lift your right foot, move it forward, and place it on the ground a few inches beyond the toes of your left foot. Then allow your weight to shift onto your right leg and mindfully lift your left foot. Then move it and place it on the ground a few inches beyond the toes of your right foot. Shift the weight of your body forward onto your left leg. And repeat. It's basic walking, of course, except with greater attention to the experience. At first, walking with attentiveness may feel awkward. Beginning practitioners sometimes even lose their balance because they're trying to be conscious of what is ordinarily an unconscious process. The awkwardness will dissipate as you become accustomed to the pace and deliberate style of the practice.

Although it is not essential to the practice, you will probably find it helpful—at least at first—to walk more slowly than usual. After many years of practice, I still like the slower pace. The slow rate helps me stay attentive and reminds me that I'm not trying to reach a goal. I think of it as sauntering.

As you move, try to retain an upright posture. Many persons walk improperly, allowing their head and upper torso to lead their body. To maintain a correct carriage as you walk, imagine the rest of your body being led forward by the belly rather than the head and chest.

Initially, you may find it helpful to coordinate your movements with your breath. On the inhalation, you can lift and move the foot. As you exhale you can place the foot and shift your weight. You'll probably discover, however, that after a while your breath and bodily movements will fall into a natural, synchronized rhythm. This natural rhythm will allow your mind and body to relax. When you sense this harmony, you can withdraw your attention from the breath. Unlike sitting, in walking practice we allow the breath to fade into the background and place our attention on other bodily sensations.

There are several places where you may focus your awareness. Some instructors recommend attending to the legs and feet while silently labeling the three-parts of each step—lifting, moving, and placing; lifting, moving, and placing. Personally, I find that technique a bit wooden and something of a distraction; it often causes me to stumble. But try it; you may find it helpful for your practice. Use it, however, only in the initial stages of learning; labeling the elements of walking should be dropped as soon as possible.

The method I prefer is to focus awareness on the sensations of your feet as they make contact with the ground. This technique is most effective when you're walking barefoot. Due to a high concentration of nerve endings, the bottoms of the feet are among the most sensitive areas of the body. Consequently, they provide an excellent anchor for the attention. Try to attend to these sensations as you walk, just as you might focus on the breath in sitting meditation. If you find yourself distracted by a thought or an emotion, you can gently return attention to the soles of the feet. If you find it helpful, you can pause to refocus your awareness and then resume your walk. As in other forms of meditation, allow your mind to be relaxed and focused.

A third technique is to direct your awareness to the sensation of your body as a whole. Rather than concentrate on a particular part, try to gain a sense of the body as a single organism. Think of the body as a fully integrated, fluidly moving being, alive to the world. Be open and attentive to whatever experiences come your way. If you get distracted, observe the distraction and allow it to pass away. This method is especially useful when you want to practice walking mindfully at a much faster pace, such as taking a walk in the woods.

Regardless of the technique you choose, your objective is to keep your attention on each moment, as time moves from one instant to the next. If at any moment you wish to stop and enjoy your environment, to watch the leaves fall or listen to a sparrow's chirrup, you should feel free to do so.

When you reach the end of your path, come to a complete stop. Stand still and observe your whole body. If you wish, you can do a brief body scan or simply take a few moments to enjoy the sensation of being alive. When you are ready, begin slowly and mindfully to turn around 180 degrees. Stop your turn when you're facing the other end of the walkway. Once again, set your intention to be mindful during the next segment and begin again.

You can walk for as long or as short a period as you like. Thirty minutes is a good time for beginning practitioners, and—as I think about it—a good time for experienced practitioners as well!

Once you've become accustomed to the basic skills of mindful walking, you're free to vary the practice in ways that you find meaningful. As you walk, you might recite a *gatha*, a short verse from the Buddhist tradition that focuses the mind on a wholesome thought. Thich Nhat Hanh, a well-known Vietnamese monk, composed this *gatha*, which I find particularly meaningful for walking practice: The mind can go in a thousand directions, but on this beautiful path, I walk in peace. With each step, a gentle wind blows. With each step, a flower blooms.

You can recite this *gatha* as you stand preparing to walk and again each time you stop to turn around on your walkway. You can also recite it as you walk, silently saying a phrase with each step: The mind can go in a thousand directions, but on this beautiful path, I walk in peace. With each step, a gentle wind blows. With each step, a flower blooms.

You may find other *gathas* that are meaningful to you or you might compose your own. One of my own that I often use is the phrase, "Just now is enough."

Walking practice can also be modified to emphasize our full attentiveness in the present moment. One way to use walking for this purpose is to stop at each step and bring your complete attention to that moment before taking another step. With each step, you become fully present before moving to the next. By so doing, you're reminding yourself that life is a series of present moments, like pearls on a string. If you fail to show up for these moments, you've missed your life. Walking can also be a way of imagining letting go. With each pace, you can envision leaving your anxieties and worries behind and taking a fresh step into a new moment. It's important to remember that you're not going anywhere. Walking meditation is not a means but an end in itself.

There are times, however, when walking does have a destination. You can be mindful as you're on your way. Anytime you walk, you can be mindful. Simply begin as you would a formal walking practice by adjusting your posture, taking a few deep breaths, and setting an intention to be present to your experience. Your pace will probably be more brisk than the formal practice, and you'll probably find it most helpful to stay aware of your entire body as it moves, rather than focusing on the feet. Try to maintain a consistent gait and remember to let your midsection lead the rest of your body. Rather than thinking about your destination, stay focused on the act of walking. You can walk mindfully as you go from your car to your work, from your office to the bathroom, and as you stroll in the mall. You can even do it as you shop for groceries. Anytime is a good time to walk mindfully, but this practice is especially helpful when you get angry. The next time you're taken with anger, try to walk mindfully. You'll discover that it cools the fires of rage.

Another variation on the practice involves using a contemplative tool that has regained popularity among many Christians in recent years. I'm referring to what is called a labyrinth. Labyrinths are intricate structures or patterns that define a pathway; they have been found in a wide range of cultures throughout history and assume a variety of different shapes. In the Middle Ages, Christians apparently began to use these pathways for spiritual development. A number of labyrinths were designed on the floors of some of the grand cathedrals of Europe, including Chartres. Although their purpose is not fully understood today, many believe the labyrinth symbolized the pilgrimage to Jerusalem and provided a surrogate experience for those who were unable to make the actual trip. Later in the 20th century, the labyrinth was rediscovered, as it were, and appropriated for use in many Christian churches and retreat centers. While it is no longer viewed so much as a substitute for going to Jerusalem, many practitioners regard it as instrument for deepening spirituality.

The labyrinth should not be confused with a maze. A maze is a kind of puzzle with many pathway options; you can get lost in a maze, and the goal is to find a way out. A labyrinth, however, has only a single route. It has twists and turns like a maze, but no branches offering alternative paths.

If you start at the entrance of a labyrinth and mindfully follow where the path leads, you will be taken to the center and then back out again. Like formal walking meditation, walking the labyrinth lacks a physical destination. The journey itself is the whole point of the exercise.

Using the labyrinth for walking meditation offers a unique perspective on this practice. You can follow the labyrinth's design using the fundamental methods involved in formal walking meditation, but the complex pathway allows the practitioner to experience different forms of consciousness and attain different insights, especially when one walks the path at the same time as others. There are now over 2,000 permanent labyrinths in the United States, so locating one shouldn't be too difficult. If you live in a city, chances are there is one nearby. A Google search on the Internet should help.

Finally, the techniques of walking meditation can be easily adapted to other activities that involve movement and repetition. Try mindfulness practice as you rake the leaves, take a jog, or walk the treadmill. Try it while you swim laps or take a stroll on the beach. The permutations are virtually endless and are only restricted by your imagination.

Walking meditation is one of the best ways I know to incorporate the practice of mindfulness into our daily lives. It helps bring the awareness we develop in sitting meditation out into the open, encouraging us to apply it wherever we are. At the same time, it's good for the body, providing us with an opportunity to burn a few extra calories and get a little extra exercise.

In our next talk, we'll be discussing the topic of mindful eating, another practice that both cultivates everyday awareness and promotes physical well-being. As part of learning that discipline, we'll investigate how to eat a tangerine. To prepare for that experience, I recommend that you find a good tangerine or a clementine and bring it with you. I'll see you there.

Consuming—Watching What You Eat
Lecture 11

Mindful eating is a way to enjoy one of the most pleasurable, yet one of the most ordinary, things we do. It's also a practice that allows us to discover—or perhaps rediscover—many wonderful things that happen right under our noses and within our bodies. Mindful eating helps us attend to our body's inner wisdom and to our natural capacity for compassion and gratitude. It also helps us appreciate our place in the greater web of life.

Eating with Mindfulness

- Like walking, consuming our food and drink is a profoundly ordinary experience whose depth is usually overlooked. Most of us, most of the time, devour mindlessly, missing out on what is potentially one of the most satisfying experiences we can have.

- To introduce you to mindful eating, we will mindfully eat a tangerine. You can perform this exercise with any kind of food, but this meditation is designed specifically for tangerines. As you'll see shortly, the practice means nothing without your participation.

Mindfully Eating a Tangerine

- First, find a quiet, well-lit location where you can sit comfortably, free from distractions. You can do this at the kitchen table, on the sofa, or in your meditation space.

- Take the tangerine in your hands and close your eyes. Allow your fingers and palms to touch the fruit's surface, carefully attending to your sensations. Take your time. Notice its shape. Feel it as if you were going to draw a picture of the fruit afterward. Observe the irregularities, the bumps and crevices, the curves and flat areas. Examine the texture of the skin.

- Now, hold the tangerine up to your nostrils. Feel it with your nose and lips and the area between them—called the philtrum. Move it around a bit and sniff. Notice your reaction to the citrusy fragrance.

- Open your eyes and hold the tangerine about 12 inches away from them, allowing your gaze to focus on the fruit. Observe the subtle shadings of color, noting the reflection of light on the surface. Find the place where the fruit was attached to the tree. These tiny details make this tangerine different from every other tangerine in the world.

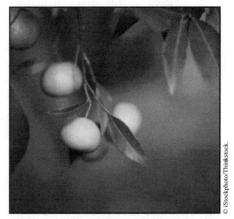

- Ponder for a few moments how this tangerine came to be in your hand. Think of the tree that produced it. Imagine how many generations of

Mindfully eating a tangerine can be a wonderful experience that deepens your awareness of the world.

tangerine trees preceded the tree from which this particular fruit came. Think of the person who planted the tree and the people who tended it. Consider all the sunshine, air, and water that were necessary to nourish that tree and produce this fruit.

- It took many years, many hands, and many physical elements for this tangerine to be with you at just this moment. And shortly, part of this fruit will become part of you, and all those years, the work of all those people and insects, and all the sunshine and water will become part of you as well.

- Now, we'll take the fruit and begin to open it. Break the skin with your thumbnail. Smell it again. The fragrance is more intense and richer. Continue to press your nail into the skin and slowly peel it back. Keep it as close to your eyes as you find comfortable.

- Feel your thumb exerting pressure on the fruit, tearing into the soft flesh. Look at the yellow-white pulp underneath. See the texture and the shades of color. Notice how the skin and pulp pull away from the fruit as your thumb slides deeper within. See the strings of pulp that cling to the tangerine sections.

- Observe the interesting shapes the peeling forms as you continue to remove it from the edible part within. Carefully finish detaching the skin and pulp, studying each detail. Feel the sensation of moisture on your thumb and fingers. See how some parts of the peeling can be more easily removed than others.

- For a few moments, hold the tangerine close to your ear as you peel. Listen to the sound of the skin tearing away from the fleshy part. When you have completely separated the peeling from the flesh, take a minute to look at and smell the skin before putting it aside.

- Now, take the edible flesh and observe. Notice the colors, the textures, the many crescent-shaped sections of the fruit. See how rough the surface appears and the filaments of pulp sticking to it. Begin to break the cluster of sections in half. Hear the sounds of separation and watch as the sections try to cling to one another. Notice the pulpy part in the center.

- Gently remove one section of the cluster. Observe the patterns on the section's translucent skin. Peel away a bit of skin to reveal the orange, juicy flesh. The section comprises even more parts within. See how tightly packed they are—how nicely arrayed—each part about to burst.

- Take the section and place it in your mouth, letting it rest on your tongue. Don't bite it just yet. Close your eyes. Let your tongue examine the fruit. Use your tongue to move the tangerine section to your molars and softly bite into it, but don't bite completely through. Just chew the flesh slightly to allow the fruit to release its juices. Let the liquid flow from the fruit and swish it around in your mouth a bit. Taste it.

- Now, continue to chew slowly and thoroughly. Then, allow the fruit to slide down your throat and swallow. For a few seconds, concentrate on the lingering sensations in your mouth. Notice how the sensations that were so intense just a few moments ago are now fading away. Examine your response to that impermanence.

- When you're ready, pick up another slice and repeat the process, all the while concentrating on your sensations and reactions—trying to savor the experience without judgment or evaluation. Do this for each section of the tangerine until it's gone. Pause between each section. Don't pick up another section until you have completely finished with the one that's in your mouth.

Eating Mindfully as a Habit

- The value of this exercise is to reveal the possibilities available to us for using the ordinary experience of eating to deepen our awareness and act in more wholesome ways. Perhaps it would be great to eat this way all the time, but for many of us, that's not practical. We can, however, incorporate some of the methods and principles of tangerine meditation into our daily lives in relatively painless—but very meaningful—ways.

- First, let me suggest that you set a goal to practice mindful eating during one meal each week. This is a modest beginning, and as you start to see the benefits, you may want to have mindful meals with greater frequency. You'll also begin to notice how the practice of mindfulness while eating begins to affect all of your eating experiences.

- After committing yourself to a regular practice, decide if you'd like to observe it alone or with others. Eating with others provides additional richness to the experience when they are also committed to the practice. Although no one says a word, having a mindful supper with friends and family can strengthen the intimacy of these relationships.

- Whether you choose to eat alone or with others, the practice of mindful eating really begins before the meal starts, as you choose and prepare your food. If you dine with company, it's an enriching practice to include them in the preparation phase.

Choosing the Menu

- It's important to give careful thought to the menu. The principal reason we eat is to nourish our bodies and minds, so making wise choices about the food that will ultimately become us is essential. The mindfulness tradition doesn't specify a particular kind of diet; it only encourages us to consume food and drink that will keep us healthy and contribute to our moment-to-moment awareness.

- Knowing what is wholesome food and what's not, however, isn't always easy. Almost daily, the media reports the shifting opinions about this or that food item. For now, we can only say that mindfulness practice entails using our best wisdom and the knowledge we have available to choose the most wholesome foods.

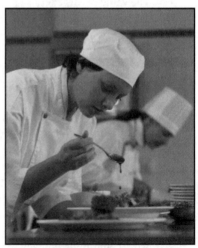

© Digital Vision/Thinkstock.

- Being conscious of what we eat also involves awareness of how food gets to our table. Unless we grow all our own food, we probably have little idea about where most of what we eat comes from or how it is produced.

Cooks everywhere—from gourmet chefs to mothers and fathers—help sustain life and bring happiness.

- We exist in a complex web of life. How we sustain our own life has a profound effect on the rest of the biosphere of which we are part. Today, we are becoming more aware that how we get our food affects the greater world in which we live.

- As an exercise in mindfulness, investigate where some of your food comes from—or at least give some thought to the source of your food before you eat it, as we did in our tangerine meditation. If you're able, consider gardening, if you don't already.

The Gift of Eating

One day, a man was strolling across a field when suddenly he came face-to-face with a hungry tiger. Instinctively, he bolted, and the tiger, just as instinctively, ran after him. Knowing he had no chance to outrun the animal, the man jumped down a cliff and grabbed hold of a vine growing on the side. He looked up and saw the tiger just above him, licking his chops. He looked down below to the bottom of the cliff, where another hungry tiger was waiting for him to fall. Then, two mice—one black, the other white—began to nibble away at the vine. Just then, the man saw a juicy wild strawberry growing in the crag. He reached for it. It was incredibly delicious!

Zen Buddhists have told this parable for ages as a way to express the inexpressible essence of Zen. Like the hapless man in the story, our fate is inescapable. The jaws of death await us all, sooner or later, as time itself gnaws away at our lifeline.

That being the case, why complain or despair? Why not become fully alive to the moment we've been offered? Why not reach out and savor the wild strawberry? Every day of our lives, these moments are given to us as gifts, but we usually return them unopened. Eating, as the parable suggests, is one of these gifts.

- When the food has been bought and the menu set, you can make preparation itself a mindful practice. Work in a quiet, clean, distraction-free environment. Enjoy the sensual nature of your experience. Notice colors, textures, aromas, and tastes.

- Think about how your actions are part of the greater web of life. Reflect on the fact that other beings have given up their lives to sustain yours. If you're cooking for others—or even just for yourself—remember that what you are doing is an act of compassion. You're helping to sustain life and bring happiness.

Eating a Meal in Mindfulness

- When you are ready to begin the meal, make sure the location is quiet and uncluttered. An appropriate beginning to a mindfulness meal could be a few words encouraging reflection on the purpose of eating, the process by which the food has come to table, and the fact that many in the world are malnourished. Depending on your personal beliefs, these words may or may not make mention of God.

- When grace is concluded, the meal may begin. Eating the entire meal in silence helps create an environment conducive to moment-to-moment awareness. If you have company, eating in silence may seem awkward at first, but most people quickly become used to it.

- Eating a meal in mindfulness follows the same principles as the tangerine meditation, with just a few variations and additional options. You will, of course, eat slowly and attentively, trying to experience the richness of the moment. It will be most helpful to vary your usual eating experience to break the habits of mindless eating.

- Eat your meal at a leisurely pace, and be keenly attentive to your body to know when your hunger has been satisfied. Many of us continue to eat long after our hunger pangs have subsided. When you sense that you have eaten enough, stop.

- When everyone has finished and the mindfulness meal is over, the participants might engage in some quiet chatting, perhaps even discussing their experience.

- Like preparation, the clean up can be done in a meditative way, but it may be harder to do so because you usually want it done with as soon as possible. The mindfulness approach is to reorient your attention from getting the job finished to staying aware of what you're doing.

Questions to Consider

1. Reflect on the ways you can integrate mindfulness practices into your everyday eating experiences. What aspects of the rest of your life do you need to change in order to accommodate mindful eating?

2. Invite a like-minded friend, or group of friends, to spend an evening together cooking and enjoying a mindfulness supper using the principles suggested in this lecture.

Consuming—Watching What You Eat
Lecture 11—Transcript

One day a man was strolling across a field when suddenly he came face to face with a hungry tiger. Instinctively he bolted, and the tiger, just as instinctively, ran after him. Knowing he had no chance to outrun the animal, the man jumped down a cliff and grabbed hold of a vine growing on the side. He looked up and saw the tiger just above him, licking his chops. He looked down below to the bottom of the cliff, where another hungry tiger was waiting for him to fall. Then two mice—one black, the other white—began to nibble away at the vine. Just then, the man saw a juicy wild strawberry growing in the crag. He reached for it. It was incredibly delicious!

Zen Buddhists have told this parable for ages as a way to express the inexpressible essence of Zen. Like the hapless man in the story, our fate is inescapable. The jaws of death await us, sooner or later, as time itself gnaws away at our lifeline. That being the case, why complain or despair? Why not become fully alive to the moment we've been offered? Why not reach out and savor the wild strawberry? Every day of our lives, these moments are given to us as gifts; but usually, we return them unopened.

Eating, as the parable suggests, is one these gifts. Like walking, consuming our food and drink is a profoundly ordinary experience whose depth is usually overlooked. Most of us, most of the time, devour mindlessly, missing out on what is potentially one of the most satisfying experiences we can have. We give little attention to our consumption. An odd thing, don't you think, since we all know that we are what we eat? Is it any surprise, then, that we barely know ourselves?

Eating with mindfulness can be a great joy. Once you've had this experience, you'll see how many things you miss when you eat mindlessly. To introduce you to mindful eating, I invite you now to share a piece of fruit with me. At the conclusion of our last lecture, I asked you to have a tangerine or a clementine available as you listen to this talk. You can perform this exercise with any kind of food, but I've designed this meditation specifically for tangerines. If you don't have one, just follow along and try the exercise when you're able. As you'll see shortly, the practice means nothing without your participation. First, find a quiet, well-lit location where you can sit comfortably, free from distractions. You can do this at the kitchen table, on the sofa, or in your meditation space.

Take the tangerine in your hands and close your eyes. Allow your fingers and palms to touch the fruit's surface, carefully attending to your sensations. Take your time. Notice its shape. Feel it as if you were going to draw a picture of the fruit afterwards. It's roundish, of course, but not perfectly round. Observe the irregularities, the bumps and crevices, the curves and flat areas. Does it feel cool or warm? Is it cooler or warmer in some places than in others? Examine the texture of the skin. Is it smooth or rough or both? Does it feel hard or soft? Is it hard in some places and soft in others?

Now hold the tangerine up to your nostrils. Feel it with your nose and lips and that funny little area between them called the philtrum. Go ahead; nobody's looking. Move it around a bit and sniff. Notice your reaction to the citrusy fragrance. Do you find it pleasant or unpleasant? Does it arouse your desire to eat? Does it bring back memories?

Open your eyes and hold the tangerine about 12 inches away from them, allowing your gaze to focus on the fruit. Observe the subtle shadings of color. Note the reflection of light on the surface. See the bright areas and the shadows and the different shapes they form. Take careful notice of every detail. Look at the crevices and indentations. Find the place where the fruit was attached to the tree. Notice the simple beauty of that small spot. These tiny details make this tangerine different from every other tangerine in the world. Like this moment, this fruit is unique; there is no other just like it.

Ponder for a few moments how this tangerine came to be in your hand. Think of the tree that produced it. Wonder where it grew? California? Florida? China? Imagine how many generations of tangerine trees preceded the tree from which this particular fruit came. Think of the person who planted the tree and the people who tended it. Consider all the sunshine, air, and water that were necessary to nourish that tree and produce this fruit. Reflect on the bees that pollinated the flowers that became this tangerine. Think of the person who picked it or the person operating the machinery that harvested it. They had friends and families. They were people just like you and me, with pains and pleasures, hopes and ambitions. Think of the people who transported it to the store where you bought it. Think of the people who sold it to you. It took many years, many hands, and many physical elements for this tangerine to be with you at just this moment. And shortly, part of this fruit will become part of you, and all those years, the work of all those people and insects, and all the sunshine and water will become part of you as well.

Now, we'll take the fruit and begin to open it. Break the skin with your thumbnail. Smell it again. The fragrance is more intense and richer. Continue to press your nail into the skin and slowly peel it back. Keep it as close to your eyes as you find comfortable, but watch out for errant sprays of juice! Feel your thumb exerting pressure on the fruit, tearing into the soft flesh. Look at the yellow-white pulp underneath. See the texture and the shades of color. Notice how the skin and pulp pull away from the fruit as your thumb slides deeper within. See the strings of pulp that cling to the tangerine sections. Observe the interesting shapes the peeling forms as you continue to remove it from the edible part within. Carefully finish detaching the skin and pulp, studying each detail. Feel the sensation of moisture on your thumb and fingers. See how some parts of the peeling can be more easily removed than others. For a few moments, hold the tangerine close to your ear as you peel. Listen to the sound of the skin tearing away from the fleshy part. When you have completely separated the peeling from the flesh, take a minute to look at and smell the skin before putting it aside.

Now take the edible flesh and observe. Notice the colors, the textures, the many crescent-shaped sections of the fruit. See how the rough surface appears and the filaments of pulp sticking to it. Begin to break the cluster of sections in half. Hear the sounds of separation and watch as the sections try to cling to one another. Notice the pulpy part in the center. Gently remove one section of the cluster. Observe the patterns on the section's translucent skin. Peel away a bit of skin to reveal the orange, juicy flesh. The section comprises even more parts within. See how tightly packed they are, how nicely arrayed, each part about to burst.

Take the section and place it in your mouth and let it rest on your tongue. Don't bite it just yet. Close your eyes. Let your tongue examine the fruit. How does it feel? Can you taste it? Use your tongue to move the tangerine section to your molars and softly bite into it, but don't bite completely through. Just chew the flesh slightly to allow the fruit to release its juices. Let the liquid flow from the fruit and swish it around in your mouth a bit. Taste it. Is it sweet or sour or both? Does it taste differently on different parts of the tongue? Now continue to chew slowly and thoroughly. Then allow the fruit to slide down your throat and swallow. For a few seconds, concentrate on the lingering sensations in your mouth. Notice how the sensations that were so intense just a few moments ago are now fading away. Examine your response to that impermanence. Does it leave you wanting more tangerine? Does it generate other thoughts?

When you're ready, pick up another slice and repeat the process, all the while concentrating on your sensations and reactions, trying to savor the experience without judgment or evaluation. Do this for each section of the tangerine, until it's gone. Pause between each section. Don't pick up another section until you have completely finished with the one that's in your mouth. You can turn off your media player at this point and enjoy the rest of the exercise in silence and at your leisure.

Mindfully eating a tangerine can be a wonderful experience, and I hope you found it so. The value of this exercise is to reveal the possibilities available to us for using the ordinary experience of eating to deepen our awareness and act in more wholesome ways. Perhaps it would be great to eat this way all the time, but for most of us, that's not practical. We can, however, incorporate some of the methods and principles of tangerine meditation into our daily lives in relatively painless, but very meaningful, ways.

First, let me suggest that you set a goal to practice mindful eating during one meal each week. This is a modest beginning, and as you start to see the benefits, you may want to have mindful meals with greater frequency. You'll also begin to notice how the practice of mindfulness while eating begins to affect all of your eating experiences.

After committing yourself to a regular practice, decide if you'd like to observe it alone or with others. If you wish to eat alone, perhaps you can take your lunch to a park on a nice day or find a quiet location at home or work where you can eat by yourself without distraction. Eating with others provides additional richness to the experience when they are also committed to the practice. Although no one says a word, having a mindful supper with friends and family can strengthen the intimacy of these relationships.

Whether you choose to eat alone or with others, the practice of mindful eating really begins before the meal starts, as you choose and prepare your food. If you dine with company, it's an enriching practice to include them in the preparation phase. There is great satisfaction in cooking and eating a meal with other people. This is surely one reason we find so much pleasure in holidays like Thanksgiving. In some of my courses, I assign the entire class the responsibility to plan and prepare a dinner together, which we then eat in silence. The assignment is as much an exercise in community-building as it is in mindfulness.

It's important to give careful thought to the menu. The principal reason we eat is to nourish our bodies and minds, so making wise choices about the food that will ultimately become us is essential. The mindfulness tradition doesn't specify a particular kind of diet; it only encourages us to consume food and drink that will keep us healthy and contribute to our moment-to-moment awareness. Knowing what is wholesome food and what's not, however, isn't always easy. I grew up on a diet rich in red meat and sugar, which at the time was widely considered vital to good health. We think differently now, of course, but who knows? Maybe that too will change. Almost daily, the media reports the shifting opinions about this or that food item. I'm still unsure if caffeine is good for you or not, but I keep hoping it'll end up in the healthy column. In Woody Allen's film entitled *Sleeper*, two scientists of the 22nd century discuss the diets of people of our era, perplexed by those who thought wheat germ and organic honey were healthy. One doctor of the future asks the other: Didn't they have deep fat, steak, cream pies, and hot fudge? To which the other answers that oddly those foods were "thought to be unhealthy ... precisely the opposite of what we now know to be true."

Much of the difficulty in determining the best foods for us to eat is the highly politicized nature of food production, a complicated issue that we do not have time to address here. For now, we can only say that mindfulness practice entails using our best wisdom and the knowledge we have available to choose the most wholesome foods. For doing that, I found a little book by

Michael Pollan entitled *Food Rules: An Eater's Manual* to be very helpful. Pollan suggests very simple guidelines for healthier eating. He recommends that we eat real food rather than the highly processed concoctions he calls "edible food-like substances"; that we eat mostly plants; and that we don't eat too much. Simple suggestions, of course, but due to our conditioned habits as individuals and as a culture, these are not so easy to implement.

Being conscious of what we eat also involves awareness of how food gets to our table. Unless we grow all our own food, we probably have little idea about where most of what we eat comes from or how it is produced. In the practice of mindfulness, there are good reasons for giving attention to these issues.

We exist in a complex web of life. How we sustain our own life has a profound effect on the rest of the biosphere of which we are a part. Today, we are becoming more aware that how we get our food affects the greater world in which we live. We're more sensitive to the effects of the use of pesticide on the ecosystem; to the consequences of transporting food grown at a great distance from where it is sold; and to the ethical and ecological ramifications of the industrial production of animals for slaughter. As an exercise in mindfulness, let me recommend that you investigate where some of your food comes from or at least give some thought to the source of your food before you eat it, just as we did in our tangerine meditation. If you're able, consider gardening, if you don't already. Not only does homegrown food taste better than food from stores; you'll also have the great satisfaction of learning about the many ways gardening can be a spiritual practice.

When the food has been bought and the menu set, you can make preparation itself a mindful practice. Simply bring the basic principles we've discussed so far to bear on the various tasks. Work in a quiet, clean, distraction-free environment. As you wash and chop fruits and vegetables bring your full awareness to what you are doing. Enjoy the sensual nature of your experience. Notice colors, textures, aromas, and tastes. Take a moment to listen to the sound of boiling water or garlic sizzling in olive oil. Think about how your actions are part of the greater web of life. Reflect on the fact that other beings have given up their lives to sustain yours. Think of how their lives will now be part of your life.

If you're cooking for others—or even just for yourself—remember that what you are doing is an act of compassion. You're helping to sustain life and bring happiness. Cooks everywhere—from the mothers and fathers who cook for their families, to the gourmet chefs at high-class restaurants, to the teenagers who make burritos at Taco Bell—ought to remember the great importance of what they do.

When all things are ready, the meal can begin. Make sure the location is quiet and uncluttered. You can enhance the beauty and appeal of the food by giving special attention to the aesthetics of the table, the dishes, and utensils. Start with a form of what some people call "grace." It's an excellent way to set the tone for the entire meal. You don't have to be a believer to find this custom meaningful; many people who profess atheism still say grace before meals. An appropriate beginning to a mindfulness meal could be a few words encouraging reflection on the purpose of eating, the process by which the food has come to table, and the fact that many in the world are malnourished. Depending on your personal beliefs, these words may or may not make mention of God. This Buddhist *gatha* is appropriate, I think, for anyone regardless of their religion:

> We receive this food in gratitude to all beings
> Who have helped to bring it to our table,
> And vow to respond in turn to those in need
> With wisdom and compassion.

When grace is concluded, the meal may begin.

I suggest that the entire meal be eaten in silence. Silence, of course, helps create an environment conducive to moment-to-moment awareness. If you have company, eating in silence may seem awkward at first, but most people get used to it rather quickly. You may even find silence after a hectic day to be quite refreshing.

Eating a meal in mindfulness follows the same principles as the tangerine meditation, with just a few variations and additional options. You will, of course, eat slowly and attentively, trying to experience the richness of the moment. But you may need to use certain techniques to facilitate this process, since there will be no one to guide you through the meal and set the pace. It will be most helpful to vary your usual eating experience to break the habits of mindless eating.

Here are some suggestions: Before you eat, make sure to take time to look at each bite of food and appreciate its colors, textures, and smells. When you place the food in your mouth, set your utensil down beside your plate. Chew your food carefully and mindfully. Don't pick up more food until you have completely swallowed the morsel in your mouth. If you need assistance in slowing your pace, use your non-dominant hand. If you ordinarily hold your fork with your right hand, try using the left—and vice versa. Or use different types of utensils. If you use forks, spoons, and knives, try chopsticks or no utensils at all. South Asians customarily eat their meals without any implements, using only their right hand to enjoy the tactile experience of food.

Eat your meal at a leisurely pace, and be keenly attentive to your body to know when your hunger has been satisfied. Many of us continue to eat long after our hunger pangs have subsided. When you sense that you have eaten enough, stop.

Learning to know when you are hungry and when your hunger has been appeased are especially important skills that can be developed with mindfulness. Both skills require the ability to distinguish between true bodily hunger and craving. Genuine hunger is the body's signal that it needs nutrition. Craving is the desire to eat for reasons other than nourishment. When we crave, we want food to relax, to soothe our anxieties and worries, to reward ourselves, or because we're bored or lonely. When you become aware of the desire for food, ask yourself: Do I want to eat this because I'm really hungry or am I being urged on by something else? Determining whether you are hungry or craving helps you know how to respond to your desire in wholesome ways. Eating may not be the best answer to craving. It may contribute to our already overly rich diet and fail to address the real source of our distress.

When everyone has finished and the mindfulness meal is over, the participants might engage in some quiet chatting, perhaps even discussing their experience. Or they could proceed immediately to clean-up the table and the kitchen. Like preparation, the clean-up can be done in a meditative way, but it may be harder to do so. With all the smells and colors, and the body's appetite, preparing food has an intrinsic interest that clean-up lacks. When you're at the cleaning stage, you're dealing with garbage, and you usually want it done with as soon as possible. The mindfulness approach is to reorient your attention from getting the job finished to staying aware of what you're doing. Thich Nhat Hanh put it well when he said, "There are two ways to wash dishes. The first is to wash the dishes in order to have clean dishes and the second is to wash the dishes in order to wash the dishes."

Mindful eating is a way to enjoy one of the most pleasurable, yet one of the most ordinary, things we do. It's also a practice that allows us to discover— or perhaps rediscover—many wonderful things that happen right under our noses and within our bodies. Mindful eating helps us attend to our body's inner wisdom and to our natural capacity for compassion and gratitude. It helps us appreciate our place in the greater web of life. Bon appétit!

Driving—Staying Awake at the Wheel
Lecture 12

As you drive mindfully, you will notice that you have little control over the full range of events that are unfolding before your eyes. You have slight, if any, authority over what others do. Your powers are fairly limited to the control you have over your own vehicle, but even that is not absolute. Despite your limitations, it is possible to sit back, relax, and become mindfully alert to your experiences. You'll see interesting things, scary things, things that will make you sad, things that will make you laugh—but you'll always keep going.

Driving in the United States

- Operating motor vehicles is an extremely important part of American culture. According to the Bureau of Transportation, there are more automobiles in the United States than licensed drivers. In the first decade of the 21st century, Americans drove approximately 3 trillion miles each year.

- Because we spend so much time on the road, driving represents a wonderful opportunity for us to practice mindfulness. Like walking and eating, driving is an ordinary experience whose potential for enriching our awareness of life is usually overlooked.

- Practicing mindfulness while driving is not only a choice opportunity; it's also a veritable necessity. Driving may be the most hazardous activity the average person participates in. Each year, there are well over 6 million vehicle collisions in the United States, in which 3 million people suffer injuries.

- Certainly, a major factor in many accidents is the lack of attentiveness, whether that's caused by cell phone use, eating food, engaging in conversations, or just driving under the influence of mindlessness. If there's anything we do that can benefit from the application of mindfulness, it's operating a vehicle.

- Are you a mindless driver? Take a moment to assess your ordinary driving habits. Consider how often you fail to drive completely attentive to the experience as it's happening. It's not uncommon for people to drive for miles and miles without paying full attention to the route they're taking.

- Think also about the way you drive. Do you drive aggressively? Timidly? Competitively? Do you drive lawfully, always observing speed limits and other traffic regulations? Many people don't always feel obligated to obey the rules when they're on the road. If you think of your automobile as an extension of your personality, as some psychologists suggest it is, what does your driving say about you?

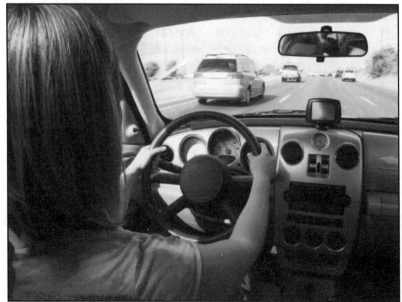

© Creatas/Thinkstock.

Each year, about 40,000 people die in vehicle mishaps. Therefore, driving mindfully is a necessity.

Driving Mindfully

- Mindful driving begins long before you enter the car. Because driving is a potentially hazardous activity, we should do all we can beforehand to ensure our journeys are safe.

- First, that means making sure the vehicle we're driving is well maintained and in good operating condition. Second, it means preparing our minds to take the responsibility of driving seriously, knowing that getting behind the wheel requires our full attention. If we're unprepared for that responsibility, we should at least be responsible enough not to drive.

- When you're ready to go, bring mindful attention to what you're doing as you approach the car. You might start by engaging in a walking meditation practice as you move toward your vehicle; then, stay attentive as you go through the usual routine of preparing to drive, such as buckling up and fixing your mirrors.

- If you have passengers, make sure everyone is prepared and safely buckled. Remember that the safety of yourself, the others in the car, and strangers on the road depends on your full awareness. Careful driving is an act of compassion. Therefore, you should focus on the experience of driving and not on the destination.

- As you prepare to leave, reflect on the value of removing potential distractions, just as you would for sitting meditation. Try driving without the radio, coffee, or any other possible distractions and study the effect of its absence on your attentiveness.

- Then, check your posture. Make sure you're sitting in a position that promotes alertness and allows you to be relaxed. Keep your hands firmly on the steering wheel, but don't clench them. They, too, should feel relaxed. Perhaps you can manage a quick body scan to release any tension you may feel. Take several deep breaths and go.

- As you begin to drive, do so normally. There is no need to slow your rate of speed as we do in walking and eating meditation. On the other hand, you might experiment with driving a bit slower than usual to see if that affects your ability to stay attentive. Slightly breaking the routine can help keep your mind focused.

Driving with Anchors

- As we do in other forms of meditation, we'll need to establish anchors as a way to stabilize our attention when it begins to wander. In driving practice, we'll use two.

- The first is the visual field available to us as we look through the car windshield and windows. You'll be paying attention to all items that come within your field of vision—other cars, pedestrians, signs and stoplights, buildings, and so on.

- Most of the time, you will anchor your attention on the visual field in general rather than on anything in particular. Occasionally, of course, it will become necessary to focus on specific things in your view as they become relevant to your driving.

- The second anchor in mindful driving is the sensation of the hands on the steering wheel. It's a good practice, both for mindfulness and for safety's sake, to keep both hands on the wheel. If you're in the habit of driving with one hand, it will take a good bit of mindfulness just to remember to use both hands.

- In mindful driving, the hands function like the feet in walking meditation. Just as you do with the feet in walking, bring your awareness to the sensations of the hands. You may feel the hardness or softness of the wheel itself, some pain or tension in your hands, or the vibrations generated by the engine and the car as it moves.

- The basic practice of driving mindfully is quite simple. It follows the observe-and-return dynamic of sitting meditation. Whenever you notice your mind drifting away from being attentive to the experience of driving, gently escort your awareness back to these two anchors, which ground you in the present.

- In driving, it's possible to create specific ways to remind yourself to return to the present moment. If you're driving in town, you can designate certain recurring markers—such as intersections, traffic lights, or stop signs—as prompters to jog your memory. If you're on the highway, telephone or light poles might serve the same function.

- Wherever you are, use markers to remind you to drop your thoughts and reacquaint yourself with the present moment. Bring your attention back to the visual field and then feel the sensations of your hands and proceed.

- Make a determination to keep your eye on the road. When the next marker appears, note how successful you were at staying attentive, return to your anchors, and continue. Over time, repeating this practice will allow your attention to remain concentrated on driving.

Nonvisual Sensations

- As you begin to master the basic technique, you can start to work with other aspects of your experience. Keeping the mind focused on the visual field and the sensations of the hands affords the occasional opportunity to attend to other aspects of your bodily experience. Every so often, you can take a moment to check your posture and make adjustments if necessary. You can notice if any areas of your body are contracted or tense and allow them to relax.

- A good time to review your bodily experience is whenever you pull up to a red light. You can also concentrate attention on specific physical functions involved in operating the vehicle, such as using your foot to brake or rotating your head to scan your field of vision.

- As you continue with the practice, you can add the sensation of hearing to the experiences you observe. As you drive, you can spend a moment listening to the sound of your engine. This practice not only keeps your attention in the present, but it can also alert you if there is something wrong with your car.

- Driving involves all sorts of other interesting sounds when you take time to listen: the humming of the tires on the road, the whir of the air conditioning or heater, and the clamorous noises of traffic. As with sitting meditation, try to stay attentive to the sensations themselves; if you find yourself drifting off into thought about the sensations, gently escort attention back to your anchors.

- Once you've become comfortable returning awareness to your field of vision and observing your bodily sensations, you can begin to give systematic attention to your emotions. Being aware of the emotional aspect of your experience is extremely important in driving practice because emotions play an extremely important role in driving.

- Out on the road, we're apt to have many occasions to feel anger, frustration, fear, and surprise. Think of how often you've found yourself getting angry at other motorists or at traffic delays. Driving can be an emotionally charged experience, and it can certainly take its toll on our general sense of well-being.

- As in other forms of meditation, our aim in driving practice is to observe these emotions arising without judgment and allowing them to fall away, preserving our equanimity. You don't have to act on these emotions, just witness them. Of course, it takes a great deal of practice to permit such powerful emotions as anger and fear to arise and fall without reacting in a negative way.

- Almost everyone feels irritation, if not outright rage, when we come upon some kind of traffic delay, even if it's relatively brief. The mindfulness approach is to acknowledge the situation and recognize our limited powers to change it. You can welcome these moments as an opportunity to think about things you haven't had the time to contemplate—permitting your reflections to run as deep as you like.

- Even as you allow these ruminations in stalled traffic, you should frequently return to the visual field and maintain touch with your present situation. It's certainly fine to ponder the future and recall the past, but always do so with the awareness of what you're doing.

- Of course, driving isn't just about dealing with maniacs, idiots, and traffic jams. It can also be about having pleasurable experiences. It's a fascinating world out there, and driving is one way to see it. However, in order to see it, you have to be awake. You have to marshal your capacities for attention and train your mind to see what is occurring in each moment.

Driving as a Metaphor

- Driving, in fact, is a kind of metaphor for the journey through life. You're moving through the world on pathways generally established by others who've come before you. Occasionally, you may go off the beaten path and discover something very interesting or something very terrifying. You may stop for a while, but eventually you'll keep going.

- As you're traveling along, you may have a general idea about what's up ahead, but you can never be certain. There are always surprises and possible dangers, even along your habitual routes. There are delays and detours, smooth pavement and potholes, nice people and not-so-nice people. You can unwittingly take a wrong turn and travel down a road that will change your life forever—or you can stick to the main road and never deviate from it.

Questions to Consider

1. How does ordinary driving affect you? How does it influence your emotions and your ability to pay attention? What past experiences have shaped your experience of driving? How does driving reflect the rest of your life?

2. Schedule 30 minutes to devote yourself to driving mindfully. Don't plan a destination. Simply have the single purpose to drive in complete awareness for that amount of time.

Driving—Staying Awake at the Wheel
Lecture 12—Transcript

Americans love cars. According to the Bureau of Transportation, there are more automobiles in the United States than licensed drivers. And we love to drive.

In the first decade of the 21st century, Americans drove approximately 3 trillion miles each year. Many of you, I'm sure, have been listening to these lectures as you've been driving. It hardly needs to be said then: Operating motor vehicles is an extremely important part of our culture.

Because we spend so much time on the road, driving represents a wonderful opportunity for us to practice mindfulness. Like walking and eating, driving is an ordinary experience whose potential for enriching our awareness of life is usually overlooked.

But practicing mindfulness while driving is not only a choice opportunity; it's a veritable necessity. Driving may be the most hazardous activity the average person participates in. Each year, there are well over 6 million vehicle collisions in the United States, in which 3 million people suffer injuries. Automobile accidents are the leading non-disease-related cause of death in the United States. Car accidents are the number one cause of death for young people ages 15–24. Each year, 40–45 thousand people die in vehicle mishaps. That's the equivalent of over a dozen 9/11s or about 200 commercial jet crashes each year. Can you imagine the public outcry if a jet plane crashed every other day? Yet, the same number of people die each year on the nation's roads.

Certainly a major factor in many accidents is the lack of attentiveness, whether that's caused by cell phone use, eating food, engaging in conversations, or just driving under the influence of mindlessness. In fact, distracted driving is the leading cause of vehicle collisions. Some studies suggest that 80 percent of all car accidents are caused by distracted driving. If anything we do can benefit from the application of mindfulness, it's operating a vehicle.

Are you a mindless driver? Take a moment to assess your ordinary driving habits. Consider how often you fail to drive completely attentive to the experience as it's happening. If you're in the car as you hear me speak, simply note where your mind has been for the last 15 minutes. It's not uncommon for people to drive for miles and miles without paying full attention to the route they're taking. Ever get to your destination and wonder, "How did I get here?"

Think also about the way you drive. Do you drive aggressively? Timidly? Competitively? When I'm on the highway, I sometimes notice the urge to accelerate as another car begins to pass me, as if I'm in a race. Do you drive lawfully, always observing speed limits and other traffic regulations? Based on what I see, what others tell me, and my own adventures as a youth, many people don't always feel obligated to obey the rules when they're on the road. We can even purchase technology to help us speed without getting caught. If you think of your automobile as an extension of your personality, as some psychologists suggest it is, what does your driving say about you?

I'd like to introduce you to some simple techniques to begin to incorporate mindfulness practice into your driving routines. Many of the fundamental skills I'll mention we've already discussed in previous lectures, but we're now taking those abilities and applying them to the special context of driving. I hope you'll find these practices make your time in the car more enjoyable, more enlightening and, most of all, safer.

Mindful driving begins long before you enter the car. Since driving is a potentially hazardous activity, we should do all we can beforehand to ensure our journeys are safe. First, that means making sure the vehicle we're driving is well-maintained and in good operating condition. Second, it means preparing our minds to take the responsibility of driving seriously, knowing that getting behind the wheel requires our full attention. If we're unprepared for that responsibility, we should at least be responsible enough not to drive.

When you're ready to go, bring mindful attention to what you're doing as you approach the car. You might start by engaging in a walking meditation practice as you move toward your vehicle. Then stay attentive as you go through the usual routine of preparing to drive. Be aware of all the small things that you might otherwise overlook: Listen to the sound of unlocking the car; feel the muscular effort it takes to open the door; be aware of your movements as you get into your seat; notice any scent in the car's interior; attend to the sensations as you reach over your shoulder to get the seat belt; listen to the clicking sound as you buckle it; be mindful of adjusting the mirrors to fit your vision; put your key in the ignition and hear the sound of the engine starting. Attending to these routine procedures can begin to ground our attention in the present moment.

If you have passengers, make sure everyone is prepared and safely buckled. Remember that the safety of yourself, the others in the car, and strangers on the road depends on your full awareness. Careful driving is an act of compassion. This is also a good time to remind yourself that you should focus on the experience of driving and not the destination. The destination is mindfulness.

As you prepare to leave, reflect on the value of removing potential distractions, just as you would for sitting meditation. Will eating and drinking, using the cell phone, reading, applying make-up, shaving, or engaging in conversations pose hazards to your driving or create possible distractions? Even at the risk of silencing my own voice, I ask you to consider whether or not listening to the radio or the CD player constitutes a hazardous diversion. If you suspect that any of these activities take your mind away from being fully present to driving, then consider refraining from them. If you're not sure, just conduct an experiment. Try driving without the radio, the coffee, or any other possible distractions, and study the effect of its absence on your attentiveness. Now, I'm putting my concerns about distracted driving in very soft language, asking you to think about it and make a choice. But there is one growing practice that seems to deserve a stronger tone: texting. Ladies and gentlemen, I implore you, do not text and drive!

Now check your posture. Make sure you're sitting in a position that promotes alertness and allows you to be relaxed. Keep your hands firmly on the steering wheel, but don't clench them. They too should feel relaxed. Perhaps you can manage a quick body scan to release any tension you may feel. Take several deep breaths, and go.

As you begin to drive, you'll do so normally. There is no need to slow your rate of speed as we do in walking and eating meditation, unless of course your speed violates the law. On the other hand, you might experiment with driving a bit slower than usual to see if that has an effect on your ability to stay attentive. As we've discussed with other forms of meditation, just slightly breaking the routine can help keep our minds focused.

As we do in other forms of meditation, we'll need to establish anchors as a way to stabilize our attention when it begins to wander. In driving practice, we'll use two. The first is the visual field available to us as we look through the car windshield and windows. For simplicity, I'll refer to this as "keeping your eye on the road," although it means more than merely looking at the road. You'll be paying attention to all items that come within your field of vision—other cars, pedestrians, signs and stop lights, buildings, and so on. Most of the time, you will anchor your attention on the visual field in general rather than on anything in particular. Occasionally, of course, it will become necessary to focus on specific things in your view as they become relevant to your driving. As you come to an intersection, for example, you'll concentrate on the stop sign rather than potential distractions such as a bus stand advertisement.

The second anchor in mindful driving is the sensation of the hands on the steering wheel. It's a good practice, both for mindfulness and safety's sake, to keep both hands on the wheel. If you're in the habit of driving with one hand, as I have been, it will take a good bit of mindfulness just to remember to use both hands. These days, I fortunately have my seven-year-old daughter in the back seat to remind me when I revert back to my old ways. She keeps a close eye on me as I drive and yells "Both hands on the steering wheel!" as it becomes necessary. Yes, it can be annoying, but I'm really grateful to her for helping me pay better attention.

In mindful driving, the hands function like the feet in walking meditation. Just as you do with the feet in walking, bring your awareness to the sensations of the hands. You may feel the hardness or softness of the wheel itself, some pain or tension in your hands, or the vibrations generated by the engine and the car as it moves. Just be attentive to whatever sensations show up.

The basic practice of mindful driving is quite simple. It follows the observe-and-return dynamic of sitting meditation. Whenever you notice your mind drifting away from being attentive to the experience of driving, gently escort your awareness back to these two anchors. As we practice in sitting meditation, our goal is to be aware of the moment when our mind slips away from present experience and, without judgment or commentary, return attention to where it belongs. Coming back to the anchors grounds your awareness in the present—and that's where you want to be.

In sitting meditation, we're usually left on our own to remember when to return to the breath. Thus, our mind can easily get caught up in daydreaming for long periods of time before it realizes it's gone astray. In driving, however, it's possible to create specific ways to remind yourself to return to the present moment. If you're driving in town, you can designate certain recurring markers, such as intersections, traffic lights, or stop signs as prompters to jog your memory. If you're on the highway, telephone or light poles might serve the same function. Or you can simply get a sticky note and write on it the words "Wake up!" Then post the note on the console just above the speedometer where you'll see it whenever you check your speed. Wherever you are, use these markers to remind you to drop your thoughts and reacquaint yourself with the present moment. Bring your attention back to the visual field, and then feel the sensations of your hands and proceed. Make a determination to keep your eye on the road. When the next marker appears, note how successful you were at staying attentive, return to your anchors, and continue. Over time, repeating this practice will allow your attention to remain concentrated on driving.

As you begin to master the basic technique, you can start to work with other aspects of your experience. Keeping the mind focused on the visual field and the sensations of the hands affords the occasional opportunity to attend to other aspects of your bodily experience. Every so often, you can take a moment to check your posture and make adjustments if necessary. You can notice if any areas of your body are contracted or tense and allow them to relax.

A good time to review your bodily experience is whenever you pull up to a red light. The brief time it takes for the light to turn green is an ample period to do a quick body scan. You can also concentrate attention on specific physical functions involved in operating the vehicle, such as using the foot to brake or accelerate, or rotating your head to scan your field of vision.

As you continue with the practice, you can add the sensation of hearing to the experiences you observe. As you drive, you can spend a moment listening to the sound of your engine. This practice not only keeps your attention in the present, but it can also alert you if something's wrong with your car. One of the first things a mechanic does to diagnose a malfunctioning auto is to listen to it. My brother, who is a mechanic, actually uses a specialized stethoscope to help ferret out problems. Of course, it takes a specially trained ear to be able to determine the nature of a problem just by listening, but simply being acquainted with the sound of a properly functioning vehicle helps anyone know when something is askew. Driving involves all sorts of other interesting sounds when you take time to listen: the humming of the tires on the road, the whirr of the air conditioning or heater, and the clamorous noises of traffic. As with sitting meditation, try to stay attentive to the sensations themselves; if you find yourself drifting into thought about the sensations, gently escort attention back to your anchors.

Once you've become comfortable returning awareness to your field of vision and observing your bodily sensations, you can begin to give systematic attention to your emotions. Being aware of the emotional aspect of your experience is extremely important in driving practice because emotions play an extremely important role in driving. Out on the road, we're apt to have many occasions to feel anger, frustration, fear, and surprise. Think of how often you've found yourself getting angry at other motorists. George Carlin once observed there are only two kinds of drivers: maniacs and idiots. The maniacs are the ones who are driving faster than you, and the idiots are the ones who are driving slower. And both types drive you mad. You, apparently, are the only sane driver out there! Or remember the many frustrations you've had when you've encountered delays due to road construction or accidents caused by other drivers who weren't paying attention. Or recall the fears you've had when you had to drive during a thunderstorm or a blizzard. Driving can be an emotionally charged experience, and it can certainly take its toll on our general sense of well-being.

As in other forms of meditation, our aim in driving practice is to observe these emotions arising without judgment and allowing them to fall away, preserving our equanimity. You don't have to act on these emotions, just witness them. Of course, it takes a good deal of practice both on and off the cushion to permit such powerful emotions, as anger and fear, to arise and fall without clutching onto them and reacting in a negative way. You may find it helpful to employ some of the techniques I discussed in the earlier lecture on working with thoughts. Take that maniac, for instance. As she swooshes past you on a narrow two-lane highway, leaving your teeth rattling and your nerves frayed, you might be inclined to shout, curse, or gesture rudely. Instead, wish her a safe journey. Remind yourself that you don't really know what's driving her apparent recklessness. Maybe she has a legitimate emergency. Remember that holding onto your anger toward her will do nothing but disturb your own peace of mind and put your own safe driving at risk. Driving around angry is not very wise.

But what do you do when you come upon the slow driver? Once again, you can shout, curse, gesticulate wildly, or blow your horn like Gabriel at the Last Judgment. Or you can approach the situation calmly. Let the slight delay remind you to return to mindfulness. Take some breaths. Allow your body to relax. Think of the person ahead of you. As best you can, suspend judgments about the way others drive. Maybe he's new to area and unfamiliar with the road; maybe he has just received some terrible news. Whatever his reason, little is accomplished by acting on your anger. You're better served by allowing your frustration to fall away and serenely take the first opportunity to pass him safely. Driving mindfully means driving kindly.

Just about everyone feels irritation, if not outright rage, when we come upon some traffic delay, even if it's relatively brief. What's the mindful approach to these situations? It's the same as all situations we encounter: Accept it and learn from it. We acknowledge the situation and recognize our limited powers to change it. Then we try to make a virtue of necessity. You say to yourself, Here I am. This is the way it is. Now, how do I redeem this experience so that it's not an utter waste of precious time? Your response doesn't have to be anything profound, although it can be. You can welcome these moments as an opportunity to think about things you haven't had time to contemplate: What color should I paint the upstairs bathroom? What would be a good gift for Dorothy and Gordon's 50th anniversary? Should I be investing in treasury bonds?

Or you can permit your reflections to run deeper. What does your anxiety about getting to where you're going tell you about yourself? Does it seem you're always rushing from one place to another? Where are you really headed? I mean, really, what is your ultimate destination? When it comes time to draw the bottom line and sum up your life, is this frustration on Interstate 95—as infuriating as it is—going to make a big difference? Probably not, but a lifetime of getting exasperated at all the things that inconvenience you probably will.

Yet even as you allow these ruminations in stalled traffic, you should frequently return to the visual field and maintain touch with your present situation. It's certainly fine to ponder the future and recall the past, but always do so with the awareness of what you're doing.

Of course, driving isn't just about dealing with maniacs and idiots and traffic jams. It can also be about having pleasurable experiences. It's a fascinating world out there, and driving is one way to see it. But in order to see it, you have to be awake. You have to marshal your capacities for attention and train your mind to see what is occurring moment by moment. If you get to your destination wondering "How did I get here?" you've missed out.

Driving, in fact, is a kind of metaphor for the journey through life, which is one reason road movies and novels are such popular genres. You're moving through the world on pathways generally established by others who've come before you. Occasionally, you may go off the beaten path and discover something very interesting or something very terrifying. You may stop for a while, but eventually you'll keep going. As you're traveling along, you may have a general idea about what's up ahead, but you can never be certain. There are always surprises and possible dangers, even along your habitual routes. There are delays and detours, smooth pavement and potholes, nice people and some not-so-nice. You can unwittingly take a wrong turn and travel down a road that will change your life forever. Or you can stick to the main road and never deviate from it.

As you move along, you notice that you have little control over the full range of events that are unfolding before your eyes. You have slight, if any, authority over what others do. You can't stop the huge semi from dangerously pulling out in front of you. Your powers are fairly well limited to the control that you have over your own vehicle, but even that is not absolute. It can breakdown or skid out of your control. But despite your limitations, it is possible to sit back, relax, and become mindfully alert to your experiences, whatever they may be. You'll see interesting things and scary things, things that will make you sad, things that will make you laugh. But you'll keep going. Bon voyage.

Insight—Clearing the Mind
Lecture 13

Insight into transience is central to mindfulness practice. How we respond to the fact of impermanence determines whether we suffer or find lasting happiness in the world. The mindfulness tradition tells us that change is nothing to fear and that it is possible to live a life of contentment amid a world of constant flux. However, to overcome our fear of change and to find equanimity in its midst requires clearly gazing into it. It is here that words must stop, and we must return to the silence of meditation.

The Element of Insight

- We've all had moments when things suddenly become clear. The haze dissipates, and what was there all along becomes obvious. The solution to the problem you've been pondering unexpectedly presents itself. The issue you've been struggling with dissolves, your heart catches fire with inspiration, and immediately you know what you must do. Sometimes we wonder how we could have missed what is now so plainly apparent.

- Mindfulness practice promises these unmistakable moments when something within you moves and you see things differently. Appropriately enough, the mindfulness tradition calls these moments "insights," or "clear gazing," to translate the Buddhist word *vipassana*.

- The element of insight distinguishes mindfulness practice from forms of meditation that seek only to calm the mind. In mindfulness, stilling the mind is essential, but it is only a precondition for a deeper purpose: to gain insight into the way the world is and to live our lives accordingly. We cannot coerce insights, but we can use meditation to clear the way for them to arise.

- If you have been continuing with a daily mindfulness practice, you have already been doing the necessary groundwork for insight. In fact, you may have already experienced insights and started to feel that a whole new world is opening up to you.

- Meditation helps us to be more attentive to our lives. At the same time, it enables us to develop a new relationship with our experience, characterized by acceptance and relinquishment. The qualities of attention, acceptance, and relinquishment are what prime our minds for insight.

- We learn through meditation that just because a thought arises does not mean we have to believe it. If we simply accept the fact that it has arisen and let it go, without aversion or attachment, the mind remains clear, spacious, and ready to see what is there.

- When a mind is so full of thoughts and ideas about the way things are and the way things should be, it lacks the flexibility and openness to see the world in a new way. The problem with such a mind is not that it has ideas and opinions; the difficulty is the way it clings to these thoughts with such tenacity.

- Meditation practice enables us to recognize our ideas and beliefs, accept them for what they are, and remain unattached to them. We allow our thoughts and sensations to arise and then allow them to go their own way.

The Beginner's Mind

- It requires constant practice to prevent ourselves from becoming experts. Staying a beginner means having to start over and over again. One way to stay a beginner—or become one—is to practice **not-knowing**, which begins with an honest assessment of what we really know and what we really can know.

- Most of what we as individuals profess as "knowledge" is perhaps better categorized as "belief." Everyone "knows" the world is a sphere, but how many of us have actually taken the trouble to verify that for ourselves? Consider how much of what we think we know has been received on the basis of this sort of faith.

- It is impossible as well as unnecessary to take the time to verify everything we claim to know, but recognizing that so much of what we call knowledge is founded on implicit trust in authorities rather than on immediate personal experience ought at least to make us cautious about asserting anything with too much conviction.

- Most of us feel great pressure to be knowledgeable—or at least appear that way. We learn early in our careers how to speak with the authority to convince others and ourselves that we know what we're talking about. Sometimes, of course, we do know what we're talking about.

- The truth is that we really know less than we think, and much of what we profess to know is actually belief, opinion, and conjecture. This is especially true when it comes to facing the great questions in life: From whence have we come and why? Does life have a meaning or purpose? What happens when we die?

- Knowledge—or even just the illusion of knowledge—provides us with a hedge against the terrors of uncertainty. It furnishes us with the pleasant feeling that we are actually in control of our lives.

- To practice not-knowing means finding the courage to be at ease with uncertainty and mystery. Essentially, one overcomes the fear of the unknown by becoming more familiar with it. Certainly, meditation helps us with this.

- In our practice, all manner of thoughts and feelings arise, and we are encouraged simply to be with them. Rather than making us feel secure by answering all our questions, mindfulness practice invites us to become free from attachment to security, free from the frantic need to know, and free from the ego's desire to appear knowledgeable.

- The Buddha was renowned for refusing to answer questions. Unlike many other sages of his era, and even sages of our era, the Buddha did not feel compelled to provide a comprehensive worldview that could explain any question that might arise in the mind.

- Not-knowing does not mean one necessarily lacks knowledge or that we're required to forget everything or to suspend all interpretations of a situation. Not-knowing does not mean that we are confused. Rather, it is a consciously chosen attitude that we take to allow us to see things more clearly. It is the acknowledgement that we may not understand everything we need to know to handle a particular situation.

- Maintaining a beginner's mind, practicing not-knowing, relaxing attachments to thoughts, being humble, learning to live with uncertainty—these are all interrelated aspects of clearing the way for insight. Insight comes when our minds are ready. This must be why moments of crisis are often times of great spiritual development.

- Such cognitively disorienting occasions as death, divorce, and addiction carry the potential to disrupt old habits of mind and to open us to new ways of seeing. These are often times when uncertainty, not-knowing, and humility are thrust upon us. If we are wise and attentive, these critical times can be gifts of great value.

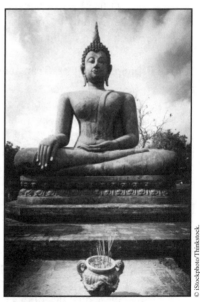

For Zen Buddhists, seeking to understand the true nature of Zen is the same as wanting to know the true nature of reality.

- When we speak of insight in the mindfulness tradition, we are speaking of something more than just discovering a solution to a problem—although a mindful insight may lead to that. We're speaking of something more than just a profound thought that suddenly occurs to us—although insight may coalesce into profound thinking.

- Insight in mindfulness is understood as an immediate experience of clarity about the nature of reality. There is nothing supernatural about insight. It is the ordinary, natural experience of seeing the world as it is, devoid of the heavy overlay of preconceptions and beliefs that clutter our perceptions of it.

- Insight pertains more to the function of perception than to thinking. Thinking, of course, precedes insight and may proceed from it, but insight itself is distinguishable from thinking. The very same sense is conveyed by the original meaning of the English word "insight," which is "to see into."

Three Principal Insights: Transience

- While there are an infinite number of possible insights into human existence, Buddhism focuses on three that pertain to the heart of our experience of reality. These are known as the three marks, or characteristics, of existence.

- The three insights are transience, or impermanence; not-self, or the "illusion and insubstantiality of the self"; and dukkha, a word that is usually translated as "suffering" but whose meaning is rich and deep.

- Insight into these three qualities is regarded by Buddhists as essential to freedom and happiness. In addition, Buddhism argues that these qualities of our experience are interrelated and so to gain insight into one is to also see the other two.

- When the tradition insists that these three characteristics must be grasped by insight, we must bear in mind that these are not regarded as beliefs to which one gives assent, nor are they simply concepts to be grasped by the intellect. They are considered facts about the nature of existence that must be apprehended by direct personal experience.

- Transience, or impermanence, is the name for the insight that is probably the easiest to understand. Everyone acknowledges that things change, but the mindfulness tradition contends that most of us fail to acknowledge the depth of change without qualification, and hence we live resisting the impermanence over which we have no control.

- When it comes to the reality of change, we often look for ways to believe we are somehow exempt from it. Perhaps the chasm between what we believe to be true and how we live our lives can be explained by a lack of genuine insight.

- We grasp the idea of impermanence conceptually, but impermanence has not yet grasped us in the way that insight makes possible—in the manner that revolutionizes our whole way of life.

- Meditative practice makes it possible to sharpen perceptive attention to such a degree that one can have a direct knowledge of the momentary arising and passing away of all reality. When viewed this way, any perception of stability or permanence is only apparent.

- A deep, penetrating awareness of the world reveals that all things are concatenations of events happening so rapidly that they seem to be stable or changing only very slowly.

- If you have a chance, spend a few moments outside and contemplate an ordinary tree—or simply imagine one. To the casual observer, a tree appears to be a more or less stable thing, but looking deeper, we can see it is a grand spectacle of ever-changing processes happening in swift succession at every level of its existence. From this perspective, a tree is not—and cannot be—the same from moment to moment.

- Change is so far-reaching, so thoroughgoing, that ultimately we can say there are no "things" in the world at all. No item in our experience—no thought, feeling, or physical object—endures long enough from one moment to the next for us to say it is a "thing," an entity that has its own existence in space and time.

- Our minds, conditioned as they are by our language, tend to reify, or regard as concrete things, matters that are better understood as events or occurrences. The danger arises only when we forget that talking and thinking about "things" is a mere convenient contrivance. The true reality of the world of existence is something that cannot be easily captured by our thought and language—but it can be grasped by insight.

Important Terms

not-knowing: A beginning practice that starts with an honest assessment of what one really knows and what one really can know.

vipassana: The Buddhist word for "insights" or "clear gazing," these are unmistakable moments when a person sees things differently.

Questions to Consider

1. Choose a simple object, like a vase or chair, to look at. Take a moment to become mindful of your breathing. Then, place your attention on the object. Try to observe the object as clearly and as naïvely as possible without the usual overlay of conceptual thought. How does this approach differ from your usual manner of observation?

2. Reflect on how much of what you think you know is based on belief and faith and how much is founded on personal experience.

Insight—Clearing the Mind
Lecture 13—Transcript

We've all had moments when things suddenly become clear. The haze dissipates and what was there all along becomes obvious. The solution to the problem you've been pondering for days unexpectedly presents itself. The thing you've always been told was true, but which you only half-believed— or even disbelieved—now becomes as real as your own existence. The issue you've been struggling with dissolves, and your heart catches fire with inspiration, and immediately you know what you must do. Sometimes we wonder how we could have missed what is now so plainly apparent.

Mindfulness practice promises moments such as these. They may not always appear amid fireworks and the 1812 Overture. Perhaps they are more like the quiet and gradual "dawn's early light" than the "rocket's red glare." But they are unmistakable moments when something within you moves and you see things differently. Appropriately enough, the mindfulness tradition calls these moments "insights," or "clear gazing," to translate the Buddhist word *vipassana*. The element of insight distinguishes mindfulness practice from other forms of meditation that seek only to calm the mind. In mindfulness, stilling the mind is essential, but it is only a precondition for a deeper purpose: to gain insight into the way the world is and to live our lives accordingly. These insights do not always come as we're sitting on the cushion; they may appear at any time. Yet meditation prepares the mind to receive them. We cannot coerce insights, but we can clear the way for them to arise.

If you have been continuing with a daily mindfulness practice, you have already been doing the necessary groundwork for insight. In fact, you may have already experienced insights and started to feel that a whole new world is opening up to you. Here's why: Meditation helps us to be more attentive to our lives. At the same time, it enables us to develop a new relationship with our experience, characterized by acceptance and relinquishment. We learn through meditation that just because a thought arises does not mean we have to believe it. It's just a thought, and given the erratic nature of the mind, it's probably not a keeper. If we simply accept the fact that it has arisen and let it go, without aversion or attachment, the mind remains clear, spacious, and ready to see what is there. The qualities of attention, acceptance, and relinquishment are what prime our minds for insight.

The role of meditation in preparing us for insight is well-illustrated in the story of a Japanese university professor who went to visit a Zen master to inquire about the true nature of Zen. Now, asking about the true nature of Zen is more than just asking about the beliefs and practices of a particular religion. For Zen Buddhists, seeking to understand the true nature of Zen is the same as wanting to know the true nature of reality. When the professor made his request, the Zen master said nothing in response but simply poured the visitor a cup of tea. When the cup was filled, the master continued to pour, until it overflowed. The professor begged the master to stop. "It's full! It won't hold anymore!" "Precisely," said the master, "and your mind is like this teacup, full of your own opinions and conjectures. How can you see Zen unless you first empty your cup?"

Zen masters are fond of this sort of prank, just as professors are fond of their opinions and conjectures. Of course, it's more than just a prank; it's a fine object lesson, the kind of concrete demonstration that Zen specializes in. The master graphically illustrates the problem of a mind conditioned to mindlessness. When it is so full of thoughts and ideas about the way things are and the way things should be, the mind lacks the flexibility and openness to see the world in a new way. Perhaps it lacks the capacity to see the world at all, since its view is filtered through a rigid mass of beliefs and concepts. The problem with such a mind is not that it has ideas and opinions; the difficulty is the way it clings to these thoughts with such tenacity. Someone who seems to have grasped this idea, at least according to one statement attributed to him, is former president George Herbert Walker Bush, who is reported to have said: "I have opinions of my own—strong opinions—but I don't always agree with them." Far from being a linguistic gaffe, Bush cogently articulates the mindfulness view!

Meditation practice enables us to recognize our ideas and beliefs, accept them for they are, and remain unattached to them. We allow our thoughts and sensations to arise and then allow them to go their own way. In this manner, we maintain what Shunryu Suzuki called "beginner's mind," the mind of openness and flexibility, the mind that can be taught and can view things afresh. Suzuki said, "In the beginner's mind there are many possibilities, but in the expert's mind there are few." It requires constant practice to prevent ourselves from becoming experts. Staying a beginner means having to start over and over again.

One way to stay a beginner—or become one—is to practice not-knowing. Not-knowing begins with an honest assessment of what we really know and what we really can know. Most of what we as individuals profess as "knowledge" is perhaps better categorized as "belief." Everyone "knows" the world is a sphere, but how many of us have actually taken the trouble to verify that for ourselves? How many of us would even know how to verify it? Would it not be more accurate for us to say that we believe the earth is a sphere because we have faith in people and books who tell us this is true?

Consider how much of what we think has been received on the basis of this sort of faith. I'm not suggesting that we ought to take the time to verify everything we claim to know; that would be impossible as well as unnecessary. But recognizing that so much of what we call knowledge is founded on implicit trust in authorities rather than on immediate personal experience ought at least to make us cautious about asserting anything with too much conviction.

Yet most of us feel great pressure to be knowledgeable—or at least appear that way. In my job, it's very hard to admit that really and truly you don't know, especially if it is something you're "supposed" to know. This is probably why the whipping boy in the Zen story is a professor. We learn early in our careers how to speak with the authority to convince others and ourselves that we know what we're talking about. Sometimes, of course, we do know what we're talking about. But the truth is, we—and I mean all of us, not just we professors—we really know less than we think and much of what we profess to know is actually belief, opinion, conjecture, and BS, to use the philosophically precise term.

When it comes to facing the great questions in life, this is especially true: From whence have we come and why? Does life have a meaning or purpose? What happens when we die? I've often thought that one of the functions of conventional religion is to mask the mystery of existence by disguising it with intelligible concepts to assuage our fears of the unknown. Knowledge—or even just the illusion of knowledge—provides us with a hedge against the terrors of uncertainty. It furnishes us with the pleasant feeling that we are actually in control of our lives. One of the reasons I'm uncomfortable with both theism and atheism is that they assert too much about the nature of reality. They place more confidence in human knowledge than is warranted. Neither theism nor atheism is very comfortable with uncertainty, and they rush headlong to hide it.

To practice not-knowing means finding the courage to be at ease with uncertainty and mystery. Essentially, one overcomes the fear of the unknown by becoming more familiar with it. Certainly meditation helps us with this. In our practice, all manner of thoughts and feelings arise, and we are encouraged simply to be with them. Rather than making us feel secure by answering all our questions, mindfulness practice invites us to become free from attachment to security, free from the frantic need to know, and free from the ego's desire to appear knowledgeable.

The Buddha was renowned for refusing to answer questions. Unlike many other sages of his era, and even sages of our era, the Buddha did not feel compelled to provide a comprehensive worldview that could explain any question that might arise in the mind. In one famous incident, a monk named Malyunkyaputta came to the Buddha threatening to leave the order unless the Buddha settled a group of metaphysical issues, including whether or not the universe came into existence at a particular time or whether it always existed; whether the universe was finite or infinite; and whether the soul is identical to the body or whether it is separate from the body. The Buddha flatly told the monk that he would not resolve these issues because knowing the answers was not pertinent to living a virtuous and happy life; indeed, becoming obsessed with discovering the answers to these questions could actually encumber the pursuit of happiness and freedom. In this way, the Buddha urged his disciple to accept a world in which some things are uncertain and attachment to security is an obstacle to well-being.

Not-knowing does not mean one necessarily lacks knowledge or that we're required to forget everything or to suspend all interpretations of a situation. Not-knowing does not mean that we are confused. Rather, it is a consciously chosen attitude that we take to allow us to see things more clearly. It is the acknowledgement that we may not understand everything we need to know to handle a particular situation. As Saint John of the Cross says in *The Dark Night of the Soul*, the wise "never presume to be right about anything." That does not mean they are not right, only that they are keenly aware of the limitations of what they know. Call it humility.

Maintaining a beginner's mind, practicing not-knowing, relaxing attachments to thoughts, being humble, learning to live with uncertainty—these are all interrelated aspects of clearing the way for insight. Insight comes when our minds are ready. This must be why moments of crisis are often times of great spiritual development.

The loss of a job, the death of a loved one, an illness, the acknowledgement of an addiction, divorce—these can all be cognitively disorienting occasions that carry the potential to disrupt old habits of mind and open us to new ways of seeing. These are often times when uncertainty, not-knowing, and humility are thrust upon us. If we are wise and attentive to these critical times they can be gifts of great value.

When we speak of insight in the mindfulness tradition, we are speaking of something more than just discovering a solution to a problem, although a mindful insight may lead to that. We're speaking of something more than just a profound thought that suddenly occurs to us, although insight may coalesce into profound thinking. Insight in mindfulness is better understood as an immediate experience of clarity about the nature of reality. It is not a revelation from on high; there is nothing supernatural about insight. It is the ordinary, natural experience of seeing the world as it is, devoid of the heavy overlay of preconceptions and beliefs that clutter our perceptions of it. As I mentioned earlier, the term usually translated as insight literally means "clear gazing." Thus, insight pertains more to the function of perception than to thinking. Thinking, of course, precedes insight and may proceed from it. But insight itself is distinguishable from thinking. The very same sense is conferred by the original meaning of the English word "insight," which is "to see into."

Buddhism customarily speaks of three principal insights made possible by the development of mindfulness. While there are an infinite number of possible insights into human existence, Buddhism focuses on three that pertain to the heart of our experience of reality. These are known as the three "marks," or characteristics, of existence. Insight into these three qualities is regarded by Buddhists as essential to freedom and happiness. The three are transience, or impermanence; not-self, or the "illusion and insubstantiality of the self"; and *dukkha*, a word that is usually translated as "suffering" but whose meaning is so rich that I'm choosing to use the original term to keep its depth ever-present in the discussion. Buddhism argues that these three qualities of our experience are interrelated and so to gain insight into one is to also see the other two.

When the tradition insists that these three characteristics must be grasped by insight, we must bear in mind that these are not regarded as beliefs to which one gives assent, nor are they simply concepts to be grasped by the intellect. They are considered facts about the nature of existence that must be apprehended by the direct personal experience. We'll discuss each of these qualities and explain how mindfulness practice clears the way for their realization. We'll begin with transience and in the next lecture we'll cover not-self and *dukkha*.

Transience, or impermanence, is the name for the insight that is probably the easiest to understand. Everyone acknowledges that things change. We even have a popular maxim that says "the only thing that doesn't change is change itself." But truthfully, how thoroughly do we accept this adage? The mindfulness tradition contends that most of us fail to acknowledge the depth of change without qualification, and hence we live resisting the impermanence over which we have no control. In the *Mahabharata*, the great epic of India, Yudhishthira, one of the story's heroes, is put through a battery of riddles by a spirit disguised as a crane. In the culminating question, the spirit asks: "What is the most amazing thing in the world?" Yudhishthira replies, "The most amazing thing in the world is that every day we see death strike and yet we live as if it will not happen to us." When it comes to the reality of change, we often look for ways to believe we are somehow exempt from it.

Perhaps the chasm between what we believe to be true and how we live our lives can be explained by a lack of genuine insight. The fact of transience, in other words, simply has not been brought home to us with sufficient clarity and depth. We grasp the idea of impermanence conceptually, but impermanence has not yet grasped us in the way that insight makes possible, in the manner that revolutionizes our whole way of life.

From the point of view of insight, change is not merely what happens to an entity over the course of time. Change is not simply the birth, growth, decay, and death of an organism, the kinds of changes that are ordinarily perceptible. Birth, growth, decay, and death also occur at every instant in a manner difficult to discern without the skills of meditation.

Meditative practice makes it possible to sharpen perceptive attention to such a degree that one can have a direct knowledge of the momentary arising and passing away of all reality. When viewed this way, as the constant coming and going of transitory events, any perception of stability or permanence is only apparent. A deep, penetrating awareness of the world reveals that all things are concatenations of events happening so rapidly that they seem to be stable or changing only very slowly.

If you have a chance, spend a few moments outside and contemplate an ordinary tree. If you're unable to do so, simply imagine one. To the casual observer, a tree appears to be more or less a stable thing, but looking deeper, we can see it is a grand spectacle of ever-changing processes happening in swift succession at every level of its existence. Consider the leaves. At any given moment, each one of them is in a process of growth or decline. Perhaps the leaf is just budding or about to die and fall away. If it's in its prime, it may be actively engaged in photosynthesis as its chlorophyll interacts with the light of the sun, transforming carbon dioxide into sugar and oxygen. Within the tree, sap may be flowing through its xylem and phloem carrying water and nutrients throughout the tree's body. The nutrients themselves are likely to be the decaying remains of animals and plants, including former parts of the tree itself.

On the outside, minute cells comprising the bark are dying and sloughing off as new cells are born to replace the old. At an even deeper level, we may imagine the vast number of atoms and their subatomic components that make up these cells and systems. These invisible constituents are themselves in a wild, mind-boggling state of constant transformation. From this perspective, a tree is not—and cannot be—the same from moment to moment.

Change is so far-reaching, so thoroughgoing, that ultimately we can say there are no "things" in the world at all. No item of our experience—no thought, feeling, or physical object—endures long enough from one moment to the next for us to say it is a *"thing."* By *"thing,"* I simply mean an entity that has its own existence in space and time. Because change occurs so rapidly and so thoroughly, and because all items of experience are dependent on other items, like photosynthesis depends on the sun, it is misleading and technically wrong to call a tree a thing. There is nothing about a tree that warrants saying it has its own existence, since it depends so much on what is not-tree, like air, light, soil, and water, and since no particular form of it endures over time, not even a moment, however that would be defined. To call a tree a thing is merely a function of our language and thinking processes.

Our minds, conditioned as they are by our language, tend to reify, or regard as concrete things, matters that are better understood as events or occurrences. It is certainly more convenient to say, "Look at that tree over there" than to say "Look at that complex concatenation of successive events engaged in the processes of photosynthesis, the transport of nutrients, the death and birth of new cells, and the swirl of electrons." The danger arises only when we forget that talking and thinking about "things" is a mere convenient contrivance. The true reality of the world of existence is something that cannot easily be captured by our thought and language. But it can be grasped by insight.

Insight into transience is central to the mindfulness practice. As we shall see in our next lecture, how we respond to the fact of impermanence determines whether we suffer or find lasting happiness in the world. The mindfulness tradition tells us that change is nothing to fear and that is possible to live a life of contentment amid a world of constant flux. But to overcome our fear of change and to find equanimity in its midst requires clearly gazing into it. It is here that words must stop, and we must return to the silence of meditation.

Wisdom—Seeing the World as It Is
Lecture 14

Transience, dukkha, and not-self are interrelated marks of existence. The failure to apprehend that people are subject to impermanence and insubstantiality gives rise to dukkha, and the experience of dukkha reinforces our misapprehensions. By imputing permanent selfhood where there is none, we effectively believe ourselves to be individual entities whose fragile existences must be propped up by possessions, achievements, beliefs, and relationships—but that is an illusion. Paradoxically, when we awaken to reality, we discover that the only way to find happiness is to relinquish these feverish efforts to protect and empower the mistaken belief we call the self.

The Quest for Happiness

- Like Aristotle, Mencius, and a great many other thinkers, the Buddha thought that the quest for lasting happiness was the principal impulse of human activity. Aristotle said happiness was the one thing we seek for itself and not as a means to something else; whether we're aware of it or not, happiness is the true aim of all we do. The Buddha would have agreed.

- Neither the Buddha nor Aristotle, however, conceived of happiness in the way we're apt to think of it these days—as a pleasurable experience. The Buddha understood happiness as an enduring reality that is not contingent on fleeting pleasures. This kind of contentment is what all beings truly want and seek.

- While he regarded the desire for happiness to be natural and wholesome, the Buddha did see serious problems with the ways we try to satisfy that yearning. Because we lack wisdom, because we fail to see the world as it is, we inevitably go about the pursuit of happiness in the very ways that sabotage its fulfillment.

- Without awakening to the true nature of reality—without insight into the three marks of existence—we seek contentment in the wrong places and through the wrong means. Because we can never find it, our thirst for satisfaction intensifies and worsens.

Acquisition

- Most of us seek happiness in two basic ways: the first is by acquisition, which is the preferred method in the modern world, and the second is by aversion, which is trying to avoid unpleasant situations. Both techniques are based on what Sigmund Freud called the **pleasure principle**—grasping for the things that we enjoy and evading the things we don't.

- The quest for contentment through acquisition usually leads us to try to enhance our lives by surrounding ourselves with things we believe will give us pleasure: homes, cars, clothing, trophies, and other commonly accepted markers of well-being and achievement.

- Acquisitiveness, however, need not focus on material items. One can seek happiness by having unique and interesting experiences—including spiritual experiences—or by holding the right religious or political beliefs or by affiliating with an organization or a cause.

- If we fail to get what we want, of course, we usually suffer. Because we have made the acquisition of a particular thing the condition for our contentment, not getting it leaves us feeling sad, disappointed, frustrated, and perhaps angry—thinking we've missed the very thing that would have made us happy.

Life's Two Tragedies

- A lot of our remembrance of the past is a reflection on the times we didn't get what we wanted—the first tragedy of life. Tragedy two appears when we actually get what we want.

- Getting what we want may indeed bring us great pleasure, but the pleasurable feelings won't last. When the initial pleasure subsides, disappointment sets in. Disappointment comes in exact proportion to how much happiness we expected our acquisition to provide.

- Desires, whether they are fulfilled or frustrated, only beget more desires. There is no end to our desires when we think that fulfilling our wishes is the way to happiness.

Aversion

- Alongside acquisition, we also seek satisfaction by avoiding unpleasant situations, things, or people. Aversion is actually just the opposite of acquisition; both are manifestations of desire. As with acquisition, the problem with trying to find your happiness through avoidance is the nature of reality. Reality simply does not allow us to evade unwanted experiences.

Getting what we want may indeed bring us great pleasure, but the pleasurable feelings won't last.

- We might be able to escape a few unwanted experiences, but the evasive life often comes at a cost. Even if we can successfully ward off some terrifying experiences, we cannot avert them all—particularly the most unpleasant ones: sickness, old age, and death.

Three Principal Insights: Dukkha

- If our strategy has been to flee from unpleasant circumstances, when they come to meet us, as they surely will, our suffering will be great indeed. These difficult situations are all encompassed by the Buddhist word **dukkha**, which denotes the fundamental frustrating, insatiable quality of our mindless existence.

- Usually translated into English as suffering or dissatisfaction, the meaning of dukkha is actually far richer than a single English word, or even a cluster of English words, can express. You might find it translated as illness, anguish, sorrow, unease, distress, unsettledness, lamentation, pain, grief, despair, and disappointment.

- Dukkha does not merely characterize episodes or aspects of existence. It does not simply suggest that life has a lot of sorrow and anguish, although it does mean that. Rather, the term dukkha indicates that sorrow and anguish, suffering and disappointment permeate existence.

- Dukkha is pervasive, subtle, and insidious—not merely episodic. Like impermanence, there are no exceptions to dukkha in the conditioned world of life as we ordinarily know it. Dukkha names every aspect of experience in which there is the slightest twinge or possibility of anxiety, fear, or disappointment.

- In its full sense, dukkha is not a readily apparent fact of life but a challenge for individuals to discover for themselves by means of introspection and observation. As with the facts of transience, the surface of dukkha can be grasped conceptually, but its depth can only be seen by insight.

An Exercise in Dukkha

- Schedule an appointment with disappointment. Determine to spend an entire day trying to be mindful of all your disappointments and frustrations—no matter how small. If you find this approach too demanding, take some time at the end of a day for reflection.

- As you prepare for the day or reflect back on it, consider the potential sources of routine disappointment: When you're on the road, how's the traffic? Does anyone say something to hurt your feelings? After you've tallied up your disappointing experiences, reflect on how you reacted to them.

- With continued observation and mindfulness practice, the reality of dukkha becomes clearer, and we begin to gain insight into its source and its cure. Eventually, we realize that dukkha is the result of one thing: the fact that the world does not always conform to our desires and expectations.

- The world's not to blame, of course. Reality just is what it is. The problem is with our desires and expectations. We simply expect too much from the world.

- Insight lets us see that the whole approach to contentment through acquisition or aversion is fundamentally misguided. Rather than bringing the satisfaction we so deeply want, acquisition and aversion only serve to frustrate us and increase our anguish and disappointment.

- Instead of questioning these methods themselves, we foolishly think in our mindless state that we simply haven't acquired or averted the right thing or enough things.

Three Principal Insights: Not-Self

- The third mark of existence—and the most difficult to grasp both by intellect and by insight—is **not-self**, which is sometimes compared to "insubstantiality." Not-self is even difficult for those within the tradition to understand, yet it is central to the Buddhist worldview.

- By observing the radical depth of transience, we have already begun to make our acquaintance with the mark of not-self. Insight into impermanence reveals that nothing maintains sameness or identity over successive moments or exists independently of other realities.

- Consequently, the idea of a thing, an entity enduring through time and having its own separate existence, is potentially a misleading habit of the mind. Ultimately, there is no such thing as a thing.

- This idea sounds fine as long as we're considering trees and other items in the world, but when it comes to the human person, we become a bit more apprehensive.

- As we observed in the previous lecture, people want to exempt themselves somehow from the reality of impermanence, even against evidence to the contrary. One of the ways we try to make an exception for ourselves is through the concept of the soul or a permanent self.

- Almost every religious and many philosophical worldviews posit an immortal soul or some version of an unchanging self in which the personality has a core identity that endures even if the body dies.

- Even some modern views in psychology maintain the existence of a "true self" that underlies so many false selves or masks of our personality.

- Not-self is nothing more than a denial of the idea of an immortal soul or an enduring self. It simply means that human beings are not exempt from the quality of impermanence; our every aspect is subject to change.

- Not-self does not mean that human beings do not really exist or are unreal. We exist and are real, but we do not exist in the way we're accustomed to think. Problems arise when we reify the concept of the self—when we begin to think of the self as a real thing.

- If we take the concept of self as referring to something real and permanent, we mobilize the rest of our lives to accommodate it. On the basis of a self, we create all manner of self-centered desires, and on the basis of those desires, we and others suffer. That is dukkha.

- In view of the tendency of the idea of the self to cause damage, the mindfulness tradition, as well as other religious and philosophical traditions throughout the world, maintains that it is in our best interest—and in the best interest of everyone—to relinquish our attachment to self and to live without putting ourselves at the hub of the universe.

- No matter how wholesome it may be, relinquishing the idea of self may be the most difficult thing a person can do. We are so attached to this sense of self that we believe giving it up will mean our demise. However, many thinkers and traditions throughout history have suggested that this is precisely the way to lasting happiness.

- What we must realize, according to the Buddhist mindfulness tradition, is that all we are letting go of is a fiction, a fabrication of the mind that causes us to suffer. It is not our true identity; it is not who we really are.

- We should also realize that letting go of the self, or ego if you prefer, does not mean we are on a crusade to destroy it. If we simply refrain from acting as if it were real, the self—a thought like any other—will fall away of its own accord. Paradoxically, if we try to annihilate the self, we will only empower it.

An Exercise in Not-Self

- During a sitting meditation practice, spend some time reflecting on these questions. When I refer to myself, what exactly do I mean? When I use the word "I," to what does that refer? Is there anything about me that endures or is permanent? If so, what is it? How do I know it's there? Is there anything about me that does not rely on something else for its existence?

dukkha: A Buddhist term that basically means "suffering" and that denotes the fundamental frustrating, insatiable quality of the mindless existence of human beings.

not-self: A term that is sometimes compared to "insubstantiality." This is the third mark of existence that is central to the Buddhist worldview—and the most difficult to grasp both by intellect and by insight, even for those within the tradition.

pleasure principle: A term introduced by Sigmund Freud that describes the way in which people grasp for the things they enjoy and evade the things they don't.

Questions to Consider

1. Why is getting what we want so often unable to provide us with satisfaction?

2. Do you agree that belief in a permanent, substantial self leads to the experience of what the Buddha called dukkha?

Wisdom—Seeing the World as It Is
Lecture 14—Transcript

In Oscar Wilde's play, *Lady Windermere's Fan*, Dumby tells Lord Darlington: "In this world there are only two tragedies. One is not getting what one wants, and the other is getting it."

Whether Wilde realized it or not, Dumby's comical pronouncement succinctly captures the quintessence of *dukkha*, one of the three qualities of existence according to the Buddhist mindfulness tradition. The other two qualities, transience and not-self, help us to understand why Dumby's observation is right on target.

Like Aristotle, Mencius, and a great many other thinkers, the Buddha thought that the quest for lasting happiness was the principal impulse of human activity. Aristotle said happiness was the one thing we seek for itself and not as a means to something else; whether we're aware of it or not, happiness is the true aim of all we do. The Buddha would have agreed. Neither the Buddha nor Aristotle, however, conceived of happiness in the way we're apt to think of it these days, as "a pleasurable experience." The Buddha understood happiness as an enduring reality that is not contingent on fleeting pleasures. This kind of contentment—this happiness—is what all beings really, truly want. And all beings, in their many and various ways, seek it.

While he regarded the desire for happiness to be natural and wholesome, the Buddha did see serious problems with the ways we try to satisfy that yearning. Because we lack wisdom, because we fail to see the world as it is, we inevitably go about the pursuit of happiness in the very ways that sabotage its fulfillment. Without awakening to the true nature of reality—without insight into the three marks of existence—we seek contentment in the wrong places and through the wrong means. Because we can never find it, our thirst for satisfaction intensifies and worsens. It's like trying to put out a fire with gasoline.

Most of us seek happiness in two basic ways: The first is by acquisition, which is the preferred method in the modern world, and the second is by aversion, which is trying to avoid unpleasant situations. Both techniques are based on what Freud called the "pleasure principle," grasping for the things that we enjoy and evading the things we don't.

The quest for contentment through acquisition usually leads us to try to enhance our lives by surrounding ourselves with things we believe will give us pleasure: home, cars, clothing, trophies, and other commonly accepted markers of well-being and achievement. Acquisitiveness, however, need not focus on material items. One can seek happiness by having unique and interesting experiences—including spiritual experiences—or by holding the right religious or political beliefs or by affiliating with an organization or a cause. One can look for lasting contentment in gaining knowledge or performing deeds. One can seek it through the love of other beings, both human and divine. There is no end to the ways we can pursue contentment by means of getting and having.

If we fail to get what we want, of course, we usually suffer. Because we have made acquisition of a particular thing the condition for our contentment, not getting it leaves us feeling sad, disappointed, frustrated, and perhaps angry, thinking we've missed the very thing that would have made us happy.

A lot of our remembrance of the past is reflection on the times we didn't get what we wanted. I still feel a stab of pain in my chest when I recall not getting selected to be an astronaut in our eighth-grade space program—over 40 years ago! Tragedy one.

Tragedy two appears when we actually get what we want. We marry our sweetheart, buy our dream home, get the promotion, win the marathon, and finally take the Mediterranean cruise. Now, we're happy, right? Well, perhaps, for a while. Getting what we want may indeed bring us great pleasure, but the pleasurable feelings won't last. Back at the dream house, the plumbing starts to leak and the microwave is on the fritz; what's left of the cruise is just fading memories and photographs; the new job brings a bigger salary, to be sure, but now you have more anxieties and less time to spend with your family. When the initial pleasure subsides, disappointment sets in. And disappointment comes in exact proportion to how much happiness we expected our acquisition to provide.

The greatest disappointment in my life was probably receiving my Ph.D. That's right: the very thing I carry around as my ego's trump card! Ever since my college days, I desperately wanted to have the title "Dr." attached to my name. I am not even sure why, but I wanted it like nothing else. When the day finally came to receive my diploma, amidst all the fanfare and festivities, I couldn't help but notice a slight discontentment. For several months afterwards, I got increasingly depressed. It took me a while, but I finally realized I had expected that the degree would somehow radically transform my life, that my self-confidence would soar and I would command great respect and the admiration of everyone, that I would be capable of superior intellectual feats. The disappointment came when none of that happened. There was no radical transformation as I had hoped. I felt some satisfaction in attaining my long-held ambition, but that satisfaction didn't last long. It was soon forgotten in a slew of new goals and new expectations. I had burdened that single achievement with so much expectation that nothing could have possibly satisfied me.

Desires, whether they are fulfilled or frustrated, only beget more desires. There is no end to our desires when we think that fulfilling our wishes is the way to happiness. It's like that old kid's trick: What would wish for if you could be granted one wish? Why, I'd wish for a million more.

Alongside acquisition, we also seek satisfaction by avoiding unpleasant situations or things or people. Aversion is actually just the flip-side of acquisition; both are manifestations of desire. As with acquisition, the problem with trying to find your happiness through avoidance is the nature of reality. Reality simply does not allow us to evade unwanted experiences.

Sure, we might be able to escape a few, like dodging the class bully or using that web site that keeps telemarketers from calling. But the evasive life often comes at a cost, like having to live your life in terror. Having mentioned the eighth grade and the class bully floods my mind with vivid memories of what such a life is like. Even if we can successfully ward off some terrifying experiences, we cannot avert them all, particularly the most unpleasant ones: sickness, old age, and death. If our strategy has been to flee from unpleasant circumstances, when they come to meet us, as they surely will, our suffering will be great indeed.

These situations I have been describing are all encompassed by the Buddhist word, *dukkha*. That single term denotes the fundamental frustrating, insatiable quality of our mindless existence. Usually translated into English as suffering or unsatisfactoriness, the meaning of *dukkha* is actually far richer than a single English word, or even a cluster of English words, can express. You might find it translated as illness, anguish, sorrow, unease, distress, unsettledness, lamentation, pain, grief, despair, and disappointment. Certainly all of these terms can be associated with *dukkha*, and certainly we can agree that life brings an abundance of such experiences.

But *dukkha* does not merely characterize episodes or aspects of existence. It does not simply suggest that life has a lot of sorrow and anguish, although it does mean that. Rather, the term *dukkha* indicates that sorrow and anguish, suffering and disappointment permeate existence. *Dukkha* is pervasive, subtle, and insidious, not merely episodic. Like impermanence, there are no exceptions to *dukkha* in the conditioned world of life as we ordinarily know it. *Dukkha* names every aspect of experience in which there is the slightest twinge or possibility of anxiety, fear, or disappointment.

In its full sense, *dukkha* is not readily an apparent fact of life but a challenge for individuals to discover for themselves by means of introspection and observation. The Buddha himself hinted at this when he said that the truth he attained is "profound, hard to see and hard to understand, peaceful and sublime, unattainable by mere reasoning, subtle, to be experienced by the wise." As with the facts of transience and not-self, the surface of *dukkha* can be grasped conceptually, but its depth can only be seen by insight. With insight, the prevalence of *dukkha* is made clear and a way beyond it is revealed. But insight into *dukkha* is usually gradual and cannot be forced. Mindfulness practice only removes the obstacles that inhibit clear gazing.

This is an exercise that may help. Schedule an appointment with disappointment. Determine to spend an entire day trying to be mindful of all your disappointments and frustrations, no matter how small. If you find this approach too demanding, then take some time at the end of a day for reflection. Whichever approach you choose, be very attentive to your experiences of disappointment. You'll probably need to be more sensitive than usual because we often condition ourselves to ignore many of our disappointments.

As you prepare for the day or reflect back on it, consider the potential sources of routine disappointment. For many of us, the day begins when the alarm goes off. How does that make you feel? Then we go to the bathroom and look in the mirror. Are you pleased with what you see? If you leave the house for the day, what is the process of getting ready like? As smooth and as uncomplicated as you want? When you're on the road, how's the traffic? How do you feel when you realize you're running late to work and the gas tank is on empty? When you get to where you're going, be attentive to your interactions with others. Does someone say something to hurt your feelings or slight you in any way? How do you feel when a colleague receives lavish praise? Be honest! Does the sandwich you have for lunch taste as good as you anticipated? What's it like standing in a long line at Starbucks to get your afternoon caffeine fix? You get the idea. After you've tallied up your disappointing experiences, reflect on how you reacted to them. Small, minor irritations may not warrant a great response, but how do you handle a day's worth of little frustrations? As you go about your life, try to remain as attentive as you can to these moments of discontentment.

With continued observation and mindfulness practice, the reality of *dukkha* becomes clearer, and we begin to gain insight into its source and its cure. Eventually, we realize that *dukkha* is the result of one thing: the fact that the world does not always conform to our expectations and desires. The world's not to blame, of course. Reality just is what it is. The problem is with our desires and expectations. We simply expect too much from the world.

Insight lets us see that the whole approach to contentment through acquisition or aversion is fundamentally misguided. Rather than bringing the satisfaction we so deeply want, acquisition and aversion only serve to frustrate us and increase our anguish and disappointment. Instead of questioning these methods themselves, in our mindless state we foolishly think that we simply haven't acquired or averted the right thing or enough things.

Many years ago, I came across a little boy about three, bitterly crying and frantically running down the aisles of Target, screaming, "I need something! I need something!" When his parents finally caught up with him, they could get no more out him than what he said: He needed something. Yet, he had no idea what it was. I knew just how he felt. We all think we need something, and we're frantically running up and down the aisles, looking for it, believing that when we get, we'll be happy and the tears will stop.

The third mark of existence—and the most difficult to grasp both by intellect and by insight—is not-self. Not-self, which I sometimes call "insubstantiality," is also the element that is most apt to be misunderstood by those who view it from outside. It's even difficult for those within the tradition. The great Buddhist philosopher Nagarjuna compared not-self to a poisonous snake and said one must know how to handle it or risk being bitten and killed. Yet not-self is central to the Buddhist worldview, so we're going to take our chances.

By observing the radical depth of transience, we have already begun to make our acquaintance with the mark of not-self. Insight into impermanence reveals that nothing maintains sameness or identity over successive moments or exists independently of other realities. Consequently, the idea of a thing, an entity enduring through time and having its own separate existence, is a potentially misleading habit of mind. Ultimately, there is no such thing as a thing.

This idea sounds fine as long as we're considering trees and other items in the world. But when it comes to the human person, we become a bit more apprehensive. As we observed in the previous lecture, people want to exempt themselves somehow from the reality of impermanence, even against evidence to the contrary. One of the ways we try to make an exception for ourselves is through the concept of the soul or a permanent self. Almost every religious and many philosophical worldviews posit an immortal soul or some version of an unchanging self in which the personality has a core identity that endures even if the body dies. Even some modern views in psychology maintain the existence of a "true self" that underlies so many false selves or masks of our personality.

Not-self is really nothing more than a denial of the idea of an immortal soul or an enduring self. It simply means that human beings are not exempt from the quality of impermanence; every aspect is subject to change. Not-self does not mean that human beings do not really exist or that we're unreal. We are real; we exist. But we do not exist in the way we're accustomed to think. Just as a tree is a complex symphony of events, so too are we. Just as a tree is in constant state of flux, so too are we. Just as "tree" is a convenient term indicating an amalgam of ever-changing events, so too is the word "self."

But unlike the word "tree," the term "self" or "soul"—if we take it to mean something substantial, fixed, or immortal—can have serious, unwholesome consequences for the way we live. Problems arise when we reify the concept of the self, that is, when we begin to think of the self as a real thing. When we regard the self as something more than a mere convenient concept, when we start taking it seriously and literally, we are apt to think and act in ways that will cause us and others to suffer. If we forget that the idea of self is a fabrication of the mind, we experience *dukkha*. When virtually everything you think and do is for yourself, and there isn't one, is it any wonder you suffer?

If we take the concept of self as referring to something real and permanent, we mobilize the rest of our lives to accommodate it. If the self is real, it needs protection; it needs to be guarded against those other selves out there that might take away its precious possessions or threaten its existence. If the self is real, it would make sense to stockpile resources and seek increasing amounts of power to prevent the other selves from harming it. It would make sense to surround the self with allies who will help protect it from enemies. It would make sense to provide the self with as many comforts and pleasures as possible. After all, this is who you are. And so it goes. On the basis of a self, we create all manner of self-centered desires, and on the basis of those desires, we and others suffer. That is *dukkha*.

Does it seem preposterous that a mistaken conception could wreak so much havoc in our lives? Consider what would happen if one evening, as you're getting out of your car, you mistook the garden hose lying on the lawn for a poisonous snake about to strike. Imagine the fear welling up inside, how your heart would begin to race, your breath become shallow. Think of how your consciousness would now perceive the beautiful hedge of roses as an ugly obstacle to your escape. Envision how your desire has been suddenly focused on only one thing: getting away. Your fear might cause you to harm others. It might even give you a heart attack and cause you to die—all because of an illusion, a misapprehension.

In view of the tendency of the idea of the self to cause damage, the mindfulness tradition, as well as other religious and philosophical traditions throughout the world, maintains that it is in our best interest—and in the best interest of everyone—to relinquish our attachment to self, to live without putting ourselves at hub of the universe.

Yet, no matter how wholesome it may be, relinquishing the idea of self may be the most difficult thing a person can do. We are so attached to this sense of self that we believe giving it up will mean our demise. Yet many thinkers and traditions throughout history have suggested that this is precisely the way to lasting happiness. What we must realize, according to the Buddhist mindfulness tradition, is that all we are letting go of is a fiction, a fabrication of the mind that causes us to suffer. It is not our true identity; it is not who we really are. We should also realize that letting go of the self, or ego if you prefer, does not mean we are on a crusade to destroy it. There is nothing to destroy. The self is a thought like any other, a habit of mind. If we simply stop supporting it, if we refrain from acting as if it were real, if we see it as a fiction, the self will fall away of its own accord. Paradoxically, if we try to annihilate the self, we will only empower it.

In a sense, all practices of mindfulness work toward dropping the thinking and acting that condition and bolster the illusion of self. But there are some exercises that specifically address the insight of not-self. Here are a few. Remember, none of these exercises can cause insight; they may only clear the way.

During a sitting meditation practice, spend some time reflecting on these questions. When I refer to myself, what exactly do I mean? When I use the word "I," to what does that refer? Where is and what is this "I"? Is there anything about me that endures or is permanent? If so, what is it? How do I know it's there? Is there anything about me that does not rely on something else for its existence?

Transience, *dukkha*, and not-self are interrelated marks of existence. The failure to apprehend that the world and human persons are completely subject to impermanence and insubstantiality gives rise to *dukkha*, and the experience of *dukkha* in turn reinforces our misapprehensions. By imputing permanent selfhood where there is none, we effectively believe ourselves to be separate, individual entities whose fragile existences must be propped up by possessions, achievements, beliefs, and relationships to convince ourselves that we are safe, protected from the vagaries of life. But this is an illusion. None of these things give the security, the sense of well-being, the contentment that we really desire, and neither can trying to avoid unpleasant and unwanted things and situations. Although it may allow us transitory pleasures, conditioned existence simply will not satisfy our deepest longings for true happiness. When we gain wisdom, when we awaken to the world "as it is," we discover, paradoxically, that the only way to find happiness is to relinquish our feverish efforts to protect and empower this mistaken belief we call the self.

Compassion—Expressing Fundamental Kindness
Lecture 15

S ome of the noblest aspirations of the human heart include the ability to see wrong and try to right it, to see suffering and try to heal it, and to see war and try to stop it. These phrases also offer a precise description of the essence of compassion. For most of us, the skill to be compassionate toward difficult people comes at the end of a very long road. Mindfulness can guide you through working with the easier cases and help you gradually progress to the harder ones.

Compassion versus Pity

- **Compassion** is the desire to alleviate suffering—or dukkha, to use the richer term. Compassion entails the courage to face dukkha, the wisdom to gaze into it deeply, and the resolve to respond to it in a way that brings relief.

- More than just a sentiment, compassion is born of a brave consciousness and a strong will. It may arise as tenderness in the heart, but it requires the support of a tough mind.

- Compassion is not pity, although the two are sometimes confused. **Pity** is simply feeling sorry for someone who has to endure suffering, but pity keeps its distance from suffering. Pity can't get past the element of fear; it's afraid of pain and suffering and wants to flee from their presence.

- Compassion doesn't keep its distance; it literally means "to experience or endure with." Compassion is willing to be with suffering up close because it has learned to accept rather than resist suffering.

- Words are sometimes used to hide our discomfort with suffering. Sometimes we just don't know what to say, but it's better to keep quiet than to utter vacuous words. The compassionate person does not flee from pain or silence.

- Even without words, one can bring comfort to another by merely being physically present and mindfully attentive. Such gestures can strengthen others by conveying that it is possible neither to resist nor run away from suffering.

- The capacity for compassion is in our deepest nature as human beings. To be sure, some of us manifest the face of compassion more plainly than others. Many consider motherhood to be the prime exemplar of compassion.

- In the Tanakh—the Hebrew Bible—the word translated as compassion derives from the same root syllable from which the word for womb comes. In fact, the word for womb, *rehem*, is itself occasionally translated as compassion. Both words are related etymologically to *ar-Rahman*, meaning "the exceedingly compassionate," one of the Qur'an's 99 most beautiful names for God.

- When we fail to act in a compassionate way, as we often do, we have either been conditioned to ignore suffering, or we have suppressed the desire to relieve it. Our frequent failure to be compassionate does not mean that compassion is not a basic part of who we are; it simply means that our fundamental nature has been obscured and needs to be gently revealed.

- Much in our modern culture works to separate us from our basic compassion and, hence, alienate us from one another and from ourselves. Our love of competition, our fear of pain and suffering, our quest for pleasure, and our endless forms of distraction all function to enshroud compassion.

- As we continue with daily sitting practice, occasional body scans, walking meditation, and mindful eating, we subtly counteract those deadening aspects of our culture. Whether we recognize it or not, mindfulness practice quietly subverts those forces and gently eases their effects on us.

The Cultivation of Compassion

- Being able to see dukkha is the prerequisite to deeper compassion, but perceiving the deeper expressions of suffering isn't easy and requires the skills of attentiveness that mindfulness practice sharpens.

- Seeing the extensive and subtle nature of dukkha permits us to be more adept at identifying it and becoming more familiar with it. That familiarity, in turn, helps us to accept it as present-moment experience, which we need not run from or resist.

- Compassion requires the willingness to look at suffering, tragedy, and pain without aversion or attachment. Recognizing the subtle nature of dukkha also enables us to see how its clearly evident manifestations, such as war and conflict, are interrelated with its less-apparent forms, such as greed, fear, and disappointment.

- Common to all experiences of dukkha are self-centered desires that often outstrip the capacity of reality to satisfy them. Insight into the conditions that give rise to suffering is necessary to being able to respond to that suffering constructively.

- Recognizing dukkha in our own experience is critical to seeing it in the lives of others. Unless you understand the nature of your own suffering, you can do little to help others with theirs.

- Paradoxically, then, you can take your conditioned tendency to focus on you and use it to turn outward toward others in compassion. As we go further into our practice, however, we begin to see that this is hardly a paradox at all, as we come to understand that there is not your suffering and the suffering of others—there is only suffering.

Compassion and Empathy

- Being compassionate toward others is based on empathy, or what the Buddha called "putting yourself in the place of others." Knowing that you want to be happy and free from suffering, you can infer that other beings want this as well, and you can treat them accordingly.

- The first step in being compassionate toward others thus involves imaginatively entering into the interiority of another person, sharing his or her inner life in a profound way by recognizing that they are like you.

- The world's religions and philosophies almost uniformly endorse this empathetic precept and make it the cornerstone of their ethics. It is the basis of what we in the West call the Golden Rule: "Do unto others as you would have them do unto you."

- In East Asia, many follow the same principle as it was formulated by Confucius over 2,500 years ago: "Never impose on others what you would not choose for yourself." If you do a little research, you might be surprised by how widely and frequently this simple idea is articulated in the world's wisdom traditions.

- Despite its ubiquity, most of us find it difficult to remember to be empathetic, which may be a clue as to why the principle is so repeatedly articulated in the traditions.

- It's not that empathy is particularly difficult for us. Sometimes, it arises within us spontaneously, perhaps more than we ordinarily recognize—unless we're paying attention. Just as often, however, we neglect to practice empathy because the illusion of self gets in the way.

- Your conditioned tendency to regard the universe as revolving around you makes it easy to forget that the rest of the world thinks the universe revolves around them. When you're so absorbed in seeking your own happiness by means of the usual frantic and misguided methods, you're too preoccupied to appreciate that others are seeking the same freedom from suffering that you are.

- If we can just look around—at our world and at each other—taking some time to stop the futile climbing up and sliding down, we can see what a state we're really in. That awareness changes our whole attitude toward the world and toward each other.

Empathy in Practice

- When you're not feeling particularly empathetic with some of your fellow human beings, there is a simple practice to remind you of the common humanity we all share beneath the labels and identifications that divide us. Any time you discover yourself being annoyed by or feeling alienated from someone, recite the words "just like me."

- If you're seeking an ideal location for testing your progress on the mindfulness path, there's no better place than an airport. Where else do you have such wonderful opportunities to experience the subtle manifestations of dukkha, to practice patience and anger management, to observe other people, and even to meditate?

- Let's say you find yourself waiting in one of the several airport queues you have to go through to get to where you're going. Just ahead of you as you're rushing to get through security is a bumbling passenger who has no clue how to negotiate this procedure expeditiously.

- As you watch the bumbling passenger, it is the perfect time to practice your skills of empathy. Say to yourself: "Just like me. Here is a person who forgot to empty his pockets: It's so easy to get flustered going through these stressful queues that I can understand how someone could overlook that step."

- You don't know what is ailing the pushy woman behind you or the slow man in front of you in line. What you do know is they are seeking happiness just like you—and probably doing so in the same misguided ways as you.

- "Just like me" is a versatile practice. It can be performed just about anywhere, at any time. You can practice as you read about or watch events in the news, taking a moment to ponder why others behave the way they do, trying to imagine how you would react in a similar situation, reflecting on the ways we share a common humanity.

- "Just like me" is extremely effective for establishing empathy with others, particularly those we find difficult to like. Empathy and compassion do not require that we feel affection for the other. We can have compassion for our worst enemies.

- Ultimately, the full pursuit of compassion practice requires that we cultivate empathy for some very tough characters, including those whom we know to be the perpetrators of horrendous violence and abuse. Compassion cannot be selective.

- There is one very tough character you'll have to work with before you can go any further with this practice: yourself. For some of us, it may be harder to muster compassion for ourselves than for others.

- There is a saying attributed to the Buddha: "You can search throughout the entire universe for someone who is more deserving of your love and compassion than you are yourself, and that person is not to be found anywhere. You yourself, as much as anybody, deserve your love and compassion."

Important Terms

compassion: The desire to alleviate suffering.

pity: Feeling sorry for someone who has to endure suffering.

Questions to Consider

1. Recall a time when you were the recipient of another's compassion. What effects did that experience have on your state of mind?

2. Do you accept the idea that compassion is an inherent part of who we are? Why or why not? Either way, compassion needs cultivation.

Compassion—Expressing Fundamental Kindness
Lecture 15—Transcript

When Robert Kennedy was assassinated in 1968, his brother Edward eulogized him as a "good and decent man, who saw wrong and tried to right it, saw suffering and tried to heal it, saw war and tried to stop it." Even at my tender age, I found the younger Kennedy's words deeply moving as I watched the funeral on TV.

When I first heard them, I was in no position to know if those words were an accurate characterization of the person they were intended to describe. That didn't matter. What moved me then, and still moves me now, is how those phrases seem to express some of the noblest aspirations of the human heart, something I intuitively recognized as a child: to see wrong and try to right it; to see suffering and try to heal it; to see war and try to stop it. It was not until many years later that I recognized in those haunting words a precise description of the essence of compassion.

Compassion is the desire to alleviate suffering—or *dukkha*, to use the richer term. Compassion entails the courage to face *dukkha*, the wisdom to gaze into it deeply, and the resolve to respond to it in a way that brings relief. Compassion is not merely a feeling. More than just a sentiment, it is born of a brave consciousness and a strong will. It may arise as tenderness in the heart, but it requires the support of a tough mind.

Compassion is not pity, although the two are sometimes confused. Pity is simply feeling sorry for someone, feeling bad because someone has to endure suffering. But pity keeps its distance from suffering. Pity often sounds like this: "So sorry things aren't going so well for you; and thank goodness it's not me!" Pity can't get past the element of fear; it's really afraid of pain and suffering and wants to flee from their presence. Compassion doesn't keep its distance. Compassion literally means "to experience or endure with." Compassion is willing to be with suffering up close, because it has learned to accept rather than resist suffering.

People in distress can usually tell if they are being treated with pity or with compassion. I worked as a chaplain in a hospital in Maine during my days in graduate school and was often with patients as they received visitors. I learned that I could tell when guests were uncomfortable seeing their loved one in the bed, and I'm sure this did not pass unnoticed by the patient. Ill-at-ease visitors usually felt compelled to talk, often about anything other than the illness. If the sickness or injury was brought up, the visitor often spoke hollow words, assuring the patient that everything would be all right. The uneasy guest occasionally looked at his or her watch during the conversation and sometimes took the first opportunity to depart. These visitors weren't uncaring; they merely found it hard to be in the presence of suffering.

On the other hand, those who seemed to me to bear the face of compassion did not appear eager to direct the conversation away from the patient's pain and anguish. Yet, they may not have had much to say about it. Words are sometimes used to hide our discomfort with suffering. Sometimes we just don't know what to say, but it's better to keep quiet than to utter vacuous words. The compassionate person does not flee from pain or silence. In many cases, the person who seemed to bring the greatest relief to the patient was the one who was willing simply to stay by the bedside and listen when necessary. Even without words, one can bring comfort to another by merely being physically present and mindfully attentive. Such gestures can strengthen others by conveying that it is possible neither to resist nor run away from suffering.

Compassion is not something we have to learn. It is what we are. The capacity for compassion is in our deepest nature as human beings. To be sure, some of us manifest the face of compassion more plainly than others. For me, the clearest and most common expression of compassion can be seen in a mother's love for her child. As the recipient of that love as a child, I wasn't always appreciative of my own mother's attention and selflessness. Having always had them, it was difficult for me to think of life without them or even imagine what great care they expressed. But I came to view maternal love more clearly when I watched my wife nurture our young daughter and witnessed up close the power of that bond. Amazement would not be too strong a word for my reaction.

I'm certainly not the only one to consider motherhood as the prime exemplar of compassion. In the Tanakh, the Hebrew Bible, the word translated as compassion derives from the same root syllable from which the word for womb comes. In fact, the word for womb, *rehem*, is itself occasionally translated as compassion. Both words are related etymologically to *ar-Rahman*, meaning "the exceedingly compassionate," one of the Qur'an's 99 most beautiful names for God.

Please don't think I'm romanticizing motherhood by this example. I'm fully aware that mothers, like everyone else, do not always exhibit their compassionate natures. I'm also aware that fathers can be as compassionate as mothers, although the social construction of modern masculinity makes the expression of compassion more difficult for males.

When we fail to act in a compassionate way, as we often do, we have either been conditioned to ignore suffering, or we have suppressed the desire to relieve it. Our frequent failure to be compassionate does not mean that compassion is not a basic part of who we are; it simply means that our fundamental nature has been obscured and needs to be gently revealed.

Much in modern culture works to separate us from our basic compassion and hence alienate us from one another and from ourselves. Our love of competition, our fear of pain and suffering, our quest for pleasure, and our endless forms of distraction all function to enshroud compassion. But as we have been continuing with our daily sitting practice, our occasional body scans, walking meditation, and mindful eating, we have been subtly counteracting those deadening aspects of our culture. Whether we've recognized it or not, our mindfulness practice has been quietly subverting those forces and gently easing their effects on us.

Let's refresh our memories about the skills we are acquiring through the exercises we've already studied and show how they contribute to the cultivation of compassion. Then, we'll discuss some methods specifically designed for helping us to express our compassionate nature.

Being able to see *dukkha* is the prerequisite to deeper compassion. As Ted Kennedy said of his brother: "He saw wrong. He saw suffering. And he saw war." For anyone with a TV or access to the Internet, it's easy to see the overt manifestations of *dukkha*. But perceiving the deeper expressions of suffering isn't easy and requires the skills of attentiveness that mindfulness practice sharpens. Seeing the extensive and subtle nature of *dukkha* permits us to be more adept at identifying it and becoming more familiar with it. That familiarity, in turn, helps us to accept it as present-moment experience, which we need not run from or resist. Compassion requires the willingness to look at suffering, tragedy, and pain without aversion or attachment. Recognizing the subtle nature of *dukkha* also enables us to see how its clearly evident manifestations like war and conflict are interrelated with its less apparent forms such as greed, fear, and disappointment. Common to all experiences of *dukkha* are self-centered desires that often outstrip the capacity of reality to satisfy them. Insight into the conditions that give rise to suffering is necessary to being able to respond to that suffering constructively.

Recognizing *dukkha* in our own experience, as has been our focus up to this point, is critical to seeing it in the lives of others. Unless I understand the nature of my own suffering I can do little to help you with yours.

Paradoxically, then, I can take my own conditioned tendency to focus on me and use it to turn outward toward others in compassion. As we go further into our practice, however, we begin to see that this is hardly a paradox at all, as we come to understand that there is not my suffering and your suffering. There is only suffering.

Being compassionate toward others is based on empathy, or what the Buddha called "putting yourself in the place of others." Knowing that I want to be happy and free from suffering, I can infer that other beings want this as well. Knowing that about others, I ought to treat them accordingly. The first step in being compassionate towards others thus involves imaginatively entering into the interiority of another person, sharing his or her inner life in a profound way by recognizing that they are like me.

This basic empathetic principle is hardly a revelation to any of us. The world's religions and philosophies almost uniformly endorse this precept and make it the cornerstone of their ethics. It is the basis of what we in the West call the Golden Rule: "Do unto others as you would have them do unto you." In East Asia, many follow the same principle as it was formulated by Confucius over 2500 years ago: "Never impose on others what you would not choose for yourself." If you do a little research, you might be surprised by how widely and frequently this simple idea is articulated in the world's wisdom traditions. Just Google "Golden Rule." In its many versions, this precept boils down to the practice of empathy.

Despite its ubiquity, most of us find it difficult to remember to be empathetic, which may be a clue as to why the principle is so repeatedly articulated in the traditions. I don't think this is because empathy is particularly hard for us. Sometimes, it arises within us spontaneously, perhaps more than we ordinarily recognize, unless we're paying attention. But just as often, we neglect to practice empathy because the illusion of self gets in the way. My conditioned tendency to regard the universe as revolving around me makes it easy to forget that the rest of you think the universe revolves around you! When I'm absorbed in seeking my own happiness by means of the usual frantic and misguided methods, I'm too preoccupied to appreciate that you're seeking the same freedom from suffering that I am. If I can just stop a moment, I can realize that we're really all in the same boat. This humorously profound poem by David Budbill aptly captures the power of a moment of insight and empathy. It's called "Bugs in a Bowl."

Han Shan, that great and crazy, wonder-filled Chinese poet of a thousand years ago, said:

We're just like bugs in a bowl. All day going around never leaving their bowl.

I say, That's right! Every day climbing up
the steep sides, sliding back.

Over and over again. Around and around.
Up and back down.

Sit in the bottom of the bowl, head in your hands,
cry, moan, feel sorry for yourself.

Or. Look around. See your fellow bugs.
Walk around.

Say, Hey, how you doin'?

Say, Nice Bowl!

If we can just "look around," as Budbill says, at the bowl and each other, taking some time to stop the futile climbing up and sliding down, we can see what a state we're really in. That awareness changes our whole attitude towards our bowl and our fellow bugs.

In the time I spent as a chaplain, I had occasions to be with the families of patients who were in the Intensive Care Unit. These were times I spent in the waiting rooms as family members anticipated word on their loved one's condition. As the patient lay in critical condition, quartered away elsewhere in the ICU, anxious relatives waited in uncertainty, never knowing if the doctor would be walking through the door with news of improvement or decline—or perhaps even death.

The days could be long, and waiting often seemed interminable. Although they could be grim places to visit, I sometimes saw things in the ICU waiting rooms that heartened me immensely. These were times—and they were not rare—when I observed how the medical crisis would draw family members closer to one another. In the space created by the grave situation they shared, members of a family seemed to become more sensitive and kinder to one other, offering to get a cup of coffee for one, recommending that another go home for some much needed rest, speaking in soft and gentle tones. I even witnessed how members of two or three different families—all total strangers, but united by trying circumstances—suddenly overcame any awkwardness to talk and commiserate with one another. I can well imagine that in other circumstances, these individuals would have remained within the safe confines of their own family without reaching beyond it to invite conversation with someone from another family. Sometimes, of course, families did stay isolated from one another. But just as often, their common lot freed them to cross the imaginary barriers separating them. I often saw solidarity emerge between different families as members of one would share the joy of good news received by another or share the grief when the news was unwelcome.

While observing this outpouring of compassion in the ICU was encouraging, I was also a bit saddened that it required such a liminal experience to bring it out. Why couldn't we be this way all the time, caring for one another as if we were always in the waiting room of the ICU? After all, life itself isn't that different from such places. We're all subject to sickness and death; we're all liable to receive bad news about a loved one at any time; we all spend a great deal of time in uncertainty.

Fortunately, there are ways to encourage a deeper empathy with others even when our circumstances are less dire than in the hospital. When you're not feeling particularly empathetic with some of your fellow human beings, here's a simple practice to remind you of the common humanity we all share beneath the labels and identifications that divide us. Any time you discover yourself being annoyed or feeling alienated from someone, recite the words, "Just like me."

Let's say you're at an airport, which by the way is one of the greatest places on earth to practice mindfulness. Where else do you have such wonderful opportunities to experience the subtle manifestations of *dukkha*, to practice patience and anger management, to observe other people, and even meditate? If you're seeking an ideal location for testing your progress on the mindfulness path, there is no better place than an airport. The bigger and busier, the better! Thank your lucky stars when your flight has been delayed or even canceled; now you have an unrivaled opportunity to attend to what's really important in life!

Okay, so let's say you find yourself waiting in one of the several airport queues you have to go through to get to where you're going. Just ahead of you, as you're rushing to get through security, is a bumbling passenger who has no clue how to negotiate this procedure expeditiously. You know the one: the man or woman who forgets to empty their pockets and sets off the scanner; the one who neglects to pack the travel-size containers of shampoo and lotion and whose suitcase has to be hand-inspected as a consequence; the one who leisurely removes his shoes and belt, completely oblivious that other people have planes to catch in the next ten minutes. Or consider the passenger behind you who's in such a hurry she's practically pushing you and your things out of the way, cursing under her breath.

Need I continue? I could! I could finish this lecture and part of the next one simply by cataloguing all the potential annoyances you can experience waiting to go through airport security. I'm not a person who needs to make an "appointment with disappointment" to be aware of frustrations! But I'll spare you all that.

What I want to say is this: Now is the time to practice your skills of empathy. As you watch the bumbling passenger, you say to yourself: "Just like me. Here is a person who forgot to pack travel-size containers. I could have done that. How many times have I been in such a hurry that I've forgotten things while packing?" Or the fellow who forgets to empty his pockets: You say, "Just like me. It's so easy to get flustered going through these stressful queues that I can understand how someone could overlook that step." And the guy who takes his time with his shoes: You say, "Just like me. Perhaps he suffers from such physical pain that he can't move any faster. I too have struggled with debilitating pain." And the pushy woman behind you: "Just like me. Perhaps she's late for a flight and eager to get home to her sick child. I've been late for flights, and I know I'd be in a rush if my sick daughter were waiting for me."

True, you don't really know if the pushy lady has a sick child or if the slow fellow has arthritis. Maybe, maybe not. You don't know. What you do know is that they are seeking happiness just like you—and probably doing so in the same misguided ways as you. By the way, each of these examples I've cited come from my own experiences. Not only have I been personally annoyed by the pushy woman and the bumbling man, I have actually been the pushy woman and the bumbling man, becoming a nuisance for someone else! Empathy, indeed!

"Just like me" is a versatile practice. It can be performed just about anywhere, at any time. You can practice as you read about or watch events in the news, taking a moment to ponder why others behave the way they do, trying to imagine how you would react in a similar situation, reflecting on the ways we share a common humanity. You can practice as you drive, wait in line in the grocery, or endure poor service at a restaurant.

"Just like me" is extremely effective for establishing empathy with others, particularly those we find difficult to like. Empathy and compassion do not require that we feel affection for the other. We can have compassion for our worst enemies. Ultimately, the full pursuit of compassion practice requires that we cultivate empathy for some very tough characters, including those whom we know to be the perpetrators of horrendous violence and abuse.

Compassion cannot be selective. For most of us, the skill to be compassionate for such persons comes at the end of a very long road. For now, let's try to work with the easier cases and gradually progress to the harder ones.

There is, however, one very tough character you'll have to work with before you can go any further with this practice: yourself. For some of us, it may be harder to muster compassion for ourselves than for others. There is a saying attributed to the Buddha: "You can search throughout the entire universe for someone who is more deserving of your love and compassion than you are yourself, and that person is not to be found anywhere. You yourself, as much as anybody, deserve your love and compassion." In the next lectures, we will continue our discussion of compassion, beginning with compassion for oneself and then moving outward to consider every being in the world.

Imperfection—Embracing Our Flaws
Lecture 16

The effects of perfectionism are everywhere. We observe perfectionism in the way we readily heap blame and criticism on ourselves, even for the most minor mistakes. We see it in the ways we treat our bodies, condemning them for being too thin or too fat or too old. We notice it in the way we make excessive demands of ourselves, expecting to be wildly successful in our careers or to be model friends or ideal parents. We must come to accept our imperfections—and our inner critic—in order to better understand the world and others.

Checklist for Perfectionism

- Most human beings are afflicted with at least a touch of perfectionism—or perhaps with more than just a touch. If any or all of the following descriptions apply to you, you may be a perfectionist.

    o When you make a mistake, you find it hard to forget. You think about it over and over again—until you make another mistake to take its place or until you get praised for something.

    o Any error—or perceived error—that you make is completely your fault. You think that if you had only been more attentive or thought things out more thoroughly, the misstep wouldn't have occurred.

    o You're constantly comparing yourself with others and you feel painfully vulnerable and totally defeated when you think you've come up short against someone else.

- You're always telling yourself you must try harder. You believe that if can't do something flawlessly, you shouldn't do it at all.

- If you make a mistake in front of others, you think you'll die of embarrassment.

- You're extremely reluctant to ask for help, believing that to do so is to reveal your weakness as person.

- You do everything you can to keep others from seeing this weaker side, and what's worse is that you try to hide this side from yourself, making it extremely difficult to admit your mistakes.

Perfectionist Mindsets

- Perfectionism is the practice of trying to live up to impossible ideals and then feeling worthless when we don't. It's a textbook recipe for dukkha. Perfectionism is not the same as the mere desire to do well by striving to meet high standards.

- Unlike the simple aspiration to excel at what one does, perfectionism involves an insidious attachment to an unrealistic view of the self. Perfectionists believe they can be perfect and must be perfect, and if they can't, they consider themselves utter failures.

- In response to that judgment, perfectionists may become extremely self-critical and attempt virtually anything to rid themselves of the negative feelings those thoughts precipitate.

- One response might be self-punishment, which could be anything from constantly berating oneself to inflicting physical harm. Another might be to turn to intoxicating substances or overeating to silence those voices of derision. Still another is to submit to a grueling regimen in order to make oneself the ideal person one thinks one must be.

- This affliction is one of the major reasons we find it difficult to extend compassion to ourselves. Because we often hold ourselves to unrealistic standards, we sometimes find it hard to believe that we actually deserve compassion.

- What lies beneath resistance to self-compassion is a completely egocentric belief that, even though perfection is out of reach for most mortals, you are different—you are not like the ordinary person. Some religious traditions attribute this overweening attitude to a desire to be like God.

Perfectionism and Spirituality

- Over 1,600 years ago, Saint Augustine observed that the self longed to experience the pleasure of having godlike powers and assuming God's place at the center of the universe. Augustine suggested that this endeavor to be God was precisely what alienated us from the divine, other people, and ourselves; in other words, it was the very thing that caused us to suffer.

- Aspiring to live up to the image of a wholly self-sufficient and perfect being that is beyond reproach can drive us to great misery. Like other forms of suffering, perfectionism stems from an unrealistic view of the self, and it is perhaps the principal obstruction to our practice of self-compassion.

- Developing one's spirituality can hold out the promise of relief for the perfectionist, but at the same time, it can add fuel to the flames when the path becomes another form of achievement.

- Spiritual discipline can provide a means for sinners to receive punishment and a way for the saints to attain sanctity. Neither of these are goals of the mindfulness path, but that doesn't mean that people won't seek mindfulness as a way to purge themselves of guilt or to reach sainthood.

- To put it in more secular terms, some may seek mindfulness as a method of self-improvement. Mindfulness is for awareness—not expiation, sainthood, or self-improvement.

- On a spiritual pathway, perfectionism can manifest as an obsession with doing everything right. When you learn that perfectionism may hinder your capacity to show compassion to yourself, then you'll most likely eliminate perfectionism.

- Trying to be perfect takes a massive amount of energy, and in the end, it's a futile effort. Therefore, why not just accept the fact that perfection is completely unrealistic and yet you still want to be perfect? Be mindful of both your imperfection and your perfectionism. After all, perfectionism is part of your imperfection.

- You probably see the flaws in human nature everywhere—in other people—and you probably already believe that imperfection is a human quality. The difficulty is in accepting that you're human like everyone else. For some reason, you think you're exceptional.

- In a scriptural story, Siddhattha Gotama—the man who became the Buddha—is depicted as a king's son who is naïve about the fact that sickness, old age, and death apply to him, too. Eventually, he accepts his own participation in the human experience.

- We perfectionists need to come to the same awareness. There are no exemptions from human nature: We'll get sick, we'll get old, we'll die, and we'll make thousands of mistakes along the way.

- If we need help with this insight, the practice of "just like me" can be very effective. When introduced, that exercise was to show how extending empathy to others could rouse compassion for them, but we can also practice the exercise with the reverse goal in mind—to awaken compassion for ourselves.

- Seeing others act in less-than-perfect ways gives us the opportunity to recall to ourselves that we, too, do not always act in an ideal manner. In fact, when something about another person annoys you, let that be a signal to be extremely mindful and look within.

- We usually judge others for the very things we hate about ourselves. Try to turn those judgments of others around and make them an opportunity for extending compassion to yourself.

- Revising our views on perfection may also help. If we understand perfection as the state of being flawless or immaculate, then our striving for these qualities is sure to cause us anguish, but perhaps we can think of perfection in a way that is different from our conditioned way.

Buddhism and Perfectionism

- The Buddhist-influenced aesthetic ideal known in Japan as wabi-sabi seeks to highlight the beautiful aspects of impermanence, incompleteness, and defectiveness. Wabi-sabi values things that are rustic, asymmetrical, irregular, simple, and understated.

- Objects that are worn or in the process of decay are appreciated both for their beauty as well as the spiritual truth they express about the transience and unfinished nature of life. Many of the classical art forms of Japan reflect this aesthetic sensibility—practices such as raku pottery, ikebana flower arranging, and haiku poetry.

- Wabi-sabi invites us to look at life through a lens different from the one offered by perfectionism. The wabi-sabi view of life encourages you to feel more at home in the world, a world where all things, including yourself, could be regarded as aesthetically pleasing just for being what they are—subject to change, incomplete, and less than ideal.

- To help ease your perfectionism, consider surrounding yourself with a few items that embody the wabi-sabi aesthetic to remind yourself that so-called flaws and defects can enhance the beauty of an object. These need not be pieces of art specifically designed as expressions of wabi-sabi. Rather, just take the time to look deliberately for objects that are conventionally flawed and yet bespeak the beauty of the flawed world in which we live.

- In addition, try to embody the wabi-sabi ideal in what you do. Perhaps there is some activity you've wanted to pursue, but you've been hesitant for fear of not being able to do it right. Do it anyway.

- Give up your attachment to success and failure and, instead, focus on the pure joy of what you are doing. If you're a perfectionist, you should find at least one thing in your life about which you can relax your need to succeed.

- We can accept our common lot with humanity and we can try to rethink our understanding of perfection, but the greatest challenge may be embracing our own perfectionism. Trying to eliminate perfectionism is likely to prove counterproductive. There is a massive paradox: Wanting to get rid of perfectionism, if you think about it, is just another form of perfectionism.

- Rather than responding with belligerence to the voice that's constantly criticizing and blaming you, why not try getting to know it better? Let it speak. It will probably do so whether you want to hear it or not.

- Your inner critic is just a voice. You don't have to believe it. You don't have to do what it says. The critical voice of our perfectionism only causes us to suffer when we give it more authority than it deserves.

- Our practice of mindfulness teaches us to allow thoughts to arise and fall on their own—like all impermanent reality. The thought that tells us we must be perfect is just a thought like any other.

- Because trying to silence the critical voice hasn't worked, try to welcome perfectionism as a friend. Treat it with courtesy. Show it some compassion. Appreciate what it's trying to do for you.

- Sometimes, the inner critic says valuable things. It's probably helped you achieve some good things in your life. Sometimes, of course, what the voice of perfectionism tells us is rubbish—but don't most of our friends tell us nonsense from time to time? And we still love them.

Questions to Consider

1. Reflect on your reasons for participating in this course. Are you striving for something? What are you expecting? In what ways may striving for self-improvement thwart the objectives of mindfulness?

2. Consider something that you feel is a flaw in yourself. What will it take for you to come to regard that quality as an asset rather than as a liability?

Imperfection—Embracing Our Flaws
Lecture 16—Transcript

I've long fancied myself an excellent carpenter. I used to tell myself, there wasn't anything I couldn't build or fix—if I put my mind to it.

So when it came time to remodel the kitchen in our old 1920s home several years ago, I undertook the task myself. And I did it all. I replaced the cabinets and the counters, installed a new refrigerator and an oven. I even did the ductwork for the ventilation hood over the new range. I was so intent on doing all this myself that I went to Home Depot and took a daylong clinic on how to tile floors. When I was finished with the flooring, I was immensely pleased. It was better, I thought, than many commercial tiling jobs I've seen.

Then one morning, when I walked into my new kitchen to make a pot of coffee, I heard a slight popping noise when I stepped on my new floor. I didn't believe my ears, at first. I assumed the noise, which was ever so slight, was caused by something else—the coffeemaker perhaps. And so I went about my routine. Then I heard it again. And again, I tried to shrug it off. When it happened the third time, I stopped to investigate. My search led to a particular tile in the area near the sink. What I discovered was that stepping on one of the corners of this particular tile caused it to pop. It didn't break; it just popped, like a knuckle. It wasn't terribly loud, just annoying. And you had to step on it in just the right way.

But it drove me crazy! I tried jumping up and down on it to try to make the noise go away. It didn't. I went to the Internet to see what advice I could find. There was none. I was completely prepared to get a grout saw and chisel the offending tile off the floor and replace it. But I didn't. My wife, who is much saner about such things than I am, persuaded me to do nothing. No one else even noticed the flaw but me. My friends marveled at what a good job I had done. I could only think of the defect. My beautiful floor, totally ruined. I took it personally of course.

Unless you're Homer Simpson, you're probably afflicted with at least a touch of perfectionism. If you're like me, though, it's more than just a touch. If you're not sure that you suffer from perfectionism, see if any of these of things describes your experience. When you make a mistake, you find it hard to forget. You think about it over and over again—until you make another mistake to take its place or until you get praised for something. Any error— or perceived error—that you make is completely your fault. You think that if you had only been more attentive or thought things out more thoroughly, the misstep wouldn't have occurred. You're constantly comparing yourself with others and you feel painfully vulnerable and totally defeated when you think you've come up short against someone else. You're always telling yourself you must try harder. You believe that if you can't do something flawlessly, you shouldn't do it at all. If you make a mistake in front of others, you think you'll die of embarrassment. You're extremely reluctant to ask for help, believing that to do so is to reveal your weakness as person. You do everything you can to keep others from seeing this weaker side. And what's worse is that you try to hide this side from yourself, making it extremely difficult to admit your mistakes. If any or all of these descriptions apply to you, you may be a perfectionist.

Perfectionism is the practice of trying to live up to impossible ideals and then feeling worthless when we don't. It's a textbook recipe for *dukkha*. Perfectionism is not the same as the mere desire to do well by striving to meet high standards.

Unlike the simple aspiration to excel at what one does, perfectionism involves an insidious attachment to an unrealistic view of the self. The perfectionist believes she can be perfect and must be perfect, and if she can't, she considers herself an utter failure. In response to that judgment, the perfectionist may become extremely self-critical and attempt virtually anything to rid herself of those negative feelings those thoughts precipitate. One response might be self-punishment, which could be anything from constantly berating oneself to inflicting physical harm. Another might be to turn to intoxicating substances or overeating to silence those voices of derision. Still another is to submit to a grueling regimen in order to make oneself the ideal person one thinks one must be.

You can see the effects of perfectionism everywhere. We observe it in the way we readily heap blame and criticism on ourselves, even for the most minor mistakes. We see it in the way we treat our bodies, condemning them for being too thin or too fat or too old. We notice it in the way we make excessive demands of ourselves, expecting to be wildly successful in our careers, model friends, ideal parents, and faultless carpenters.

This affliction is one of the major reasons we find it difficult to extend compassion to ourselves. You can search the entire universe, said the Buddha, and never find a being more deserving of compassion than you yourself. Yet finding compassion for ourselves is immensely difficult for many of us. Because we often hold ourselves to unrealistic standards, we sometimes find it hard to believe that we actually deserve compassion.

What lies beneath resistance to self-compassion is a completely ego-centered belief: "Yes, it is quite true that perfection is out of reach for most mortals, but I am different. I'm not like the ordinary man or woman." Some religious traditions attribute this overweening attitude to a desire to be like God. Over 1600 years ago, Saint Augustine observed that the self longed to experience the pleasure of having godlike powers and assuming God's place at the center of the universe. Augustine suggested that this endeavor to be God was precisely what alienated us from the divine, other persons, and ourselves; in other words, it was the very thing that caused us to suffer. You don't have to believe in God to understand what Augustine meant. Aspiring to live up to the image of a wholly self-sufficient and perfect being who is beyond reproach can drive us to great misery. Like other forms of suffering, perfectionism stems from an unrealistic view of the self.

I single out perfectionism not only because it is perhaps the principal obstruction to our practice of self-compassion, but also because I suspect it is a pervasive affliction among people who would be interested in a course such as this one. A spiritual path is sometime attractive to perfectionists, and therein lies a great danger.

Developing one's spirituality can hold out the promise of relief for the perfectionist, but at the same time it can add fuel to the flames when the path becomes another form of achievement. Spiritual discipline can provide a means for the sinner to receive his punishment and a way for the saint to attain her sanctity. Neither of these are goals of the mindfulness path, but that doesn't mean that persons won't seek mindfulness as a way to purge themselves of guilt or to reach sainthood. Or to put it in more secular terms, some may seek mindfulness as a method of self-improvement. Mindfulness is for awareness, not expiation, not sainthood, and not self-improvement.

On a spiritual pathway, perfectionism can manifest as an obsession with doing everything right. You have to follow the instructions to the letter; you must muster all your energy to follow the discipline correctly; it is essential to make tangible progress. When you learn that perfectionism may hinder your capacity to show compassion to yourself, then, by God, you'll eliminate perfectionism! The tendency to make spirituality just one more thing at which to excel led Saint John of the Cross to suggest that "Spiritual accomplishments are not only worthless but can actually become vices."

At some point, you just have to say, "Enough!" Trying to be perfect takes a massive amount of energy and in the end, it's a futile effort. So why not just accept it? I mean, why not just accept that perfectionism is completely unrealistic, and yet you still want to be perfect? Be mindful of both your imperfection and your perfectionism. After all, perfectionism is part of your imperfection. Trying to be perfect may be our greatest flaw.

You probably don't need to work too hard on recognizing that imperfections lie within our humanity. If you're like me, you see the flaws in human nature everywhere—in other people. You probably already believe that imperfection is a human quality. The difficulty is in accepting that you're human like everyone else. For some reason, you think you're exceptional.

Most of you will already be familiar with the life story of the Buddha as it has been passed down by tradition. According to an ancient narrative, Siddhattha Gotama—the man who became the Buddha—lived his early life in lavish surroundings. His father, King Suddhodana, had endeavored to shield Siddhattha from all unpleasant experiences. According to the traditional legend, Suddhodana, on the advice of his counselors, kept his son shielded from the realities of life outside the royal palace and ensured his every experience was a pleasant one. According to the counselors, exposure to suffering in the world might upset the young prince and prompt him to renounce his right to the throne and seek an end to anguish by becoming a holy man. But despite his father's efforts, Siddhattha managed to encounter the harsh facts of life at age 29, when he saw sickness, old age, and death for the first time. This dramatic episode ultimately spurred Siddhattha to leave his father's household and seek a spiritual path—the very thing his father had tried to prevent!

What's always intrigued me about this story was the claim that Siddhattha was oblivious to sickness, old age, and death until he was 29 years old. Even if his father had been wealthy enough to keep his son in pleasure palaces year round, it's hard for me to imagine that Siddhattha could have been as totally naïve about the realities of life as the tradition suggests. He never saw an old person until he was 29? Never got sick? Never had a pet that died? Sounds too far-fetched. What finally made this story plausible for me—indeed, what made it completely compelling—was the realization that the tale is more allegory than history. I'd been reading it too literally. When we're told that Siddhattha sees sickness, old age, and death for the first time at 29, I don't think that means he was completely unacquainted with these facts of life until that age. What we should understand is that at age 29, Siddhattha really sees sickness, old age, and death. And here, I mean "seeing" in the same sense as insight, clear gazing. For the first time, the Buddha-to-be understands that these aspects of life are not abstractions; they are concrete realities that pertain to him.

In the scriptural story, Siddhattha keeps asking his companion: Will this happen to me? Am I also subject to this? Will I die? What sends Siddhattha Gotama on his quest for Buddhahood is his unqualified acceptance of his own participation in the human experience. He finally realizes that even being a king's son does not provide him a magical exemption from the infirmities of all human beings. We perfectionists need to come to the same awareness. There are no exemptions from human nature: We'll get sick, we'll get old, we'll die, and we'll make thousands of mistakes along the way.

And if we need help with this insight, the practice of "just like me" can be very effective. When I introduced that exercise in the last lecture, it was to show how extending empathy to others could rouse compassion for them. But we can also practice the exercise with the reverse goal in mind—to awaken compassion for ourselves.

Seeing others act in less than perfect ways gives us the opportunity to recall to ourselves that we too do not always act in an ideal manner. In fact, when something about another person really, really annoys you, let that be a signal to be extremely mindful and look within. We usually judge others for the very things we hate about ourselves. Try to turn those judgments of others around and make them an opportunity for extending compassion to yourself.

Revising our views on perfection may also help. If we understand perfection as the state of being flawless or immaculate, then our striving for these qualities is sure to cause us anguish. But perhaps we can think of perfection in something other than our conditioned way.

Zen Buddhism is known for its simple, clean, and very beautiful temples and gardens. Zen novices are often charged with keeping the grounds in shape, and it takes a lot of work. The work is not meant to be just busywork; it's an integral part of the discipline. One day a young monk was given the task of cleaning the rock garden in the temple courtyard. It was autumn, and he had to work for hours raking leaves and picking up broken sticks and branches. After painstaking effort, he finally thought the garden was good enough to be shown to the chief monk. After one look, the abbot said, "It's not perfect." Crestfallen and tired, the young monk went back to work. On hands and knees, he sifted through the tiny pebbles looking for twigs and fragments of leaves. When he felt the garden simply could not be improved, he fetched the abbot. "Still not perfect," the abbot said. Then the elder monk reached up to a nearby tree and gave it a hardy shake, letting a few leaves flutter to the ground. "Now," he said, "it's perfect."

The abbot's gesture reflects the Buddhist-influenced aesthetic ideal known in Japan as wabi-sabi. Wabi-sabi seeks to highlight the beautiful aspects of impermanence, incompleteness, and defectiveness. Wabi-sabi values things that are rustic, asymmetrical, irregular, simple, and understated. Objects that are worn or in the process of decay are appreciated both for their beauty as well as the spiritual truth they express about the transience and unfinished nature of life. Many of the classical art forms of Japan reflect this aesthetic sensibility, practices such as *raku* pottery, *ikebana* flower arranging, and haiku poetry.

Wabi-sabi invites us to look at life through a lens different from the one offered by perfectionism. The wabi-sabi view of life encourages me to feel more at home in the world, a world where all things, including myself, could be regarded as aesthetically pleasing just for being what they are: subject to change, incomplete, and less than ideal. I compare it to the way putting on my old, threadbare blue jeans after work makes me feel at home.

To help ease your perfectionism, consider surrounding yourself with a few items that embody the wabi-sabi aesthetic to remind yourself that so-called flaws and defects can enhance the beauty of an object. These need not be pieces of art specifically designed as expressions of wabi-sabi. Rather, just take the time to look deliberately for objects that are conventionally flawed and yet bespeak the beauty of the flawed world in which we live.

I'd also recommend that you try to embody the wabi-sabi ideal in what you do. Perhaps there is some activity you've always wanted to pursue, but you've been hesitant for fear of not being able to do it right. Do it anyway. Years ago, I decided to take voice lessons even though some of my friends had assured me that I couldn't carry a tune. For some reason, I'd always wanted to learn to sing 19th century classical German songs. Don't ask me where that idea came from; I've no clue. I disregarded my friends' admonitions and signed up for voice lessons anyway. But before I began, I gave myself permission not to succeed. I allowed myself to accept that, possibly, my friends were right. But at the same time, I didn't allow their opinion to deter me. For once, I allowed myself to try something I wanted to do, but I totally relaxed any expectation of success. And I had one of the most enjoyable experiences of my life. Was I perfect? Hardly. Was I as bad as my friends thought? Not at all. I was told by my teacher that I was actually pretty good. But that didn't matter. I had simply given up attachment to success and failure and focused on the pure joy of what I was doing. I wish I could say that I approached all aspects of my life with the same degree of non-attachment. But I don't. Yet having had this experience, allowed me to know that I'm capable of it. If you're a perfectionist, you should find at least one thing in your life about which you can relax your need to succeed.

We can accept our common lot with humanity and we can try to rethink our understanding of perfection, but the greatest challenge may be embracing our own perfectionism. Trying to eliminate perfectionism is likely to prove counterproductive. There is a massive paradox here: Wanting to get rid of perfectionism, if you think about it, is just another form of perfectionism.

Rather than responding with belligerence to the voice that's constantly criticizing and blaming you, why not try getting to know it better? Let it speak. It will probably do so whether you want to hear it or not. Your inner critic is just a voice. You don't have to believe it. You don't have to do what it says. The critical voice of our perfectionism only causes us to suffer when we give it more authority than it deserves. Our practice of mindfulness teaches us to allow thoughts to arise and fall on their own, like all impermanent reality. The thought that tells us we must be perfect is just a thought like any other.

Since trying to silence the critical voice hasn't worked, try to welcome perfectionism as a friend. Treat it with courtesy. Show it some compassion. Appreciate what it's trying to do for you. Sometimes, it says valuable things. It's probably helped you achieve some good things in your life. Sometimes, of course, what the voice of perfectionism tells us is rubbish. But don't most of our friends tell us nonsense from time to time? And we still love them.

You'll recall Mara from an earlier lecture in which we mentioned the story of the Buddha's awakening under the Bodhi tree. Mara, you'll remember, is the mythological tempter, the spirit who tried to keep the Buddha from reaching enlightenment. He's sometimes called a demon and the god of death or evil. He is also understood to be an aspect of our own minds. The Buddha, of course, was not deterred by Mara's frightening visions and nasty accusations and pressed onward to realize his goal. This achievement is sometimes referred to as the "defeat of Mara." But interestingly, Mara didn't just go away after his so-called defeat; he returned on many occasions to visit the Buddha. Usually, Mara continued to taunt the Buddha, trying to insinuate that the awakening experience he had wasn't authentic. On one such visit, however, the Buddha welcomed Mara like an old friend, bowed before him, and asked about his health. Despite the protests of his disciples, the Buddha invited Mara in for tea, and the two sat down for refreshment and quiet conversation. Mara confided that he was tired of playing the evil role and was considering another occupation. The Buddha listened with compassion and shared his own experiences, citing some of the drawbacks about being a Buddha. At the end of the day, Mara bade farewell to the Buddha and returned home. No doubt they met again on a later occasion.

If you're old enough, you may remember an old Looney Tunes cartoon featuring Sam Sheepdog and Ralph Wolf. Sam was in charge of protecting a flock of sheep, and Ralph spent the day using any devious means possible to procure one of the hapless animals for his supper. Sam and Ralph fought tooth and claw throughout the day until 5:00, when the whistle blew, signaling the end of work. Then the pair got their lunchboxes, punched the clock, and walked off, arm-in-arm, to the pub.

As the stories of the Buddha and Mara and Sam and Ralph remind us, just because you're enemies doesn't mean you can't also be friends!

Wishing—May All Beings Be Well and Happy
Lecture 17

To act, we must call upon our wisdom. Seeing suffering and being willing to heal it does not guarantee that we will act wisely. To be wisely compassionate requires especially that we attend carefully to our own lives and treat ourselves with compassion. What we learn through self-compassion provides important clues for the compassionate treatment of others. Thus, we return to the importance of the Golden Rule. Learning to practice compassion for ourselves and others is a lifetime endeavor, but it is one of the most important things we can do.

The Good and the Bad

- Sometimes it isn't easy to wish others well. Every now and then—perhaps more often than we'd like to admit—we can feel that those who suffer get what they deserve.

- It's especially easy to feel this way about those who have been the source of great suffering to others. We may even take special delight in thinking that those who have caused harm are getting what they deserve.

- However, life is a bit more complicated and less clear cut than we often think it is. It's not always easy to discriminate between good and bad. The differences between all of us are matters of degree rather than quality. There are things we might call "good" and "bad" in each one of us. No one is wholly good, and no one is wholly evil.

- When we see deeply into the life of those we're inclined to despise, we can recognize that whatever vile acts they may commit do not completely express all that they are. We can understand that their hatred and greed arise from fear, self-centeredness, ignorance, and misunderstanding—the very things that afflict all of us from time to time.

- If we ever lose sight of the moral ambiguity that pervades the human condition, we run great risks. Without insight into our own propensity to act in unwholesome ways, we become blind to our own faults. Without insight into the goodness of others, it becomes all too easy to hate them, especially when we feel our hatred is justified by their wrongdoings.

- However, these reactions distort the reality of what we are and lead us to behave unskillfully—in ways that cause suffering to ourselves and others. They incline us to forget how much the personalities of all of us have been shaped by circumstances beyond our control.

- The dangers inherent in forgetting that we're all capable of both wholesome and unwholesome actions have led sages throughout history to urge us to love our enemies, as well as ourselves and our neighbors. This admonition can be considered as one of humanity's truly great moral developments.

- Although loving our enemies may be one of the most difficult things we can possibly do—rivaled perhaps only by loving ourselves—it is clearly one of the most beneficial practices we can perform.

- It's easy to see how hatred lies at the root of much of human misery, but what we seem to find difficult is accepting that we cannot end hatred by hating. Hating those who hate may feel cathartic and even righteous, but it brings us no closer to a solution to what is a very deep problem. Only love and compassion for others can end hostility and hatred; we can never transform an enemy into a friend with hate.

- We also forget what hating others does to us as individuals. Hatred is a manifestation of our false self; it is not what we truly are. To allow ourselves to be consumed by hatred distorts us, wounds us, and scars us.

- Hatred causes us to misperceive the world, confusing the beautiful and the ugly, the true and the false, the skillful and the unskillful.

Hatred is sure to cause us to suffer and is itself a manifestation of suffering.

Alternatives to Hatred

- While it is not difficult to grasp how hatred can perpetuate animosity between people and disfigure our own basic goodness, it is also not easy to find alternatives. How does one erase a lifetime of conditioning in which we have been encouraged to detest others? Hatred can become a habit that is not simple to break.

- Fortunately, the mindfulness tradition offers many practices to help change this pattern, including some we've already discussed. There is one exercise that is particularly effective in awakening the natural compassion that lies within us; this discipline is known as **metta meditation**.

- "Metta" is a Buddhist term that usually translates as "loving-kindness." This ancient practice has long been the cornerstone for cultivating compassion in the Buddhist tradition. It is a great tool for helping us to wish others well and arouse our resolve to alleviate pain and suffering.

- Like other mindfulness techniques, metta meditation requires commitment, regular practice, and patience. It works by reconditioning our mind and opening our hearts. The intention of this practice is to awaken our determination to ease suffering wherever we may find it.

- Metta practice does not discriminate between those who deserve our compassion and those who do not. Compassion is something all beings deserve, even those responsible for horrendous crimes against humanity.

- Metta meditation is a series of wishes for the happiness of all beings. It begins with the recitation of aspirations for oneself and loved ones and concludes with the same aspirations for all beings—without exception.

Metta Meditation in Practice

- This guided meditation is a form of the practice that has been developed and personalized over the years. Feel free to work with this practice and adapt it in ways most suitable to you. For example, alter the wording of the aspirations or change the people for whom they are intended.

- At the mention of each category, try to picture a particular person and keep him or her in your imagination; the practice is more effective when we're thinking of particular individuals. At the end, however, we do get more generic, and it'll be difficult to create a concrete image.

- As you read each aspiration, try to form a sincere intention based on the wish. Be especially attentive to those you have difficulty wishing well.

- Make yourself comfortable, and follow the instructions. You may assume a traditional meditation position or simply sit on the sofa. You may find it helpful to close your eyes.

- In your mind, form an image of yourself, and wish for yourself the following: May I be well and happy. May I be well and happy. May I have no fears or sorrows. May I be healthy and free from illness. May I live calmly and peacefully.

- Now, imagine your parents, and make the following aspirations: May my parents be well and happy. May my parents be well and happy. May they have no fears or sorrows. May they be healthy and free from illness. May they live calmly and peacefully.

- If you have one, think of your spouse or life companion. May my spouse be well and happy. May my spouse be well and happy. May he or she have no fears or sorrows. May he or she be healthy and free from illness. May my spouse live calmly and peacefully.

- If you have a child or children, hold their image before your mind. May my children be well and happy. May my children be well and happy. May they have no fears or sorrows. May they be healthy and free from illness. May my children live calmly and peacefully.

- Imagine one of your relatives, a brother or sister, aunt or uncle, or any family member to whom you're close. May my relatives be well and happy. May my relatives be well and happy. May they have no fears or sorrows. May they be healthy and free from illness. May my relatives live calmly and peacefully.

- Think of one of your older benefactors, a teacher or other elder. May my teachers and elders be well and happy. May my teachers and elders be well and happy. May they have no fears or sorrows. May they be healthy and free from illness. May my teachers and elders live calmly and peacefully.

- Consider a friend. This is a person for whom you feel great affection. May my friends be well and happy. May my friends be well and happy. May they have no fears or sorrows. May they be healthy and free from illness. May my friends live calmly and peacefully.

- Now, call before your mind a person for whom you have no strong feelings, a neutral person. Although you do not know this person well, you know that he or she shares a common bond in being human. May my acquaintance be well and happy. May my acquaintance be well and happy. May he or she have no fears or sorrows. May he or she be healthy and free from illness. May this person live calmly and peacefully.

- Imagine an enemy or person you strongly dislike. Although this person is an enemy, he or she is just like you—with pains and frustrations, desires and hopes. May my enemies be well and happy.

May my enemies be well and happy. May they have no fears or sorrows. May they be healthy and free from illness. May my enemies live calmly and peacefully.

- Consider all human beings. Dwell a moment on their pain and anguish. Suffering afflicts every one of us, and everyone wishes to be free of it. May all people be well and happy. May all people be well and happy. May they have no fears or sorrows. May they be healthy and free from illness. May all people live calmly and peacefully.

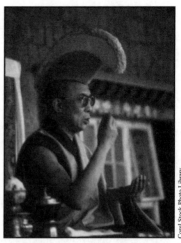

Tenzin Gyatso, the 14th Dalai Lama, said: "If you want others to be happy, practice compassion. If you want to be happy, practice compassion."

- Now, think of all living beings, from the lowliest single-cell organisms to the highest forms of intelligence. Every one of them wants to live and be happy. May all living beings, everywhere and without exception, be well and happy. May all living beings, everywhere and without exception, be well and happy. May all living beings, everywhere and without exception, have no fears or sorrows. May all living beings, everywhere and without exception, be healthy and free from illness. May all living beings, everywhere and without exception, live calmly and peacefully.

Loving-Kindness Meditation

- Many people have a hard time believing that simply wishing can free others from fear, illness, and other forms of anguish. However, medical studies have been conducted that support the claim that prayer has a tangible, empirical effect on the health of those prayed for.

- Whether or not you believe in the effects of this practice, it is important to consider the fact that relieving a little of the hostility of just one person—yourself—will make that world a little better for everyone.

- Perhaps if your enemies were truly happy and free from suffering, then they wouldn't be your enemies. After all, what makes them such difficult people derives from their own struggle with dukkha—the very thing that makes you a difficult person for them. Plus, it's a little harder to get angry at someone for whom you've been wishing happiness.

- Loving-kindness meditation is a way to cultivate the mind and heart to produce wholesome actions. The practice doesn't, however, tell us in advance specific ways to act. Rather, the practice sensitizes us to the manifestations of suffering and prepares us to respond when the opportunity arises.

Important Term

metta meditation: An ancient practice that has long been the cornerstone for cultivating compassion in the Buddhist tradition. "Metta" is a Buddhist term that usually translates as "loving-kindness."

Questions to Consider

1. How is the well-being of others related to our personal happiness?

2. How is it possible to be compassionate toward another without feelings of affection?

3. Do you agree with the Buddha's contention that hostility cannot be ended with hostility?

Wishing—May All Beings Be Well and Happy
Lecture 17—Transcript

Sometimes it isn't easy to wish others well. Every now and then, perhaps more often than we'd like to admit, we can feel that those who suffer get what they deserve.

It's especially easy to feel this way about those who have been the source of great suffering to others. We may even take special delight in thinking that those who've caused harm are getting their just deserts. Who doesn't feel a surge of glee when the Wicked Witch of the West melts before our eyes after Dorothy accidentally splashes her with water? "What a world! What a world!"

But back in Kansas, life is a bit more complicated and less clear-cut. It's not always easy to discriminate between the innocent farm girls and the evil sorceresses. Blue gingham dresses and pointy hats just aren't reliable indicators of moral condition. The differences between witches and farm girls—and the differences between all of us—are always matters of degree rather than quality. There are things we might call "good" and "bad" in each one of us. No one is wholly good; none is wholly evil. When we see deeply into the life of those we're inclined to despise, we can recognize that whatever vile acts they may commit do not completely express all that they are. We can understand that their hatred and greed arise from fear, self-centeredness, ignorance, and misunderstanding—the very things that afflict all of us from time-to-time. There is probably enough within each of us to make us both a Dorothy and a wicked witch.

If we ever lose sight of the moral ambiguity that pervades the human condition, we run great risks. Without insight into our own propensity to act in unwholesome ways, we become blind to our own faults. Without insight into the goodness of others, it becomes all too easy to hate them, especially when we feel our hatred is justified by their wrongdoings. But these reactions distort the reality of what we are and lead us to behave unskillfully, in ways that cause suffering to ourselves and others. They incline us to forget how much the personalities of all of us have been shaped by circumstances beyond our control. Who knows how Dorothy might have turned out had she been raised in a gloomy castle surrounded by flying monkeys instead of the loving arms of Auntie Em?

The dangers inherent in forgetting that we're all capable of both wholesome and unwholesome actions have led sages throughout history to urge us to love our enemies, as well as ourselves and our neighbors. I consider this admonition to be one of humanity's truly great moral developments. Although loving our enemies may be one of the most difficult things we can possibly do (rivaled perhaps only by loving ourselves), it is clearly one of the most beneficial practices we can perform.

It's easy to see how hatred lies at the root of much of human misery, but what we seem to find difficult is accepting that we cannot end hatred by hating. Hating those who hate may feel cathartic and even righteous, but it brings us no closer to a solution to what is a very deep problem. As the Buddha put it: "In this world, hostility is never appeased by hostility; only in the absence of hatred does hatred cease." Only love and compassion for others can end hostility and hatred. We can never transform an enemy into a friend with hate.

We also forget what hating others does to us as individuals. Hatred is a manifestation of our false self; it is not what we truly are. To allow ourselves to be consumed by hatred distorts us, wounds us, and scars us. It causes us to misperceive the world, confusing the beautiful and the ugly, the true and the false, the skillful and the unskillful. Hatred is sure to cause us to suffer and is itself a manifestation of suffering.

While it is not difficult to grasp how hatred can perpetuate animosity between people and disfigure our own basic goodness, it is also not easy to find alternatives. How does one erase a lifetime of conditioning in which we have been encouraged to detest others? Hatred can become a habit that is not so simple to break.

Fortunately, the mindfulness tradition offers many practices to help change this pattern, including some we've already discussed. But there is one exercise that is particularly effective in awakening the natural compassion that lies within us. This discipline is known as metta meditation. "Metta" is a Buddhist term that usually translates as loving-kindness. This ancient practice has long been the cornerstone for cultivating compassion in the Buddhist tradition. I know of no better tool for helping us to wish others well and arouse our resolve to alleviate pain and suffering. Like other mindfulness techniques, metta meditation requires commitment, regular practice, and patience. It works by reconditioning our mind and opening our hearts. The intention of this practice is to awaken our determination to ease suffering wherever it we may find it. Metta meditation does not discriminate between those who deserve our compassion and those who do not. Compassion is something all beings deserve, even those responsible for horrendous crimes against humanity. Metta meditation is a series of wishes for the happiness of all beings. It begins with the recitation of aspirations for oneself and loved ones and concludes with the same aspirations for all beings, without exception.

You may practice this exercise at any time and place where you can find peace and quiet. To help you learn the practice, I'll first offer it as a guided meditation. You'll find that the exercise is quite simple and can be easily remembered. What I'll present is a form of the practice that I have developed for myself over the years. It's structured in a way that I have found particularly meaningful, although you may not find my version as compelling as I do. That's perfectly fine. I invite you to work with this practice and adapt it in ways most suitable to you. Feel free to alter the wording of the aspirations or change the persons for whom they are intended. You may find that some of the persons mentioned in my version are not applicable in your situation. For example, I mention spouses and children, but of course not everyone has a spouse or a child. In these cases, simply think of someone else. For the most part, though, I'll mention people with whom we all have relationships: ourselves, parents, relatives, elders, friends, and enemies. If you dislike the word "enemy," substitute another term to indicate a person whom you find difficult to like. Perhaps you prefer "adversary" or "rival." I will also mention what I call a "neutral" person. Lacking a better term, I mean simply someone for whom you have no strong feelings, neither a friend nor an enemy; he or she could the cashier at the grocery or a teller at the bank.

At the mention of each category, try to picture a particular person and keep him or her in your imagination. When I mention friends, for instance, think of a specific friend. The practice is more effective when we're thinking of particular individuals. At the end, however, we do get more generic, and it'll be difficult to create a concrete image. As I recite each aspiration, try to form a sincere intention based on the wish. Be especially attentive to those you have difficulty wishing well.

Now, we will begin. Make yourself comfortable, and follow my instructions. You may assume a traditional meditation position or simply sit on the sofa. You may find it helpful to close your eyes. In your mind, form an image of yourself, and wish for yourself the following: May I be well and happy. May I be well and happy. May I have no fears or sorrows. May I be healthy and free from illness. May I live calmly and peacefully.

Now imagine your parents and make the following aspirations: May my parents be well and happy. May my parents be well and happy. May they have no fears or sorrows. May they be healthy and free from illness. May they live calmly and peacefully.

If you have one, think of your spouse or life-companion. May my spouse be well and happy. May my spouse be well and happy. May he or she have no fears or sorrows. May he or she be healthy and free from illness. May my spouse live calmly and peacefully.

If you have a child or children, hold their image before your mind. May my children be well and happy. May my children be well and happy. May they have no fears or sorrows. May they be healthy and free from illness. May my children live calmly and peacefully.

Imagine one of your relatives, a brother or sister, aunt or uncle, or any family member to whom you're close. May my relatives be well and happy. May my relatives be well and happy. May they have no fears or sorrows. May they be healthy and free from illness. May my relatives live calmly and peacefully.

Think of one of your older benefactors, a teacher or other elder. May my teachers and elders be well and happy. May my teachers and elders be well and happy. May they have no fears or sorrows. May they be healthy and free from illness. May my teachers and elders live calmly and peacefully.

Consider a friend. This is a person for whom you feel great affection. May my friends be well and happy. May my friends be well and happy. May they have no fears or sorrows. May they be healthy and free from illness. May my friends live calmly and peacefully.

Now call before your mind a person for whom you have no strong feelings, a neutral person. Although you do not know this person well, you know that he or she shares a common bond in being human. May my acquaintance be well and happy. May my acquaintance be well and happy. May he or she have no fears or sorrows. May he or she be healthy and free from illness. May this person live calmly and peacefully.

Imagine an enemy or person you strongly dislike. Although this person is an enemy, he or she is just like you, with pains and frustrations, desires and hopes. May my enemies be well and happy. May my enemies be well and happy. May they have no fears or sorrows. May they be healthy and free from illness. May my enemies live calmly and peacefully.

Consider all human beings. Dwell a moment on their pain and anguish. Suffering afflicts every one of us and everyone wishes to be free of it. May all people be well and happy. May all people be well and happy. May they have no fears or sorrows. May they be healthy and free from illness. May all people live calmly and peacefully.

Now think of all living beings, from the lowliest single cell organisms to the highest forms of intelligence. Every one of them wants to live and be happy. May all living beings, everywhere and without exception, be well and happy. May all living beings, everywhere and without exception, be well and happy. May all living beings, everywhere and without exception, have no fears or sorrows. May all living beings, everywhere and without exception, be healthy and free from illness. May all living beings, everywhere and without exception, live calmly and peacefully.

I practiced sitting and walking meditation for many years before I took up the loving-kindness exercise. I was very reluctant to try it. Initially, the practice seemed to be an affront to my masculinity. The practice of loving-kindness just sounded and felt kind of sissy.

As I noted in an earlier lecture, the expression of compassion can be very difficult for males under modern ideals of masculinity. Sitting and walking meditation, on the other hand, took a kind of manly discipline—so I thought. But even beyond my fears that my masculinity might somehow be compromised, the exercise seemed to be just so much wishful thinking. I felt exactly the way one of my students reacted after I taught the practice to a class several months ago. When it was over he said: "So what? Nothing changes. People aren't going to be happy and free from fear just because you wish it for them. It's more effective to act than to wish." Twenty years ago, I would have completely agreed.

For some reason—and I can't recall it now—I overcame my reluctance and tried the practice anyway. Maybe I was just in an experimental mood. I started reciting the aspirations just before I practiced sitting. It was awkward at first, but I persisted. Continued practice with sitting and walking meditation had at least made me aware that I couldn't pass judgment until I had given the exercise a fair shake. After some time, and it wasn't too long, I began to see results. But the results were nothing I could see on the faces of the people who had been the subjects of my meditation. I couldn't tell if they were any happier or freer from suffering, but I could tell a considerable difference in me. I felt happier and noticed that I was freed from suffering. I noticed this change especially with respect to my enemies. The animosity I had felt towards these individuals had softened, and I discovered that I could genuinely wish them well. I didn't like them any better, and they still annoyed me sometimes, but I found I could set down the burden of hostility that I had been carrying. We don't always realize what a tremendous encumbrance animosity can be until we finally relinquish it. It occurred to me that if my enemies were truly happy and free from suffering, then perhaps they wouldn't be my enemies. After all, what makes them such difficult people derives from their own struggle with *dukkha*, the very thing that makes me a difficult person for them.

Over time, I observed that I was treating others—not just my adversaries—with a bit more kindness and understanding. Today, I'm firmly convinced of the value of this practice for revealing our fundamental compassion for others. I silently recite the metta aspirations before beginning sitting meditation, and I try to remember them when I'm dealing with an especially irritating individual. It's a little harder to get angry at someone for whom you've been wishing happiness.

I still have a hard time believing that simply wishing can free others from fear, illness, and other forms of anguish. Yet I don't disbelieve it. I have good friends and acquaintances in the medical profession who argue that prayer has a tangible, empirical effect on the health of those prayed for. They have even conducted studies to support that claim. Perhaps they're right: The world is a mysterious place. What I do know is this: Relieving a little of the hostility of just one person—myself—will make that world a little better for everyone. Knowing this, I can easily affirm the statement of Tenzin Gyatso, the 14th Dalai Lama: "If you want others to be happy," he said, "practice compassion. If you want to be happy, practice compassion."

Loving-kindness meditation is a way to cultivate the mind and heart to produce wholesome actions. The practice doesn't, however, tell us in advance specific ways to act. It doesn't tell us to go work in a soup kitchen, or make a contribution to the Red Cross, or how to make friends with our enemies. It doesn't tell us whether to vote Republican or Democrat. Rather, the practice sensitizes us to the manifestations of suffering and prepares us to respond when the opportunity arises.

To act, we must call upon our wisdom. Seeing suffering and being willing to heal it does not guarantee that we will act wisely. Very compassionate persons may still act in very foolish ways. To be wisely compassionate requires especially that we attend carefully to our own lives and treat ourselves with compassion. What we learn through self-compassion provides important clues for the compassionate treatment of others. Thus we return to the importance of the Golden Rule.

Learning to practice compassion for ourselves and others is a lifetime endeavor. But it is one of the most important things we can do. Every religious tradition affirms its centrality. Huston Smith, the prominent professor of comparative religion, writes in his autobiography about an encounter with the famous English writer Aldous Huxley toward the end of Huxley's life. Smith reports that Huxley told him: "It's rather embarrassing to have given one's life to pondering the human predicament and to find that in the end one has little more to say than, 'Try to be a little kinder.' "

Generosity—The Joy of Giving
Lecture 18

Many people that live in an affluent society own a lot of stuff—generic, inessential, space-consuming stuff. When you first acquired the material items you possess, they probably brought you a bit of pleasure—or maybe a lot of pleasure. Where is that pleasure now? Are you really happy with all that stuff? The Buddha said: "If you knew what I know about the power of generosity, you would not let a single meal go by without sharing it." Think of generosity as a way of exchanging your impermanent material goods for more lasting spiritual benefits.

Greed and Materialism

- Human beings seem to accumulate material items the way squirrels store up acorns for the winter. There was a time in our evolution as a species when collecting things conferred survival advantages: When resources were scarce, the more we had, the better we could protect ourselves against the onslaught of enemies, famine, or catastrophic weather.

- Eating copious quantities of food rich in sugar and fat served the same purpose; it helped us survive when we were uncertain when our next meal would be. In the midst of affluence, however, the evolutionary benefits we once gained from hoarding and the unrestricted consumption of sugar and fat seem now to have passed—but the old habits have not.

- Just as immoderately indulging our appetites for rich foods can be detrimental to our well-being, so too can be the acquisition of stuff. The mindfulness tradition regards our voracious appetite for wanting and accumulating inessential things to be a form of greed—one of the principal roots of dukkha.

- **Greed,** or self-centered desire for unnecessary things, is considered a defilement, a poison of the mind. It distorts our view of reality and leaves us unhappy. Whether or not we get what we want, selfish craving causes us to suffer.

- According to traditional Buddhist mythology, there is an entire realm of existence populated by beings that are consumed with greed. This is the realm of the hungry ghosts. The hungry ghosts are depicted as shadowy beings that are driven by their intense desire. They have enormous bellies but extremely narrow gullets and tiny mouths. No matter how much they try to eat, they can never consume enough to feel satisfied. When they drink, the liquid turns to fire, intensifying their thirst.

- The torture of the hungry ghosts derives not so much from the frustration of not getting what they want; they suffer because they cling to the things they mistakenly believe will bring them satisfaction and relief.

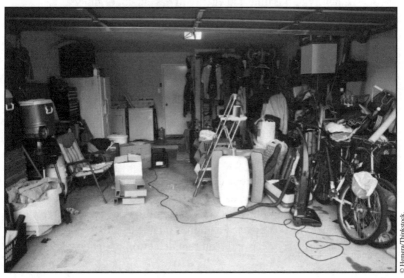

Many people that live in an affluent society own a lot of stuff that is inessential to their lives.

- The plight of the hungry ghosts closely parallels the lives of those of us who are overtaken by the defilement of greed. Like the hungry ghosts, the real problem of greedy people is our attachment to the idea that stuff will make us happy. The problem is not that there's something wrong with material things. Material things are fine and, to some extent, even necessary.

- The mindfulness tradition affirms the value of good food, adequate shelter, and a healthy body. The real issue we greedy people must face is the tremendous expectations we place on having stuff.

- Once we have provided for our basic needs, our craving continues unabated. Meeting our fundamental needs feels so good that we assume more of the same will make us feel even better.

- Despite that belief, the majority of us think that material acquisition is not really the avenue to happiness. Although many of us affirm this idea, we still surround ourselves with stuff and devote a vast quantity of our time and energy to the pursuit of things.

Beliefs versus Practices

- Although we claim to believe it, perhaps we haven't fully accepted the idea that the best things in life aren't material things. It sounds noble, and all the wisdom traditions tell us it's true, but it's very hard to embrace that claim wholeheartedly when the dominant message of our culture tells us just the opposite. It's extremely difficult to be out of step with the prevailing ethos of society.

- Perhaps we still harbor the idea that there really is something out there that will make us happy. It may be a secret belief that we hide even from our conscious awareness. Maybe we haven't truly grasped the fact that acquisition is unable to satisfy us. The roots of greed are very deep and require much effort to understand.

- Perhaps we continue with our greedy habits simply because we don't really know of any alternatives. Acquisition is so ingrained into us that we may feel bored without it.

- Whatever the reason, many of us often feel torn in opposite directions between our greedy behavior and our deeper aspirations—and we continue to suffer, partly from our selfish desires and partly from our guilt.

- The mindfulness approach to this problem follows the twofold path of seeking wisdom and practicing compassion. In the case of greed, seeking wisdom means deep insight into the transient and unsatisfying nature of the world and practicing compassion means cultivating generosity.

Mindfulness and Generosity

- The mindfulness tradition does not endorse a life of poverty and deprivation. It doesn't romanticize poverty, thinking that what the poor lack in material resources they make up in spiritual gains.

- Rather, the mindfulness tradition values simplicity. It recognizes that we must meet our basic material needs, but it also sees the danger of attachment to the world of things.

- The mindfulness tradition calmly and dispassionately recognizes that the ephemeral nature of our lives rules out any effort to find security or permanence in a world in constant change. It means we must stay on our guard to relax the tendency to latch onto things in the hope they will somehow satisfy our desires.

- As with other spiritual afflictions, the mindfulness tradition offers specific forms of practice to help neutralize the defilements of greed and attachment. The practice of generosity is the most potent antidote to greed. Generosity is fundamentally a state of mind that is manifested in particular acts of giving.

- On the simplest level, **generosity** is the willingness to give to others, but on a deeper level, generosity is the eagerness to relinquish anything that we feel is "ours." In this sense, generosity is a way to relax our tendency to become attached to things, including the principal cause of suffering: the illusion of the self.

- In the Buddhist world, generosity is one of the basic practices of the tradition. Long before Buddhists take up the disciplines of meditation, they are taught the value of *dana*, the word for generosity. As a formal practice in traditional Buddhist societies, *dana* takes the form of providing monks and nuns with food, clothing, and the basic necessities of life.

- Even beyond this, *dana* is understood as the custom of sharing with others. *Dana* practices in these cultures bring great joy to both the recipient and the giver. Families often spend days planning and preparing a single meal for the local monastics, and everyone works together to share the best of what they have with others.

- *Dana* practices are regarded as so joyful that just observing a generous act is believed to bring great happiness to the witness. In Buddhist mythology, the hungry ghosts are able to ease their torment not by eating, but by observing an act of generosity and experiencing the happiness it brings.

- By the same token, those of us who live like hungry ghosts can relieve the suffering of our incessant wanting by being generous and taking delight in the generosity of others.

- In the modern Western world, there are few opportunities for practicing *dana* in the traditional sense, but there are ample opportunities for observing it in other ways. The fundamental component in the practice of generosity is a reorientation of our thinking about wealth and giving.

- The mindfulness practice of generosity invites us to think about giving to another as a form of enrichment rather than as self-impoverishment. Consider generosity as the gift you not only give to others but to yourself as well. This is hard to do, of course, if you believe that the material world is more real or more important than the spiritual. Part of practicing generosity means relaxing that pervasive assumption.

- In addition, we don't need to attain a certain level of wealth to be generous. In fact, social research indicates that people toward the lower end of the economic scale tend to give away a greater proportion of what they have than those at the upper end.

Cultivating a Mind of Generosity

- Cultivating a mind of generosity—modest as it may seem—is a vital step in the direction of meeting the greater challenges of ensuring that the basic needs of everyone are met.

- These simple practices don't directly address the really grave issues of world hunger and the gross inequities between rich and poor, but they go a long way toward creating a mind sensitive to the needs of others and cautious about the seductions of greed.

- First, find one of your cherished possessions, and give it to someone who would appreciate it. Take time with this exercise; give it deep consideration. It doesn't have to be your most prized possession, but it should be an item you hold dear.

- Then, think about someone who would value having it. Perhaps you have a friend who has seen it and expressed appreciation for it. Then, on no particular occasion, give it to your friend. Be keenly attentive to the effects this action has on you, your friend, and your relationship.

- In addition, knowing what a sincere compliment does for us, we can imagine the goodwill it generates when we offer praise to another. Giving compliments is such an easy thing to do—if we can only remember to do it and do it with a sincere heart. Trying to make it a habit helps, but complimenting out of habit has potential pitfalls.

- Simply praising someone out of custom is disingenuous and reinforces an unwholesome state of mind, but one can help shape a mind of generosity by sincerely seeking to discover the good qualities in someone else and reflecting them back to the individual as a gift.

- It's essential, of course, that the gift of a compliment is offered with sincerity and without expectation of anything in return. A truly generous spirit gives freely—without strings attached.

- As the practice of complimenting illustrates, simply giving to others is not sufficient for cultivating true generosity. As with other forms of compassion, generosity must be exercised with wisdom. We have to maintain mindful vigilance about our motivations and practice responsible stewardship over our resources.

Important Terms

dana: The Buddhist word for generosity.

generosity: The willingness to give to others; on a deeper level, it is the eagerness to relinquish anything that one might feel is a possession.

greed: The self-centered desire for unnecessary things; it is considered to be a poison of the mind because it distorts one's view of reality and leaves one unhappy.

Questions to Consider

1. What drives the Western world's obsession with acquiring and having material objects?

2. How does practicing mindfulness help to foster a spirit of generosity?

3. Consider the material object that would be most difficult for you to part with. Why would it be hard to let it go?

Generosity—The Joy of Giving

Lecture 18—Transcript

Most of us living in this affluent society own a lot of stuff. There's no better word for it. It's stuff—generic, inessential, space-consuming stuff.

Look in your closets and your kitchen drawers. Go up to the attic. Go to the garage. And behold all your stuff. When you acquired these items, they probably brought you a good deal of pleasure—maybe some of them gave you a great deal of pleasure. Where is that pleasure now? Are you really happy with all that stuff?

We seem to accumulate stuff the way squirrels store up acorns for the winter. There was a time in our evolution as a species when collecting things conferred survival advantages, like stockpiling acorns does for squirrels. When resources were scarce, the more we had, the better we could protect ourselves against the onslaught of enemies, famine, or catastrophic weather. Eating copious amounts of food rich in sugar and fat served the same purpose; it helped us survive when we were uncertain when our next meal would be. In the midst of affluence, however, the evolutionary benefits we once gained from hoarding and the unrestricted consumption of sugar and fat seem now to have passed. But the old habits have not.

Just as immoderately indulging our appetites for rich foods can be detrimental to our well-being, so too can be the acquisition of stuff. The mindfulness tradition regards our voracious appetite for wanting and accumulating inessential things to be a form of greed, the principal roots of *dukkha*. Greed, or self-centered desire for unnecessary things, is considered a defilement, a poison of the mind. It distorts our view of reality and leaves us unhappy. As we discussed in an earlier lecture, whether or not we get what we want, selfish craving causes us to suffer.

According to traditional Buddhist mythology, there is an entire realm of existence populated by beings that are consumed with greed. This is the realm of the hungry ghosts. The hungry ghosts are depicted as shadowy beings that are driven by their intense desire. They have enormous bellies but extremely narrow gullets and tiny mouths. No matter how much they try to eat, they can never consume enough to feel satisfied. When they drink, the liquid turns to fire, intensifying their thirst. The torture of the hungry ghosts derives not so much from the frustration of not getting what they want. They suffer because they cling to the things they mistakenly believe will bring them satisfaction and relief.

The plight of the hungry ghosts closely parallels the lives of those of us who are overtaken by the defilement of greed. Like the hungry ghosts, the real problem of greedy people is our attachment to the idea that stuff will make us happy. The problem is not that there's something wrong with material things. Material things are fine and to some extent even necessary. The mindfulness tradition affirms the value of good food, adequate shelter, and a healthy body. The real issue we greedy people must face is the tremendous expectations we place on having stuff. Once we have provided for our basic needs, our craving continues unabated. Meeting our fundamental needs feels so good that we assume more of the same will make us feel even better!

Yet despite that belief, I'd wager that the majority of us—at least the majority of those who are participating in this course on mindfulness—think that material acquisition is not really the avenue to happiness. In fact, that proposition is practically a cliché. "The best things in life are not things," read bumper stickers. "You can't take it with you," they say. Yet, although many of us affirm this idea, we still surround ourselves with stuff and devote a vast quantity of our time and energy to the pursuit of things. I'm as guilty as anyone.

Why this dichotomy between our beliefs and our practices? I can imagine several responses to this question. Although we claim to believe it, perhaps we haven't fully accepted the idea that "the best things in life aren't things." It sounds noble, and all the wisdom traditions tell us it's true, but it's very hard to embrace that claim wholeheartedly when the dominant message of our culture tells us just the opposite. It's extremely difficult to be out of step with the prevailing ethos of society.

Perhaps we still harbor the idea that there really is something out there that will make us happy. It may be a secret belief that we hide even from our conscious awareness. Maybe we haven't truly grasped the fact that acquisition is unable to satisfy us. The roots of greed are very deep and require much effort to understand.

Perhaps we continue with our greedy habits simply because we don't know of any alternatives. If we don't spend our days getting things, what will we do? Acquisition is so ingrained into us that we may feel bored without it. Ever go shopping just to cheer yourself up? Whatever the reason, many of us feel torn in opposite directions between our greedy behavior and our deeper aspirations. And we continue to suffer, partly from our selfish desires, partly from our guilt.

The mindfulness approach to this problem follows the twofold path of seeking wisdom and practicing compassion. In the case of greed, seeking wisdom means deep insight into the transient and unsatisfying nature of the world and practicing compassion means cultivating generosity.

Rabbi Yisrael Meir Kagan was one of the most revered figures in modern Judaism. He ran a small store in the area of Eastern Europe known today as Belarus and lived a simple life. The story is told of an American visitor who once called upon the rabbi at his home. The visitor was surprised to discover that the home was nothing more than a room with a few books, a table, and a bench.

> The caller naturally asked, "Where's your furniture, Rabbi?"
>
> To which the rabbi responded, "Where's yours?"
>
> Surprised by the retort, the guest said, "I have no furniture. I'm just passing through."
>
> "Well," said the rabbi, "so am I."

With a flourish of wit, the rabbi succinctly conveys a spark of insight into the impermanence of existence. We're all passing through, from whence and to where, we're not sure, but about our transience there is no doubt.

When we fully, viscerally, existentially know this fact, our attitude becomes like that of Rabbi Kagan. That attitude is not aversion to the material world, but equanimity. The mindfulness tradition does not endorse a life of poverty and deprivation. It doesn't romanticize poverty, as I once did, thinking that what the poor lacked in material resources they made up in spiritual gains. That was before I really witnessed the destructiveness of destitution. Rather, the mindfulness tradition values simplicity, like that of Rabbi Kagan. It recognizes that we must meet our basic material needs, but it also sees the danger of attachment to the world of things. It calmly and dispassionately recognizes that the ephemeral nature of our lives rules out any effort to find security or permanence in a world in constant change. It means we must stay on our guard to relax the tendency to latch onto things in the hope that they will somehow satisfy our desires.

As with other spiritual afflictions, the mindfulness tradition offers specific forms of practice to help neutralize the defilements of greed and attachment. The practice of generosity is the most potent antidote to greed. Generosity is fundamentally a state of mind that is manifested in particular acts of giving. On the simplest level, generosity is the willingness to give to others. But on a deeper level, generosity is the eagerness to relinquish anything that we feel is "ours." In this sense, generosity is a way to relax our tendency to become attached to things, including the principal cause of suffering: the illusion of the self.

In the Buddhist world, generosity is one the basic practices of the tradition. Long before Buddhists take up the disciplines of meditation, they are taught the value of *dana*, the word for generosity. As a formal practice in traditional Buddhist societies, *dana* takes the form of providing monks and nuns with food, clothing, and the basic necessities of life. But even beyond this, *dana* is understood as the custom of sharing with others. I've observed both formal and informal *dana* practices in these cultures, and I'm deeply impressed by how much joy they bring to both the recipient and the giver. Families often spend days planning and preparing a single meal for the local monastics. My wife, who grew up in a devout Buddhist family in Sri Lanka, tells me that preparing and serving *dana* meals to the monks comprised some of her family's happiest moments, as everyone worked together to share the best of what they had with others. Even today, simply providing a meal for someone else brings her great happiness.

Dana practices are regarded as so joyful that just observing a generous act is believed to bring great happiness to the witness. In Buddhist mythology, the hungry ghosts are able to ease their torment, not by eating, but by observing an act of generosity and experiencing the happiness it brings. By the same token, those of us who live like hungry ghosts can relieve the suffering of our incessant wanting by being generous and taking delight in the generosity of others.

In the modern Western world, there are few opportunities for practicing *dana* in the traditional sense, but there are ample opportunities for observing it in other ways. The fundamental component in the practice of generosity is a reorientation of our way of thinking about wealth and giving. For me, the most difficult adjustment has been trying to change my belief that giving to others impoverishes me. If I hand over a $5 bill to someone else, that's $5 less I have to spend on myself. The more I give, the less I have.

The mindfulness practice of generosity, however, invites us to think about this transaction in a completely different way. Rather than seeing giving as self-impoverishment, try to think of it as a form of enrichment. Consider generosity as the gift you not only give to others but to yourself as well. This is hard to do, of course, if you believe that the material world is more real or more important than the spiritual. But part of the practice of generosity means relaxing that pervasive assumption. You may have to remind yourself that "The most important things in life aren't things." Try to think of generosity as a way of exchanging your impermanent material goods for more lasting spiritual benefits.

The story of Oseola McCarty is a fine example of someone who completely grasped the idea that generosity to others can be more enriching than having stuff. For more than 75 years in Hattiesburg, Mississippi, Oseola McCarty washed and ironed clothes. She began to do laundry work to help support her family when she was still in elementary school. In the sixth grade, however, her mother's sister became disabled, and Oseola quit school to assist the ailing aunt at home.

She continued washing and ironing but never returned to school. She always lived frugally, never owned a car, and rarely turned on her air conditioner, even during the worst parts of the steamy Mississippi summers. She never married or had children. In 1995, four years before she died, Oseola McCarty quietly donated $150,000 to The University of Southern Mississippi to establish a scholarship fund for deserving African American students. The money came from what she saved washing clothes. Ms. McCarty said, "I just want the scholarship to go to some child who needs it, to whoever is not able to help their children. I'm too old to get an education," she said, "but they can."

Oseola McCarty's story is a remarkable testament to the spirit of human generosity. It's a story that warms our heart and reminds us of the good that dwells within. It's also an astonishing story, because it defies some of our commonly held beliefs about wealth and generosity. We just don't expect to hear that a person who has the means to make such a grand contribution to the lives of others would live as simply as she did. Why didn't she take a bit of that nest egg and get a car or keep cooler in the summer? In our materialistic culture, such a life seems odd, and yet, we are not so thoroughly conditioned by our materialism that we fail to recognize her nobility. Her story reminds us that we don't need to attain a certain level of wealth to be generous. In fact, social research indicates that persons toward the lower end of the economic scale tend to give away a greater proportion of what they have than those at the upper end. Ms. McCarty helps us remember that giving is a source of great joy. Which do you think would have brought her greater happiness—spending the money on cars and other luxury items or giving it all away to benefit someone else? The Buddha said: "If you knew what I know about the power of generosity, you would not let a single meal go by without sharing it."

Here are some very simple practices that anyone can observe to help cultivate a mind of generosity. These aren't earth-shattering disciplines. They don't directly address the really grave issues of world hunger and the gross inequities between rich and poor, but they go a long way toward creating a mind sensitive to the needs of others and cautious about the seductions of greed. Cultivating such a mind, modest as it may seem, is a vital step in the direction of meeting the greater challenges of ensuring that the basic needs of everyone are met. These small examples may inspire you to think of other methods to make generosity a way of life.

The first exercise is to find one of your cherished possessions and give it to someone who would appreciate it. Take time with this exercise. Give it deep consideration. Think of something that means a lot to you. It doesn't have to be your most prized possession, but it should be an item you hold dear. Then think about someone who would value having it. Perhaps you have a friend who has seen it and expressed appreciation for it. Then, out of the blue, on no particular occasion, give it to your friend. Be keenly attentive to the effects this action has on you, your friend, and your relationship.

My first experience with this exercise was laced with irony. Many years ago, I discovered a beautiful image of the Buddha that I adored. Laying my eyes upon it, I imagined how stunning it would appear in my meditation space. I found it in a pricey Asian import store and decided to pay their inflated practices anyway, imagining the great serenity the image would inspire. I was so pleased with it that just a week later I took it with me to a lecture on Buddhism that I was giving at a local Unitarian church. At the lecture was a friend of mine who saw the statue and seemed to appreciate it as much as I did. After the lecture was over, walking back to the car with my precious Buddha cradled in my arms, my wife had the audacity to suggest that I give the image to John. "What?!" I was incredulous. I couldn't believe she was actually recommending that I give away my cherished, and not inexpensive, Buddha. But despite my initial shock, I began to think about what she was asking.

Later, it occurred to me that I had developed an attachment to this image. And then that's when I saw the irony. I bought the statue to encourage me to find the peace of mind and happiness that the image represented. I was now attached to a material representation of the individual who taught that the way to contentment was by relinquishing attachment. When that became clear, I knew that I had to give the statue to John. When my wife and I presented him with the image the next day, he was a bit shocked, but he accepted it graciously. I was glad to see the expression of delight on his face. We drove away with a feeling a great joy that I don't think I'll ever forget. And so, the Buddha that I bought to inspire happiness did just that, but not in the way I expected. I had to let him go before I found it.

Giving compliments to others probably comes more easily to some people than it does to me. I get so wrapped up in seeking praise that I often forget to express my admiration of others. Here again, the old Golden Rule provides a trustworthy guide. Knowing what a sincere compliment does for us, we can imagine the goodwill it generates when we offer praise to another. Giving compliments is such easy thing to do, if we can only remember to do it and do it with a sincere heart. Trying to make it a habit helps, but compliments out of habit have potential pitfalls. Simply praising someone out of custom is disingenuous and reinforces an unwholesome state of mind. But one can help shape a mind of generosity by sincerely seeking to discover the good qualities in someone else and reflecting them back to the individual as a gift. It's essential, of course, that the gift of a compliment is offered with sincerity and without expectation of anything in return. A truly generous spirit gives freely, without strings attached. As the Stoic philosopher Seneca said: "We should give as we would receive, cheerfully, quickly, and without hesitations, for there is no grace in a gift that sticks to the fingers."

As the practice of complimenting illustrates, simply giving to others is not sufficient for cultivating true generosity. As with other forms of compassion, generosity must be exercised with wisdom. We have to maintain mindful vigilance about our motivations and practice responsible stewardship over our resources.

Before giving to charities, for example, it's essential to understand how your contribution will be spent. Will it really be used to fund the project for which it's intended or does a great portion of it go to support exorbitant administrative costs? Giving wisely is an essential component of the generous mind.

The practice of giving wisely is humorously illustrated in the story of Nasreddin Hodja, a folk figure famous throughout the Middle East. According to legend, Nasreddin showed up at the baths dressed shabbily, and he was given poor service by the bath attendant. Nevertheless, Nasreddin rewarded him handsomely with 10 coins. The next week, Nasreddin went to the same bathhouse and got the royal treatment. When the attendant stuck out his hand for a tip, he was given a single copper penny. The attendant was dumbfounded. Nasreddin explained: "Last week's tip was for today. Today's tip was for last week." Give generously and give wisely. That's the tip for today.

Speech—Training the Tongue
Lecture 19

The link between the quality of language and the caliber of behavior is widely recognized; our words have an undeniable effect on the way we think and act. The skillful use of language involves not simply refraining from using false speech but also giving mindful attention to what we say and how we say it. Thoughtful, wholesome language can be the bearer of our compassion. The book of Proverbs reminds us: "Thoughtless words cut like a sword. But the tongue of the wise brings healing."

Wholesome Speech and Skillful Communication

- The Buddha devoted much of his teaching to the practice of skillful communication and offered very cogent ideas to guide our efforts to use language in the most beneficial ways possible.

- The Buddha taught that skillful speech should be truthful, compassionate, gentle, and edifying. When our words have all these qualities, we can know that our use of language is wholesome and conducive to the end of suffering. However, attaining these qualities is no mean feat.

- Speaking the truth is the basic condition for skillful speech, yet it is a fundamental qualification that many of us find difficult to observe. Most of us are quite capable of telling flat-out falsehoods if we think we can benefit by them, and some of us would tell them frequently if we thought we wouldn't be caught.

- Even when we don't go so far as to tell bald-faced lies, we often embellish and stretch the truth to suit our own desires. These forms of false speech can become so habitual that we even fail to recognize when they leave our lips.

The Buddha's Criteria for Wholesome Speech

- Because we're often mindless about the truthfulness of our utterances, it behooves us to pay careful attention to the content of what we say. The Buddha prescribed a simple procedure for ensuring we're speaking the truth.

Truthful Speech

- As a matter of practice, we can carefully monitor our words with mindfulness by paying attention to make sure our words comport with what we know to be true and by refraining from pretending we know when in fact we don't. We can use that same practice to help us better understand our propensity to speak falsely.

- After you observe yourself deviating from or exaggerating the truth, use your sitting practice to examine the antecedent causes underlying what you've said. If we look diligently, we'll usually find the illusion of the self lurking in there somewhere.

- The fear that often motivates a falsehood can arise from the belief that we need to appear a certain way, which is, of course, a basic expression of the ego. Likewise, embellishing the truth can serve to make ourselves seem more interesting and perhaps more important than we really are.

- As you're investigating the causes for any instances of false speech, reflect as well on the consequences. Study the effects of failing to be truthful. Take special note of the ways that dishonesty causes you to suffer.

- Whereas truthfulness is a necessary condition for skillful speech, it is not by any means the sole criterion. Just because something is truthful does not mean we should say it. Truth must be spoken compassionately. The manner in which truth is communicated is of great importance in the practice of skillful speech.

- To the provision of truthfulness, the Buddha added that wholesome speech should be delivered in a timely manner in a way that benefits the listener. For instance, we sometimes find ourselves in conversations when we have a piece of truthful information to offer, but we recognize that this particular occasion is not the best time or place to share it.

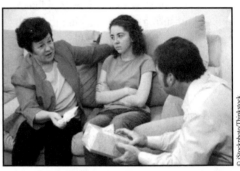

The effort to make hurtful assertions under the veil of truth still has the objective to harm.

- It might be something that is better imparted privately with the person it concerns or perhaps it's a point that needs to be said when the individual it concerns is in the proper frame of mind to receive it. In any event, it's best to maintain silence until conditions are better suited for compassionate communication.

- The Buddha made a point of saying, however, that compassionate communication does not depend on whether or not one's words would be welcomed by the hearer. If what one had to say were true, beneficial, and timely, the Buddha recommended that one speak— whether or not others would find those words agreeable.

- In short, being compassionate does not mean saying what others want to hear. It means speaking the truth in a kind of way that can help bring relief from suffering. Sometimes, the recipient may find even a compassionately delivered truth unwelcome, yet for the sake of being compassionate, one must find a way to say it.

- When hard, truthful messages have to be given, it's crucial to be clear about intent. Always ask yourself: Why am I saying this? What am I really trying to accomplish with these words? It's easy for us to fool ourselves when it comes to conversing with others—just as it's easy to fool ourselves in our internal dialogue.

- There are those who believe that the truth must be spoken regardless of consequences. These are those who think of themselves as brutally honest, and they consider their candor a noble quality. Often, however, those who pride themselves on their brutal honesty seem to get more pleasure from being brutal than from being honest.

Compassionate Speech

- Efforts to make hurtful assertions under the veil of truth are nothing more than what the Buddha called **malicious speech**. A malicious statement may be either true or false, but its objective is to harm.

- Malicious speech has been around since shortly after the first human being uttered the first word. Lately, however, it seems to have gained a new dimension with the explosion of electronic media, which has created a distance between writers and the effects of their words.

- The personal distance, the opportunity for immediate response, and the frequent anonymity afforded by the Internet is a virtual invitation for many of us to disregard the principles of propriety and vent our spleens shamelessly.

Gentle Speech

- The Buddha's third criterion for wholesome speech is gentleness. Our words should be truthful, beneficial, and timely, and they should be spoken in a mild manner. This characterization thus excludes malicious speech and what the Buddha called harsh speech.

- Malicious speech has the clear intent of hurting others, but **harsh speech** may be hurtful without any real intent to be so. Harsh speech is usually thoughtless, although it can also be malicious at times.

- Harsh speech includes profanity, sarcasm, and shouting. Essentially, harsh speech is the use of language that shows little or no regard for the feelings of others.

- Avoiding harsh speech is the negative aspect of speaking gently. The positive side involves choosing kind words and speaking them clearly and soothingly. Gentle speech means offering sincere compliments to others, helping to facilitate constructive discussion, and listening mindfully to what others have to say.

- Gentleness of speech can also mean keeping silent so that others may be heard or simply to allow high emotions to settle. The equanimity that we cultivate as we continue mindfulness practice helps us speak our words with mildness.

Edifying Speech

- Finally, the Buddha urges that our speech serve a constructive purpose. This is what is meant when we say that our words should edify. Unless our words work to provide us some real benefit, it's best to keep quiet. When a wise word can help, though—when it can ease suffering or open us to new insight—speaking is a blessing.

- Like gentleness, edifying speech has both a negative and a positive aspect. The negative side is those expressions of language that are best to avoid. The Buddha called these forms of speech **idle chatter**—the verbal equivalent of stuff, or unnecessary material possessions. It's generic, inessential language whose basic purpose is to fill airspace.

- Idle chatter often arises because silence seems so threatening. It's interesting that the English language has a great many words to describe idle chatter. They include: babble, blab, drivel, gab, jabber, jive, prattle, yakking, twaddle, and running off at the mouth.

- The most invidious form of idle chatter goes by the name of gossip, which is so pervasive that it's hard to imagine life without it. It seems almost natural to want to know about the intimate details of the lives of others.

- The phenomenon of gossip is complex, serving many functions and deriving from many causes. Certainly, part of the reason gossip is so appealing is that it lets individuals monitor social situations so they can relate to others accordingly. Sharing gossip with friends may even be a form of bonding. At least in a few ways, then, gossip may serve some important purposes.

- The perilous aspect of gossip, however, is the way it easily becomes vicious. Even when information is true, gossip has a way of shaping the truth in a negative fashion.

- Deep within most of us is the hidden—and sometimes not so hidden—capacity to enjoy hearing about the misfortunes of others, even those to whom we're close.

- What's really sad, of course, is the way that malicious gossip can cause suffering. There is now growing evidence to indicate that many teen suicides in this country have been prompted, at least in part, by vicious rumors spread by word of mouth and especially through social networks on the Internet. Perhaps less apparent is the effect of gossiping on those who perpetuate it.

- While it may be true that gossip serves some useful social functions, we ought to give thought to whether or not those functions might be better served by other, more benign means. Even when it is not malicious, idle chatter in its various forms can be a colossal waste of precious time.

Meditation and Wholesome Speech

- Wholesome speech, as taught in the Buddhist mindfulness tradition, is truthful, compassionate, gentle, and edifying. We can remember these qualities if we think of them as simple questions to ask ourselves before we speak: Why do I want to say this? Is what I want to say completely true? Will what I say result in benefit or harm? Is now the right time to say it? How may I say it to be most beneficial and effective?

- Practicing loving-kindness meditation predisposes us to being more compassionate, cultivating a frame of mind in which matters such as the effect of our words are already a prime concern. Long before we engage in conversation, our hearts are attuned to speaking compassionately.

- Sitting and walking meditation also play important roles in shaping skillful speech. These practices, of course, sharpen our skills of observation and moment-to-moment awareness. Using these techniques allows us give close attention not only to what is said but also to how we respond emotionally, mentally, and physically.

- A refined ability to monitor our own internal states makes it possible for us to avoid knee-jerk reactions and provides us with enough mental space to be more deliberate about how we respond.

- Getting to this level of self-awareness and discipline, of course, requires a great deal of practice, but learning to create a spacious mind is a powerful ally in learning to use speech skillfully. It is also an especially valuable technique in working with anger.

Important Terms

harsh speech: Speech that may be hurtful without any real intent to be so; the use of language that shows little or no regard for the feelings of others. It is usually thoughtless and includes profanity, sarcasm, and shouting.

idle chatter: Generic, inessential language whose basic purpose is to fill airspace; it is the verbal equivalent of unnecessary material possessions.

malicious speech: The Buddhist term for the practice of making hurtful assertions under the veil of truth. A malicious statement may be either true or false, but its objective is to harm.

Questions to Consider

1. What are your usual first reactions to an abusive comment? Anger, fear, or shock? What do you usually do, say, and think? Are your responses as skillful as you would like? If not, how can more skillful means be cultivated?

2. What qualities of wholesome speech—truthful, compassionate, gentle, and edifying—are most difficult for you to observe and why?

Speech—Training the Tongue
Lecture 19—Transcript

In 2011, six people were killed and 13 wounded near Tucson, Arizona, during an assassination attempt on the life of Rep. Gabrielle Giffords. In the immediate aftermath of that tragedy, many across the country connected the shooting to the level of political rhetoric at the time, which had, in their opinion, dropped well below the standards of civility and propriety.

As it turned out, there was no conclusive evidence to indicate a causal relationship between the terrible event in Tucson and the nature of public discourse in the country. But the fact that such an association was immediately and plausibly proposed as a factor in the violence indicates that the link between the quality of language and the caliber of behavior is widely recognized. Our words have an undeniable effect on the way we think and act. If unwholesome public speech can shape individual behavior in negative ways, imagine the even greater consequences of daily conversation.

Early in the series, we discussed the importance of refraining from false speech as a prerequisite to beginning meditation practice. We talked briefly about the value of curtailing harmful language to reduce the suffering of others and to promote a calm spirit conducive to the practice of mindfulness. Now that we've examined the basic components of the practice, we're in a better position to return to the subject of speech and give it a closer and more thorough consideration. We'll explore how the skillful use of language involves not simply refraining from using false speech but also giving mindful attention to what we say and how we say it. Thoughtful, wholesome language can be the bearer of our compassion. The book of Proverbs reminds us: "Thoughtless words cut like a sword. But the tongue of the wise brings healing."

Before we undertake the disciplines to cultivate the habits of wholesome speech, it's important to have a clear idea about what actually characterizes skillful communication. The Buddha devoted much of his teaching to this practice and offered very cogent ideas to guide our efforts to use language in the most beneficial ways possible. He taught that skillful speech should be truthful, compassionate, gentle, and edifying. When our words have all these qualities, we can know that our use of language is wholesome and conducive to the end of suffering. But attaining these qualities, we hardly need to be reminded, is no mean feat. "More difficult than all other acts," said the ancient Greek philosopher Pythagoras, "is the art of mastering one's own tongue."

Speaking the truth is the basic condition for skillful speech, yet it is a fundamental qualification that many of us find difficult to observe. Most of us—dare I say all of us?—are quite capable of telling flat-out falsehoods if we think we can benefit by them, and some of us would tell them frequently if we thought we wouldn't get caught. Even when we don't go so far as to tell bald-faced lies, we often embellish and stretch the truth to suit our own desires. These forms of false speech can become so habitual that we even fail to recognize when they leave our lips. Because we're often mindless about the truthfulness of our utterances, it behooves us to pay careful attention to the content of what we say. The Buddha prescribed a simple procedure for ensuring we're speaking the truth. In a discourse, he explains how to speak in a court of law if one were ever required to give testimony. He said,

> When questioned as a witness thus, "So, good man, tell what you know": knowing, [the truthful person] says, "I know"; not knowing, he says, "I do not know"; not seeing he says, "I do not see"; or seeing, he says "I see"; he does not in full awareness speak falsehood for his own ends, or another's ends, or for some trifling worldly end.

This formula is seems so simple that it's practically trivial, and it would be trivial if not for the fact that we so routinely fail to follow it. As a matter of practice, we can carefully monitor our words with mindfulness we're developing in our daily meditation practice. We pay attention to make sure our words comport with what we know to be true, and we refrain from pretending that we know when in fact we don't. We can use that same practice to help us better understand our propensity to speak falsely. After you observe yourself deviating from or exaggerating the truth, use your sitting practice to examine the antecedent causes underlying what you've said. If we look diligently, we'll usually find the illusion of the self lurking in there somewhere. The fear that often motivates a falsehood can arise from the belief that we need to appear a certain way, which is, of course, a basic expression of the ego. Likewise, embellishing the truth can serve to make ourselves seem more interesting and perhaps more important than we really are. As you're investigating the causes for any instances of false speech, reflect as well on the consequences. Study the effects of failing to be truthful. Take special note of the ways that dishonesty causes you to suffer.

Whereas truthfulness is a necessary condition for skillful speech, it is not by any means the sole criterion. Just because something is truthful does not mean we should say it. Truth must be spoken compassionately. The manner in which truth is communicated is of great importance in the practice of skillful speech.

To the provision of truthfulness, the Buddha added that wholesome speech should be delivered in a timely manner in a way that benefits the listener. For instance, we sometimes find ourselves in conversations when we have a piece of truthful information to offer, but we recognize that this particular occasion is not the best time or place to share it.

It might be something that is better imparted privately with the person it concerns or perhaps it's a point that needs to be said when the individual it concerns is in the proper frame of mind to receive it. In any event, it's best to maintain silence until conditions are better suited for compassionate communication.

The Buddha made a point, however, that compassionate communication does not depend on whether or not one's words would be welcomed by the hearer. If what one had to say were true, beneficial, and timely, the Buddha recommended that one speak—whether or not others would find those words agreeable. In short, being compassionate does not mean saying what others want to hear. It means speaking the truth in a kind way that can help bring relief from suffering. Sometimes, the recipient may even find a compassionately delivered truth unwelcome. Yet, for the sake of being compassionate, one must find a way to say it. Such a situation might arise, for example, when a family decides to confront one of its members who has developed an addiction to alcohol or other drugs. No one said compassion would be easy.

When hard, truthful messages have to be given, it's crucial to be clear about intent. Always ask yourself: Why am I saying this? What am I really trying to accomplish with these words? It's easy for us to fool ourselves when it comes to conversing with others, just as it's easy to fool ourselves in our internal dialogue. There are those who believe that the truth must be spoken regardless of consequences. These are the folks who think of themselves as "brutally honest," and they consider their candor a noble quality. But often, those who pride themselves on their brutal honesty seem to get more pleasure from being brutal than from being honest.

A relatively new expression in urban slang has appeared that tries to make it easier for someone to make ostensibly honest statements without having to take any responsibility for the suffering it may cause. The phrase is two words: "Just sayin'." Ever hear something like this: "You know, you're a pompous, arrogant, depraved moron. Just sayin'." This clever expression found its way into American English as a method to disguise an opinion with the appearance of objectivity and allow the speaker to distance him- or herself from its consequences. If pressed, one can always say: "Oh, I'm just sayin'." I don't actually believe it. That's just what the other folks say." But the disguise is thin. It's easy to see how such an expression can be used with the intent to cause another person to suffer. "Just sayin' " takes place alongside the backhanded compliment and damning with faint praise as being subtle linguistic weapons of attack.

When I was a kid, we had the fourth grade equivalent of "just sayin'." It was called a "slam book." Here's how it worked. Someone took a spiral-bound notebook and wrote the name of each person in the class at the top of a single page. Then the notebook would be passed around the class, and everyone could anonymously write their true feelings about an individual under his or her name. Now, in the fourth grade, I had a fairly high opinion of myself, and I couldn't wait see what my classmates had to say about me. Naturally, I assumed that they all shared my own high opinions. I mean, how could they not?! When the book finally came my way, I was terribly excited to read all the great things they had to say about me. What I didn't expect, however, was that the slam book would be the start of a new trajectory in my education, a new direction that began when I had to go to the dictionary to look up the word "conceited." If I had paid a bit more attention, I might have given more thought to the name "slam book." Although it was intended to hurt, I have to admit the characterization was dead-on. It was undoubtedly the most important lesson I learned in fourth grade.

These efforts to make hurtful assertions under the veil of truth are nothing more than what the Buddha called "malicious speech." A malicious statement may be either true or false, but its objective is to harm. Malicious speech has been around since shortly after the first human uttered the first word. But lately, it seems to have gained a new dimension with the explosion of electronic media. Just as the expression "just sayin' " creates a distance between the speaker and the consequences of his speech, so too has electronic media created a distance between a writer and the effects of her words. People will say things on e-mail, blogs, Twitter, and Facebook that they would never dream of saying to a person face-to-face. The personal distance, the opportunity for immediate response, and the frequent anonymity afforded by the Internet is a virtual invitation for many of us to disregard the principles of propriety and vent our spleens shamelessly.

I'll share with you a simple rule I impose on myself to prevent me from sending something into cyberspace that I might later regret. Whenever I receive an e-mail that angers or offends me in some way, I refrain from responding for 24 hours. I'll often write a response in the heat of the moment, but keep myself from sending it until the next day. Later, I review the response to see if it says what I really want to say. In the cool light of morning, I almost always delete my hastily composed email. Wouldn't the Internet be a little nicer if everyone observed that rule?

The Buddha's third criterion for wholesome speech is gentleness. Our words should be truthful, beneficial, and timely, and they should be spoken in a mild manner. This characterization thus excludes malicious speech and what the Buddha called "harsh speech." Malicious speech has the clear intent of hurting others, but harsh speech may be hurtful without any real intent to be so. Harsh speech is usually simply thoughtless, although it can be malicious at times. It includes profanity, sarcasm, and shouting. I'd probably add some more things, such as trying to dominate a conversation or loudly using the cell phone in public places. Essentially, harsh speech is the use of language that shows little or no regard for the feelings of others.

I've struggled with some forms of harsh speech most of my life, a fact I blame on my Texas upbringing. I picked up the profanity habit during the same year as the slam book. For my friends and me, profanity was not something we ever thought harmful; in fact, I definitely enjoyed it. It was only decades later that I came to believe that cussing had a negative effect on my disposition. Some of my students, on the other hand, report that cursing makes them feel better or play better on the athletic field. I don't know. For me, that's not true.

Avoiding harsh speech is the negative aspect of speaking gently. The positive side involves choosing kind words and speaking them clearly and soothingly. Gentle speech means offering sincere compliments to others, helping to facilitate constructive discussion, and listening mindfully to what others have to say. Gentleness of speech can also mean keeping silent so that others may be heard or simply to allow high emotions to settle like the jar of muddy water. The equanimity that we cultivate as we continue mindfulness practice helps us speak our words with mildness.

Finally, the Buddha urges that our speech serve a constructive purpose. This is what is meant when we say that our words should edify. Unless our words work to provide us some real benefit, it's best to keep quiet. "It's hard to improve on silence," they say. But when a wise word can help, when it can ease suffering or open us to new insight, speaking is a blessing.

Like gentleness, edifying speech has both a negative and positive aspect. The negative side is those expressions of language that are best to avoid. The Buddha called these forms of speech "idle chatter." Idle chatter is the verbal equivalent of "stuff." It's generic, inessential language whose basic purpose is to fill air-space. Idle chatter often arises because silence seems so threatening. It's interesting that the English language has a great many words to describe idle chatter. They include, babble, blab, drivel, gab, jabber, jive, prattle, yakking, twaddle, and running off at the mouth.

But the most invidious form of idle chatter goes by the name of gossip— yes, gossip, one of our favorite national pastimes. Gossip is so pervasive that it's hard to imagine life without it. It seems almost natural to want to know about the intimate details of the lives of others. The phenomenon of gossip is complex, serving many functions and deriving from many causes. But certainly part of the reason gossip is so appealing is that it lets individuals monitor social situations so they can relate to others accordingly. Sharing gossip with friends may even be a form of bonding. So, at least in a few ways, gossip may serve some important purposes. The perilous aspect of gossip, however, is the way it easily becomes vicious. Even when information is true, gossip has a way of shaping the truth in a negative fashion. Deep within most of us is the hidden—and sometimes not so hidden—capacity to enjoy hearing about the misfortunes of others, even those to whom we're close.

What's really sad, of course, is the way that malicious gossip can cause suffering. There is now growing evidence to indicate that many teen suicides in this country have been prompted, at least in part, by vicious rumors spread by word-of-mouth and especially through social networks on the Internet. Perhaps less apparent is the effect of gossiping on those who perpetuate it. I invite you to contemplate these consequences for yourself. While it may be true that gossip serves some useful social functions, we ought to give thought to whether or not those functions might be better served by other, more benign means.

Even when it is not malicious, idle chatter in its various forms can be a colossal waste of time. I mentioned in an earlier lecture how I assign students in some of my courses to practice a day of mindful speech and abstaining from media. Almost invariably, they report an epiphany upon discovering how much time they spend on trivial things. I was astonished to learn that an average college student may check his or her Facebook account about 20 or 25 times a day. Then I really sobered up when I thought about how often I check my own e-mail.

Sorry, Facebook. I know it seems I'm picking on you in this series. I don't mean to single you out. It's just you've assumed iconic status in our culture, and that makes you an easy target. And it's not really about you, or e-mail, or Twitter, or even the Internet; you're simply the means—a medium. The problem lies deep within us.

Now we've covered the basic elements of wholesome speech as taught in the Buddhist mindfulness tradition. Such speech is truthful, compassionate, gentle, and edifying. We can remember these qualities if we think of them as simple questions to ask ourselves before we speak: Why do I want to say this? Is what I want to say completely true? Will what I say result in harm or benefit? Is now the right time to say it? How may I say it to be most beneficial and effective? These are important questions, but how do you run through this slate of queries in the midst of a conversation, when words are often exchanged at a pace that sometimes seems to exceed the speed of thought?

Here is where meditation helps. Practicing loving-kindness predisposes us to being more compassionate, cultivating a frame of mind in which matters, such as the effect of our words, are already a prime concern. Long before we engage in conversation, our hearts are attuned to speaking compassionately.

Sitting and walking meditation also play important roles in shaping skillful speech. These practices, of course, sharpen our skills of observation and moment-to-moment awareness. Using these techniques allows us to give close attention not only to what is said but also to how we respond emotionally, mentally, and physically. A refined ability to monitor our own internal states makes it possible for us to avoid knee-jerk reactions and provides us with enough mental space to be more deliberate about how we respond.

Getting to this level of self-awareness and discipline, of course, requires a great deal of practice, both on and off the cushion. But learning to create a spacious mind is a powerful ally in learning to use speech skillfully. It is also an especially valuable technique in working with anger. In our next talk, we'll delve deeper into the application of this skill as we spend more time on the subject of anger. I'll see you then.

Anger—Cooling the Fires of Irritation
Lecture 20

Anger is a complex human experience involving every feature of our being: our bodies, our minds, and our emotions. The mindfulness tradition regards anger as an unwholesome state of being that is both a cause and a manifestation of dukkha. Despite its negative quality, however, the tradition also sees anger as a potential ally in the realization of freedom from suffering. If we know how to handle it skillfully, anger has much to teach us and can point the way to new insights and more wholesome ways of living.

Anger and Suffering

- **Anger** can be defined as the feeling of displeasure, usually accompanied by antagonism. It encompasses a wide range of experiences from simple irritation and annoyance to rage and fury.

- Most of the time, we experience anger as unpleasant. Our heart rate and blood pressure can increase dramatically, and our muscles can become tense and spasmodic. Our emotions become raw, and our facial expression may contort. We are unable to think clearly.

- Anger can also be dangerous. Because it clouds our thoughts, it can incite us to act in ways we later regret. In a state of anger, we can easily say and do hurtful things and even take the life of another.

- Anger is a cause of much of the world's suffering. The mindfulness tradition reminds us, furthermore, that anger itself is a form of suffering. Those who inflict pain out of anger are also the sufferers of its torment.

- Like other forms of suffering, anger is closely connected to **attachment**, the way we cling to the various items of our experience as if we can't live without them. Anger often arises when something to which we're attached is threatened or is taken away from us.

- Although anger is considered an unwholesome state because it causes and manifests suffering, the experience of anger itself is not really a problem—or, perhaps, it doesn't have to be a problem.

- Anger is nothing more than an unpleasant feeling coupled with negative thoughts and certain bodily responses. The real problem with anger is how we react to those unpleasant feelings, thoughts, and sensations.

Anger and Mindlessness

- In mindlessness, we're liable to react to anger one of two basic ways. The first is to suppress the anger—to deny it and pretend it's not there. We can get so good at this technique that it becomes automatic, and we're not even aware of it.

- The other basic reaction is to express anger immediately. Like the subjective experience of anger, the expression of anger can take a wide range of forms. The reflexive expression of anger can also become habitual.

- Both ways of reacting to anger are usually conditioned by our upbringing and other circumstances, and both have potentially hazardous consequences. The suppression of anger may allow to us to feel composed and to avoid conflict—for a while, but this strategy doesn't work for long.

- Anger that is not given attention does not go away. Eventually, unacknowledged anger may turn to rage or cynicism, erupt in violent acts, or cast us into a pit of depression and despair.

- The reflexive expression of anger tends to be a more acceptable reaction in our culture, especially for men, and it's even endorsed by some schools of psychotherapy.

Anger and Mindfulness

- From the mindfulness point-of-view, the expression of anger—whether by word or deed—often ends up reinforcing negative states of mind, and it fails to address anger's deeper causes. Just as suppressing anger may afford a temporary respite from its unpleasantness, so too may expressing it.

- Neither suppression nor expression is genuinely effective at removing the potential perils of anger or its root causes. Hostility begets more hostility.

- With practice, it's possible to find a way beyond automatically suppressing anger or reflexively expressing it. The techniques for dealing with anger more appropriately are founded directly on the basic methods of meditation.

Responding to Anger Skillfully

- The first step in the process of responding skillfully to anger when it arises is being able to know when you're angry. Many of us simply cannot identify anger as it occurs.

- Meditation is an important instrument in learning to identify anger. Of key significance is the skill of nonjudgmental observation, the basic technique of watching what happens as it happens.

- In identifying anger, the skills we gain in the body scan meditation can help us monitor how our physical natures are responding in a difficult situation. Try to note the patterns of your physical responses that coordinate with the feelings of displeasure that suggest anger.

- Identifying anger is the first step. The second is accepting it. Because it can be such an unpleasant state, we often treat anger as we do other unwanted experiences: We try to distance ourselves from it as rapidly as possible.

- At this stage of aversion, our conditioned reflexes usually come into play. We immediately suppress or express our feelings as a way to get rid of them. Both reactions intend to accomplish the same thing: to bring relief to the unwelcome experience of displeasure.

- Mindfulness practice encourages us to approach all our experiences—wanted and unwanted—with equanimity. We try neither to cling to nor run away from our experiences, regardless of their quality.

- The aversion that results in the reflexive suppression or expression of anger, however, disturbs that equanimity. Rather than seeking to eliminate the unpleasantness of anger, the equanimous approach is to allow and accept it. We might even say we should welcome it.

- However, we must also be careful here. Acceptance doesn't mean that we necessarily want anger; that could be a form of desire that is just as dangerous as aversion. Anger can still be an unwanted experience—even when you accept it.

- Acceptance is simply the willingness to be attentive to our anger to see what it wants. Just observe and treat it compassionately. This allows you to experience anger as fully as possibly. The more completely you can feel anger, the less you will fear it. When we become familiar with anger, we're less apt to try to eliminate it when it arises.

- It is crucial to realize, however, that feeling anger is not the same as acting on it. Recognizing this distinction creates the mental spaciousness that allows us to be more conscious about how we choose to respond.

- In the mindless state, we react to anger reflexively, without conscious choice, but mindfulness allows us to make a deliberate decision about the course of action we should take in the face of anger.

- As we noted when discussing skillful speech, just because our anger may urge us to respond to an insult with another insult does not mean we have to do it. We're not obliged to follow this impulsive prompting.

- Instead, we can allow angry thoughts and sensations to arise and fall away, giving us the time to consider a more appropriate response. We may need to take time away from the heat of the moment to reflect on a wise response.

- It may be that after fully experiencing your anger and assessing your options, you choose to speak sharply. You might even return insult for insult. The difference is that you have made a choice and have not reacted by impulse.

- When you create space for reflection, you will be far less likely to act in a hostile way. Over time, the insights you gain through meditation and compassion exercises will reveal that antagonistic responses are never the most suitable ones.

- In rare instances, we might decide that the appropriate response to anger is to cause bodily harm to another person. What can make such a response appropriate is when it does not arise from self-centered desires and is not carried out with hostility.

Anger and Meditation

- Meditation not only helps us deal with our anger as it arises; it can also help us

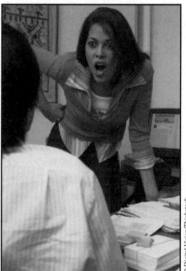

If you have difficulty knowing if you're angry, giving attention to your body is a good place to start.

cultivate a mind that is slow to anger, thus preparing us for anger before it arises.

- After practicing meditation for a significant period of time, you may begin to discover that you're less prone to getting angry, even though you've made no particular efforts to manage your anger. This occurs because our state of mind is an essential factor in determining whether or not we become angry.

- A properly cared for mind is less apt to respond to certain situations with anger—or, if it does, the degree of anger can be greatly lessened. Caring for the mind means giving it moment-to-moment attention, making an effort to keep thoughts wholesome, creating a mind of non-attachment, practicing moral integrity, and keeping the body as healthy as possible.

- Thus, one of the best ways for dealing with anger is to prevent it from arising in the first place by cultivating a mental field where it is difficult for the seeds of anger to germinate.

Studying Individual Patterns of Anger

- The process of caring for the mind is greatly enhanced by studying individual patterns of anger. Different things make different people angry.

- As you practice sitting meditation, you can study your anger experience. Make note of the things that contribute to your anger. Think about not only the things that make you mad but also the less obvious conditioning factors that might contribute to the provocation of anger.

- Anger has a lot to tell us about ourselves. Try to look beneath the anger and see what's there; it's often some kind of fear. Like pain, anger is a signal that something is wrong and needs to change.

- If we know how to experience it skillfully, anger can help us to make wholesome changes in ourselves and the society in which we live. The key is to not allow anger to develop into hostility or hatred; when that happens, anger becomes dangerous.

Working with Deep-Seated Anger

- Although we usually try to distance ourselves from anger as quickly as possible, sometimes we may find ourselves holding onto it. We can be averse to anger, but we can also get attached to it.

- Attachments to anger often manifest as grudges that we can carry for a long, long time. Life hurts us all, but some of us choose to dwell on those hurts and periodically renew their pain. As the Buddha recognized, nursing a grudge only serves to injure the one who bears it.

- The mindfulness approach to these old, festering forms of anger is forgiveness. Think of forgiveness as a form of relinquishment. To relinquish, in this sense, is to release whatever power anger holds over us.

- Forgiveness, in this sense, is rarely easy or quick. Because of its difficulty, forgiveness has to be practiced; it's less an act than a way of living. True forgiveness often comes only at the end of an inner struggle, and sometimes, it's a long one. Be wary of forgiving too quickly.

- We forgive others not so much to make them feel better, although it might. Rather, we forgive to be free—to liberate ourselves from the destructive power of anger and hatred. Holding a grudge rarely causes harm to the object of our anger, but it causes us a great deal.

- As the thoughts and feelings of anger arise, we observe them, acknowledge them, and allow them to pass away. We practice loving-kindness meditation, exercise empathy, and recognize the futility of seeking revenge. We also remember our own propensity to make mistakes. We repeat these techniques until our anger has been freed and we have been freed from its bondage.

Important Terms

anger: The feeling of displeasure, usually accompanied by antagonism; it encompasses a wide range of experiences from simple irritation and annoyance to rage and fury.

attachment: The way in which people cling to the various items of their experiences as if they can't live without them.

Questions to Consider

1. What patterns do you discern in your experiences of anger? What sorts of things evoke your anger? Do your reactions to anger follow specifiable habits? What do these patterns suggest about your beliefs about yourself?

2. In what ways does mindfulness offer more wholesome ways to respond to anger?

Anger—Cooling the Fires of Irritation
Lecture 20—Transcript

Like most parents, my wife and I surround ourselves with our young daughter's artwork. It's on display everywhere—the refrigerator, the living room walls, and in our offices.

But I keep one very special piece of her art on my desk where I can always see it. It's not a pretty picture, but to me, it's a masterpiece. Ariyana presented this particular drawing to me when she was about five, shortly after she witnessed an episode in which I allowed anger to get the better of me. The image, I was told, was me while I was angry. It looks like Edvard Munch's "The Scream," only scarier. As I said, it isn't a pretty picture, but I recognize it as a true rendering. I now keep the drawing near my work to remind of me of the dreadful consequences of succumbing to anger.

We all get angry. Anger is a complex human experience involving every feature of our being: our bodies, our minds, and our emotions. Because of its universality and complexity, theories about the causes and management of anger abound. The mindfulness tradition regards anger as an unwholesome state of being that is both a cause and a manifestation of *dukkha*. Yet despite its negative quality, the tradition also sees anger as a potential ally in the realization of freedom from suffering. If we know how to handle it skillfully, anger has much to teach us and can point the way to new insights and more wholesome ways of living.

Anger can be defined as the feeling of displeasure, usually accompanied by antagonism. It encompasses a wide range of experiences from simple irritation and annoyance on one end of the spectrum, all the way to rage and fury on the other. Most of the time, we experience anger as unpleasant. It feels bad. Our heart rate and blood pressure can increase dramatically, and our muscles can become tense and spasmodic. Our emotions get raw and set on edge, and we are unable to think clearly. Our facial expression may contort and our eyes bulge and glisten red. As my daughter's drawing reminds me, anger can make us look ugly.

Anger can also be dangerous. Because it clouds our thoughts, it can incite us to act in ways we later regret. In a state of anger, we can easily say and do hurtful things and even take the life of another. Anger is a cause of much of the world's suffering. The mindfulness tradition reminds us, furthermore, that anger itself is a form of suffering. Those who inflict pain out of anger are also the sufferers of its torment. "You will not be punished for your anger," the Buddha said, "you will be punished by your anger."

Like other forms of suffering, anger is closely connected to attachment, the way we cling to the various items of our experience as if we can't live without them. Anger often arises when something to which we're attached is threatened or taken away from us. If someone steals from me, my first response is likely anger. If I don't receive something I think I deserve, I get angry if I cling to the idea that I deserve it. If someone insults me, anger arises because a particular image of myself that I hold has been challenged. If I get angry when someone disagrees with me, I am most probably attached to an idea that I believe is true, or at least, attached to the idea that I must be right. If we look carefully at the roots of anger, we'll usually find something we're clutching.

Although anger is considered an unwholesome state because it causes and manifests suffering, the experience of anger itself is not really a problem— or perhaps I should say, it doesn't have to be a problem. Anger is really nothing more than an unpleasant feeling coupled with negative thoughts and certain bodily responses. The real problem with anger is how we react to those unpleasant feelings, thoughts, and sensations. In mindlessness, when we're not paying much attention, we're liable to react in one of two basic ways. The first is to suppress anger, to deny it and pretend it's not there. Our blood is boiling, but we keep smiling and telling ourselves and others that everything's all right. We can get so good at this technique that it becomes automatic, and we're not even aware of it. Suppressing anger becomes habitual when we grow up in an environment in which getting angry is considered unacceptable, shameful, or even immoral.

The other basic reaction is to express anger immediately. Like the subjective experience of anger, the expression of anger can take a wide range of forms.

We can fly off in a murderous rage, kick the cat, scream, curse, or do a hundred other things. The reflexive expression of anger can also become habitual.

Both ways of reacting to anger are usually conditioned by our upbringing and other circumstances, and both have potentially hazardous consequences. The suppression of anger may allow to us to feel composed and avoid conflict—for a while, but this strategy doesn't work for long. Anger that is not given attention does not go away. Eventually, unacknowledged anger may turn to rage or cynicism, erupt in violent acts, or may cast us into a pit of depression and despair. The reflexive expression of anger tends to be a more acceptable reaction in our culture, especially for men, and it's even endorsed by some schools of psychotherapy. But from the mindfulness point-of-view, the expression of anger, whether by word or deed, often ends up reinforcing negative states of mind, and it fails to address anger's deeper causes. Just as suppressing anger may afford a temporary respite from its unpleasantness, so too may expressing it. Screaming or punching a hole in the wall may bring momentary relief, but over time such behavior tends to get repeated. Hostility begets more hostility. Neither suppression nor expression is genuinely effective at removing the potential perils of anger or its root causes.

Mindfulness offers a third option. With practice, it's possible to find a way beyond automatically suppressing anger or reflexively expressing it. The techniques for dealing with anger more appropriately are founded directly on the basic methods of meditation. Let's look at how the skills developed in this practice can help us disarm anger and turn it into an ally that works to our benefit. We'll first consider how to respond to anger skillfully when it arises.

The first step in this process is being able to know when you're angry. Many of us simply cannot identify anger as it occurs. I know; I used to be one of those persons. It seems rather odd to me now, but for much of my life I had a hard time knowing when I was experiencing anger. Others would look at me and say, "You look mad. Is everything okay?" I'd respond by assuring them that I was just fine. An attachment to my self-image would not allow me to let on to others—or to myself—that I was really angry. No, I was too cool for that. It took a lot of introspection for me simply to be able to recognize anger within myself. And it took a lot of suffering before I was prompted—"forced" is probably a better word—to turn within.

Meditation was an important instrument in my learning to identify anger. Of key significance was the skill of nonjudgmental observation, the basic technique of watching what happens as it happens. Gradually, I began to know that when my breath became shallow, my neck and shoulders became tense, my heart rate increased, and my mind got muddled, I was getting angry. Sometimes, even now, I have to stop for a moment to see if I'm experiencing anger.

If you have difficulty knowing if you're angry, giving attention to your body is a good place to start. A lot of the idiomatic expressions related to anger are, with good reason, based on bodily experiences: "getting hot under the collar," "seeing red," "blowing your top," "foaming at the mouth," and "having your feathers ruffled." Here's where the skills we gain in the body scan meditation can help us monitor how our physical natures are responding in a difficult situation. Try to note the patterns of your physical responses that coordinate with the feelings of displeasure that suggest anger. With practice, carefully observing your body sensations will help you quickly recognize anger when it arises.

Identifying anger is the first step. The second is accepting it. Since it can be such an unpleasant state, we often treat anger as we do other unwanted experiences: We try to distance ourselves from it as rapidly as possible. This is aversion. It's at this stage that our conditioned reflexes usually come into play. We immediately suppress or express our feelings as a way to get rid of them. Both reactions intend to accomplish the same thing: to bring relief to the unwelcome experience of displeasure.

As we know by now, mindfulness practice encourages us to approach all our experiences—wanted and unwanted—with equanimity. We try neither to cling to nor to run away from our experiences. But the aversion that results in the reflexive suppression or expression of anger disturbs that equanimity. Rather than seeking to eliminate the unpleasantness of anger, the equanimous approach is to allow it and accept it. We might even say we should welcome it, just as the Buddha greeted Mara and invited him in for tea. But we must be careful here as well. By "acceptance" I don't mean to suggest that we necessarily want anger. That could be a form of desire that is just as dangerous as aversion. Anger can still be an unwanted experience, even when you accept it—like having the front doorbell ring just as you're sitting down for dinner. You're tired and hungry and the last thing you need is to face a stranger who wants something.

But you don't just pretend the person's not there. You have to accept the fact that you have an unexpected visitor. That doesn't mean you're pleased that your dinner has been interrupted. The kind thing to do is to ask what he wants. Maybe your caller has good news to share. Maybe he's there to warn you of some impending danger. Maybe he wants to tell you about his religion. Who knows? The same is true with anger. When it comes calling, just open the door. It may have something important to tell you, but how will you know if you don't answer? Acceptance is the willingness simply to be attentive to our anger to see what it wants. Just observe and treat it compassionately. This allows you to experience anger as fully as possibly. The more completely you can feel anger, the less you will fear it. When we become familiar with anger, we're less apt to try to eliminate it when it arises.

It is crucial to realize, however, that feeling anger is not the same as acting on it. Recognizing this distinction creates the mental spaciousness that allows us to be more conscious about how we choose to respond. In the mindless state, we react to anger reflexively, without conscious choice. But mindfulness allows us to make a deliberate decision about the course of action we should take in the face of anger. We noted in the previous lecture on skillful speech that just because our anger may urge us to respond to an insult with another insult does not mean we have to do it. We're not obliged to follow this impulsive prompting. We can allow angry thoughts and sensations to arise and fall away, giving us the time to consider a more appropriate response. We may need to take time away from the heat of the moment to reflect on a wise response.

It may be that after fully experiencing your anger and assessing your options, you choose to speak sharply. You might even return insult for insult. But the difference is that you have made a choice and have not reacted by impulse. I'm confident, however, that when you create the space for reflection, you will be far less likely to act in a hostile way. Over time, the insights you gain through meditation and compassion exercises will reveal that antagonistic responses are never the most suitable ones. In rare instances, we might decide that the appropriate response to anger is to cause bodily harm to another person. I can imagine a situation, for example, when we must physically hurt a violent oppressor who is causing harm to an innocent victim. What can make such a response appropriate is when it does not arise from self-centered desires and is not carried out with hostility. Our purpose in such a case is solely to render aid to the victim and not to hurt the perpetrator maliciously. To act this way means to separate anger from antagonism.

To sum up: When we find ourselves in a situation that provokes us to anger, the mindfulness approach encourages us to acknowledge our anger, accept it, experience its full dimensions, and respond to the situation wisely and compassionately.

Meditation not only helps us deal with our anger as it arises, it can also help us cultivate a mind that is slow to anger, thus preparing us for anger before it arises. After practicing meditation for a significant period of time, you may begin to discover that you're less prone to getting angry, even though you've made no particular efforts to manage your anger. This occurs because our state of mind is an essential factor in determining whether or not we become angry.

Let's say your air-conditioning unit breaks down in the heat of summer, and you get mad. Your anger is not simply caused by the malfunction of your air conditioning. Other factors contribute to the situation. For example, the fact that it's 95 degrees outside may have put you into an irritable state even before the air conditioning broke. You may have had an argument with a coworker earlier in the day and neglected to eat lunch because you were anxious to meet a deadline. These other factors condition your state of mind. Had they not been present, your reaction to the failure of the air conditioning may have been quite different. What if earlier in the day you had received a nice promotion and a raise and had celebrated at a nice lunch? Now the malfunction doesn't seem to be such a big deal. It might be an inconvenience, but it's nothing that warrants getting upset. The condition of our mind at any given moment thus influences whether or not we get angry and helps determine the intensity of our response.

Because hundreds of things contribute to our mental state at any given moment, it is essential to take time to care of our mind at all times. A properly cared for mind is less apt to respond to certain situations with anger, or, if it does, the degree of anger can be greatly lessened. By "caring for the mind," I mean giving it moment-to-moment attention, making an effort to keep thoughts wholesome, creating a mind of non-attachment, practicing moral integrity, and keeping the body as healthy as possible. All of these factors shape the mind and hence shape our experience. Thus, one of the best ways for dealing with anger is to prevent it from arising in the first place by cultivating a mental field where it is difficult for the seeds of anger to germinate.

The process of caring for the mind is greatly enhanced by studying our patterns of anger. Different things make different people angry. As you practice sitting meditation, you can study your anger experience. Make note of the things that contribute to your anger. Think about not only the things that make you mad but also the less obvious conditioning factors that might contribute to the provocation of anger. You may notice a greater tendency to get mad when you're hungry or tired. Anger, as I suggested, has a lot to tell us about ourselves. Try to look beneath the anger and see what's there. It's often some kind of fear. Use your mindful curiosity to investigate. Like pain, anger is a signal that something is wrong. It's an indication that something needs to change. Karl Marx called anger the "revolutionary emotion." If we know how to experience it skillfully, anger can help us to make wholesome changes in ourselves and the society in which we live. The key is not to allow anger to develop into hostility or hatred; when that happens, anger becomes dangerous.

We've discussed how mindfulness may help us respond to anger appropriately after it arises and how mindfulness may serve to make us slow to anger before it arises. Now let's consider the role of mindfulness in working with anger that's been around for a while, the kind that hasn't been treated properly. Although we usually try to distance ourselves from anger as quickly as possible, sometimes we may find ourselves holding onto it. We can be averse to anger, but we can also get attached to it. A friend of mine used to tell how his mother would get mad for some reason and resist any efforts by the other members of the family to reconcile with her. She'd turn down any conciliatory gestures and say, "No, I'd rather be angry!"

Such attachments to anger often manifest as grudges that we can carry for a long, long time. The Buddha spoke of the suffering caused by grudges. He said: *"I've been insulted!"* *"I've been hurt!"* *"I've been beaten!"* *"I've been robbed!"* Anger and hatred never cease for those who dwell on such thoughts. Life hurts us all, but some of us choose to dwell on those hurts and periodically renew their pain. But as the Buddha recognized, nursing a grudge only serves to injure the one who bears it.

The mindfulness approach to these old, festering forms of anger is forgiveness. But don't think of forgiveness solely in the narrow sense of granting pardon to someone who has offended you. Think of it as a form of relinquishment. To relinquish in this sense is to release whatever power anger holds over us. If I forgive someone for a wrong done to me, I no longer allow that offense to determine how I treat the other person. I may remember the wrong or I may forget it, but either way I have disarmed it. It no longer determines my actions, thoughts, or words.

Forgiveness in this sense is rarely easy or quick. We often say we "forgive" another person, but secretly we may still bear a grudge against him or her. Because of its difficulty, forgiveness has to be practiced. It's less an act than a way of living, a discipline, a cultivated skill. I think this is why Jesus told his students to forgive "70 times 7." True forgiveness often comes only at the end of an inner struggle, and sometimes, it's a long one. Be wary of forgiving too quickly.

We forgive others not so much to make them feel better, although it might. Rather, we forgive to be free, to liberate ourselves from the destructive power of anger and hatred. Holding a grudge rarely causes harm to the object of our anger, but it causes us a great deal. Of course, it's a lot easier to nourish the thoughts of indignation. Sometimes it's hard to surrender the delicious feeling that we've suffered unfairly. But ultimately those thoughts do us no good. We might wallow in our hurt feelings, but, really, what's the point of that? How much better it is to let them go, to follow the discipline of relinquishment. It's the harder path, to be sure, but in the end the rewards are worth it. Forgiveness is a gift we give to ourselves.

Pain—Embracing Physical Discomfort
Lecture 21

P ain, like everything else, is transient. The two guided meditations that we'll experience in this lecture are designed to give you an experiential acquaintance with the basic techniques for working with pain mindfully. These exercises will help you release your anger toward pain and accept your situation in moments of pain. As a result of these practices, you might be less inclined to feel pity for yourself by thinking your situation of pain is unfair. Throughout the world, at every moment of every hour, millions of people endure great pain. Pain is a fact of life.

Responding to Pain

- To be embodied means to be vulnerable to pain. Because of our physical nature, we are susceptible to viruses and bacteria, head-on collisions, slipping on icy sidewalks, random violence, heart attacks, beestings, and tsunamis.

- Even if by some miracle we escape the pain associated with disease and injury, we must still face the pain of getting old and watching our body wear out. Pain is a fact of life.

- Our typical response to pain is aversion. We simply don't want it, and we seek to avoid painful experiences as much as possible. As we've noted, however, aversion is an unwise strategy for living.

- Because pain is a fact of life, feverishly trying to separate ourselves from it is tantamount to separating ourselves from life itself. Instead, it is important to accept pain and other unwanted experiences as part of the greater affirmation of living life to its fullest extent.

- Mindfulness practice is a way to teach ourselves how to accept life as it is—in both its sweetness and its dreadfulness. Because pain is an immense, and often terrifying, component of life's dreadfulness, learning to respond to it in a wholesome way is an essential part of fully embracing life.

Pain versus Suffering

- Central to the mindfulness approach to pain is grasping the distinction between pain and suffering. In this tradition, pain is understood to be a name we give to a range of unpleasant sensations because what constitutes pain is highly subjective.

- Pain is usually an indication that some facet of our being requires attention. In those cases, of course, we should seek out any medical intervention that may reduce or eliminate the sensations of pain and address its root causes.

- In principle, the mindfulness tradition has no reluctance about using medication or other medical procedures to diminish pain, but it does urge us to use wisdom when doing so.

- Sometimes medication used to diminish pain can be addictive or can hinder us from seeking out the deeper causes of our distress. Sometimes medication and intervention is simply ineffective. In these cases, coping with pain by mindfulness is helpful.

- Mindfulness is perhaps an even greater ally in dealing with suffering. Suffering in this context occurs when the mind responds negatively to the sensations it identifies as pain. It's not always easy to distinguish pain from suffering.

- This distinction is important because the mindfulness tradition considers pain to be inevitable—an inescapable part of life as we know it. Suffering, on the other hand, is regarded as optional.

- In the case of pain, what generates suffering is resistance, which means wanting this moment to be other than it actually is. Resisting pain can take many forms, including responding with fear and panic, with anger, and with hatred—all of which are types of aversion.

- The more we resist the pain that is undeniably present, the greater our suffering—and the greater our suffering, the more likely we are to act in unskillful ways.

- The key to diminishing the suffering that we usually connect to physical pain is acceptance. Acceptance means confronting unwanted pain without fear or hatred. In the following guided exercises, we'll begin to work with our pain by learning to accept it for what it is, to greet it with compassion, and inquire about what it may have to teach us.

Preparing for Guided Meditations

- The following guided meditations offer instructions on ways to work with pain. Feel free to participate whether or not you are currently experiencing pain. It's beneficial to learn to work with milder forms of physical distress before trying to apply mindfulness techniques to pain's stronger manifestations.

- Before you begin these exercises, remember that it's important to let go of any attachments you may have to attaining specific results with these exercises—especially because pain is a complex phenomenon, and our responses to it are deeply conditioned.

- Accordingly, we shouldn't expect significant changes initially. The results of these exercises may become apparent only after a significant period of practice.

- Furthermore, meditating on pain may never remove the unpleasant sensations you must live with. That is simply an unrealistic hope. However, scientific studies do support the view that diligent mindfulness practice can significantly ameliorate the suffering associated with pain.

Pain and Awareness

- In the same way as you would prepare for sitting practice or a body scan, choose whichever posture you find most comfortable and most conducive to alertness. As always, make sure your environment is quiet and free from distractions.

- This first exercise is designed simply to direct your attention to the pain and allow you to feel the sensation as much as possible. Rather than trying to take our mind off the pain, in this meditation, we'll be bringing our awareness right into the painful sensation and staying with it.

- First, make sure your body is in its proper position. Make yourself as comfortable as possible, but stay alert. You may keep your eyes open or closed, as you prefer.

- Begin by taking several deep breaths, and gently bring your awareness to the sensation of breathing. With each inhale and each exhale, allow your body to settle into a deeper state of relaxation. As your body becomes more at ease, your attention becomes more focused on this present moment.

- Now, allow your attention to range throughout your body and let it alight on that part that seems most in distress at this moment. It may be an area of mild discomfort or a part that seems to be in a fair amount of pain. Once you've made your selection, stay with that area for the remainder of the exercise.

- Let your awareness approach the area slowly and cautiously. You may be a bit apprehensive about focusing your attention on this location. Sometimes we're afraid to look at painful places too closely for fear that we might be overwhelmed by unpleasant sensations or by frightening thoughts about what might be causing the pain. If you detect this sort of resistance, softly note it to yourself, let it go, and proceed.

- Your purpose is simply to observe. You're making no judgments about the pain. You have no intention to change it in any way. You neither want it to leave nor to stay. You merely want the pain to be what it is and to give it the attention it deserves.

- Let your attention come as close to the pain as possible. If your resistance to getting close becomes too great, you can always escort your awareness back to the breath and try later. When you're ready, give the painful area your full awareness and observe it with kindhearted curiosity. Silently note your observations.

- Try to define the region that feels painful. Try to gain a sense of the contours of the painful area. Observe how deeply the pain goes into your body. Imagine a three-dimensional model of your pain.

- Then, consider how you might describe the quality of your pain. Pain is experienced in a wide range of ways, and its descriptive vocabulary is immense. Choose the words that make the most sense to you. It may be, however, simply indescribable.

- Now, examine the dynamics of the pain. Most of the time, pain is changing, although it's not always easy to detect this change. Consider if the pain is fluctuating in its intensity.

- For the next few moments, simply keep your awareness on the painful area, and remain keenly observant of the sensations you feel. This time, avoid labeling the sensations and simply feel them.

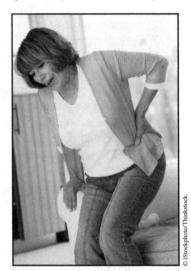

© iStockphoto/Thinkstock.

The key to diminishing the suffering that we usually connect to physical pain is acceptance.

- Now, try to become aware of your awareness of the pain. That may sound a little paradoxical, but it can be done. Simply watch yourself as you're observing your painful sensations. As you do so, see if your awareness is in pain.

- If you can become an observer of your own awareness, you may discover a place where there is no pain. Dwelling in this awareness may help mitigate the painful sensations in your body.

- You're no longer a person in pain but someone observing a person in pain. Being in this observing space may allow you to see that your pain is not you, and you are not your pain. Staying in this particular place of awareness is not easy, and it takes practice to do so—just as it takes practice to remain focused on the breath.

- Now, let's return to the breath and draw this exercise to a close. Let your attention come back to your breathing for a few moments.

- Reflect on your experience with the practice we've just completed. Did you notice any initial resistance to turning your attention to the painful area in your body? If so, what thoughts or emotions lay underneath that resistance? If you were able to give your pain a fuller attention, how did you mind respond?

Pain and Thinking

- In this second exercise, we'll incorporate more of the thinking process into the practice. It's not necessary to perform this exercise immediately after the one we've just completed; you can spend more time working with the first exercise before trying this one.

- First, take your position in the posture of your choice. Begin as you always do by relaxing your body and focusing on your inhalations and exhalations. Direct your attention to your breath, and stay attentive to what is occurring moment by moment.

- Now, permit your awareness to range over your entire body, and let it come to rest at the place of greatest discomfort. Be attentive to this location and observe the character of the sensations there as you did before.

- After you've had a chance to be aware of these sensations, turn your attention to your thoughts. Has the attention you've given this area of your body generated any mental commentary? If so, notice the character of those thoughts.

- As you become aware of these thoughts, try to relinquish them. See if you can distinguish the sensations from your thoughts about the sensations. Try to anchor your awareness in the bodily sensations alone. If a thought arises, simply observe and let it fall away.

- After some practice, see if remaining focused on the sensations and dropping thoughts alleviates the discomfort.

- Now, let's return to the breath and draw this exercise to a close. Let your attention come back to your breathing for a few moments.

- The intention of the exercise we've just concluded was to investigate the role of thinking in the experience of pain. Essentially, we wanted to see if our conditioned thought patterns worsened the unpleasant sensations we call pain.

- Next time, try to minimize any negative commentary to see if that helps. Imagine experiencing the sensation without labeling it as pain. How do you think that would change your experience?

Questions to Consider

1. Examine your history with pain. What attitudes toward pain have you developed? What habits have you created for coping with it?

2. In your experience, which strategy do you find more helpful: giving full attention to the manifestation of pain or trying to divert attention away from it?

Pain—Embracing Physical Discomfort
Lecture 21—Transcript

To be embodied means to be vulnerable to pain. Because of our physical nature, we are susceptible to viruses and bacteria, head-on collisions, slipping on icy sidewalks, random violence, heart attacks, bee-stings, and tsunamis.

Even if by some miracle we escape the pain associated with disease and injury, we must still face the pain of getting old and watching our body wear out. Pain is a fact of life.

Our typical response to pain is aversion. We simply don't want it, and we seek to avoid painful experiences as much as possible. But as we've noted many times before, aversion is an unwise strategy for living. Because pain is a fact of life, feverishly trying to separate ourselves from it is tantamount to separating ourselves from life itself.

Rainer Maria Rilke, the great Bohemian poet, suffered a long, painful illness toward the end of his life. Only just before he died was the disease diagnosed as leukemia. In a letter to a friend, he spoke of the importance of accepting pain and other unwanted experiences as part of the greater affirmation of living life to its fullest extent: "Whoever does not, sometimes or other, give his full consent, his full and joyous consent to the dreadfulness of life, can never take possession of the unutterable abundance and power of our existence."

Rilke's observation is profound, yet we find it difficult to walk the path he sets before us. How do we give full consent to the dreadfulness of life? Mindfulness practice is one way to take the course that Rilke recommends. It is a way to teach ourselves how to accept life as it is, in both its sweetness and its dreadfulness. And since pain is an immense, and often terrifying, component of life's dreadfulness, learning to respond to it in a wholesome way is an essential part of fully embracing life.

Central to the mindfulness approach to pain is grasping the distinction between pain and suffering. In this tradition, pain is understood to be a name we give to a range of unpleasant sensations. What constitutes pain is highly subjective. What hurts one person may not hurt another. Researchers are studying possible ways to identify and measure pain objectively using medical imaging, but currently the standard practice remains asking patients to self-assess their pain on a scale of 1 to 10.

Pain is usually an indication that some facet of our being requires attention. In those cases, of course, we should seek out any medical intervention that may reduce or eliminate the sensations of pain and address its root causes. In principle, the mindfulness tradition has no reluctance about using medication or other medical procedures to diminish pain, but it does urge us to use wisdom when so doing. Sometimes medication used to diminish pain can be addictive or can hinder us from seeking out the deeper causes of our distress. Sometimes medication and intervention is simply ineffective. In these cases, coping with pain by mindfulness is helpful.

Mindfulness is perhaps an even greater ally in dealing with suffering. Suffering in this context occurs when the mind responds negatively to the sensations it identifies as pain. It's not always easy to distinguish pain from suffering, but in the exercises we'll practice later, we'll try to do just that.

This distinction is important because the mindfulness tradition considers pain to be inevitable, an inescapable part of life as we know it. Suffering, on the other hand, is regarded as optional. According to the traditional narrative, the Buddha's enlightenment did not eradicate his experience of pain. Although he attained nirvana—the complete absence of suffering—the Buddha still got sick, got old, and died. He had pain for the remainder of his life, but he did not suffer as a consequence. The Buddha's story tells us—and the mindfulness tradition affirms—that we can greatly reduce the suffering associated with pain and even remove it altogether.

In the case of pain, what generates suffering is resistance, which means wanting this moment to be other than it actually is. Resisting pain can take many forms: It can be responding with fear and panic, with anger, and with hatred—all of which are types of aversion. All of these emotions express the desire to turn away from pain and distance ourselves from it. The more we resist the pain that is undeniably present in this moment, the greater our suffering; and the greater our suffering, the more likely we are to act in unskillful ways.

The key to diminishing the suffering that we usually connect to physical pain is acceptance, or what Rilke calls "full and joyous consent." Like anger, pain shows up at the door as an unwanted visitor. Acceptance means answering the door without fear or hatred. In the exercises that I'll describe shortly, we'll begin to work with our pain by learning to accept it for what it is, to greet it with compassion, and to inquire about what it may have to teach us.

The following guided meditations offer instructions on ways to work with pain. I invite you to participate in these exercises whether or not you are currently experiencing a sensation that you would identify as pain. Chances are that you are having some sort of physical discomfort, and you can treat that as you would the more intense sensation you refer to as pain. It's a good idea to learn to work with milder forms of physical distress before applying mindfulness techniques to pain's stronger manifestations. Pain can sometimes be so debilitating that it's almost impossible to introduce these methods while the sensation is occurring.

Before you begin these exercises, let me reiterate some of the standard caveats you should always bear in mind when you engage in mindfulness practice. It's important to let go of any attachments you may have to attaining specific results with these exercises. You may want a particular outcome, but to expect it is to court disappointment. Expectation is a form of attachment, and it can set the groundwork for suffering if things don't turn out the way we anticipated. Giving up expectations is especially important in working with pain. Pain is a complex phenomenon, and our responses to it are deeply conditioned.

Accordingly, we shouldn't expect significant changes initially. Working with pain, like the other practices we've discussed, requires discipline and regular implementation. The results of these exercises may become apparent only after a significant period of practice. Furthermore, meditating on pain may never remove the unpleasant sensations you must live with. That is simply an unrealistic hope. But scientific studies do support the view that diligent mindfulness practice can significantly ameliorate the suffering associated with pain. Although unrealistic expectations may contribute to greater anguish, it is important to remain open to serendipity. The mind, as we're constantly rediscovering, is capable of amazing things.

You'll prepare for these meditations in the same way as you would for sitting practice or a body scan. Choose whichever posture you find most comfortable and most conducive to alertness. If you decide to lie down, as with a body scan, make sure you have pillows, blankets, or any other props to help you become as relaxed as possible. As always, make sure your environment is quiet and free from distractions.

I will guide you through two exercises to provide a basis for your future work with pain. The exercises are similar to one another, but each has a different focus. In the first, we'll work primarily with the mental function of awareness. I'll direct you to become as deeply aware of pain as possible. This approach is at odds with our usual tendency to avoid painful sensations, but research indicates that becoming fully cognizant of pain, particularly chronic pain, is a more helpful method of reducing the suffering associated with pain. The second practice concentrates on the mental function of thinking. I'll invite you to observe your thoughts about the sensation of pain and reflect on how those thoughts condition your experience. You may discover that the way you think about painful sensations can significantly alter your experience. After you've completed these exercises, you may practice them on your own at any time or return to the lecture and let me guide you through them again.

The first exercise is designed simply to direct your attention to the pain and allow you to feel the sensation as much as possible. Rather than trying to take our mind off the pain, as we frequently do, in this meditation we'll be bringing our awareness right into the painful sensation and staying with it.

Now make sure your body is in its proper position, whether that's sitting on a chair or a cushion or lying on the floor or some other surface. Make yourself as comfortable as possible, but stay alert. You may keep your eyes opened or closed, as you prefer.

Begin by taking several deep breaths and gently bring your awareness to the sensation of breathing. With each in-breath and each out-breath, allow your body to settle into a deeper state of relaxation. As your body becomes more at ease, your attention becomes more focused on this present moment.

Your only concern is just now, breathing in and breathing out, moment by moment, breath by breath.

Now allow your attention to range throughout your body and let it alight on that part that seems most in distress at this moment. It may be an area of mild discomfort or a part that seems to be in a fair of amount of pain. Take a moment to locate that region. Once you've made your selection, stay with that area for the remainder of the exercise.

Let your awareness approach the area slowly and cautiously. You may be a bit apprehensive about focusing your attention on this location. Sometimes we're afraid to look at painful places too closely for fear that we might be overwhelmed by unpleasant sensations or frightened by thoughts about what might be causing the pain. If you detect this sort of resistance, softly note it to yourself, let it go, and proceed. Your purpose here is simply to observe. You're making no judgments about the pain. You have no intention to change it in any way. You neither want it to leave or to stay. You merely want the pain to be what it is and to give it the attention it deserves. You're approaching your pain in the way you would visit a sick friend in the hospital, with a compassionate willingness to be present no matter what happens.

Let your attention come as close to the pain as possible. If your resistance to getting close becomes too great, you can always escort your awareness back to the breath and try later. When you're ready, give the painful area your full awareness and observe it with kindhearted curiosity. Silently note your observations.

Try to define the region that feels painful. Pain has a geography. Sometimes its boundaries are sharp and well-defined; sometime they're more diffused. Try to gain a sense of the contours of the painful area. Observe how deeply the pain goes into your body. Imagine a three-dimensional model of your pain.

Then consider how you might describe the quality of your pain. Is it sharp or dull? Burning or stinging? Is it hot or freezing? Does it cramp, pound, or pulsate? Is it tight or clenching? Sore or aching? Pain is experienced in a wide range of ways, and its descriptive vocabulary is immense. Choose the words that make the most sense to you. It may be, as I've often heard, the pain is "indescribable."

Now examine the dynamics of the pain. Is it moving or does it stay in one place? Most of the time, pain is changing, although it's not always easy to detect this change. Consider if the pain is fluctuating in its intensity. Is it now strong in sensation and then weak and then strong again? Does it seem to throb, radiate, or penetrate? These descriptors suggest that the pain is moving or changing.

For the next few moments, simply keep your awareness on the painful area and remain keenly observant of the sensations you feel. This time, avoid labeling the sensations and simply feel them.

Now, try to become aware of your awareness of the pain. That may sound a little paradoxical, but it can be done. Simply watch yourself as you're observing your painful sensations. As you do so, see if your awareness is in pain. Can you discern painful sensations in the awareness itself? If you can become an observer of your own awareness, you may discover a place where there is no pain. Dwelling in this awareness may help mitigate the painful sensations in your body. You're no longer a person in pain but someone observing a person in pain. Being in this observing space may allow you to see that your pain is not you, and you are not your pain. Staying in this particular place of awareness is not easy, and it takes practice to do so, just as it takes practice to remain focused on the breath. Now, let's return to the breath and draw this exercise to a close. Let your attention come back to your breathing for a few moments.

Before we move to the next exercise, take some time to reflect on your experience with the practice we've just completed. Did you notice any initial resistance to turning your attention to the painful area in your body? If so, what thoughts or emotions lay underneath that resistance? Have you become accustomed to keeping pain out of your awareness by not thinking about it or by distracting yourself with other thoughts or seeking out diversions? If you were able to give your pain a fuller attention, how did your mind respond? Did it generate thoughts about the pain?

In the next exercise, we'll incorporate more of the thinking process into the practice. It's not necessary to perform this exercise immediately after the one we've just completed. You can spend more time working with the first exercise before trying the next. If you wish to do so, you may return to the first exercise and listen to it again, or you may choose to work with the practice on your own, without my guidance. Then come back to the second exercise at your convenience.

When you're ready to continue your practice with pain, take your position in the posture of your choice and follow my instructions as I guide you through the process. Begin as you always do by relaxing your body and focusing on your inhalations and exhalations. Direct your attention to your breath, and stay attentive to what is occurring moment by moment. Your only concern is to be present to the experience you're now having.

Now permit your awareness to range over your entire body and let it come to rest at the place of greatest discomfort.

Be attentive to this location and observe the character of the sensations there as you did before. Try to survey its geography and the kinds and intensity of feeling. See if the sensations are moving or stable. Give yourself time to become acquainted with the sensations at just this moment and at just this place.

After you've had a chance to be aware of these sensations, turn your attention to your thoughts. Has the attention you've given this area of your body generated any mental commentary? If so, notice the character of those thoughts. Do you detect thoughts of resistance or avoidance? Are there thoughts of fear or anger? As you become aware of these thoughts, try to relinquish them. See if you can distinguish the sensations from your thoughts about the sensations. Try to anchor your awareness in the bodily sensations alone, just as you would try to focus on breathing in sitting meditation. If a thought arises, simply observe and let it fall away. After some practice, see if remaining focused on the sensations and dropping thoughts alleviates the discomfort. Now, let's return to the breath and draw this exercise to a close. Let your attention come back to your breathing for a few moments.

The intention of the exercise we've just concluded was to investigate the role of thinking in the experience of pain. Essentially, we wanted to see if our conditioned thought patterns worsened the unpleasant sensations we call pain. If your discomfort was not too intense, you may have had thoughts like these: "What a nuisance this backache is! I wish it would go away." Or you may have thought: "I feel congestion in my lungs. Gosh, I hope it's not the flu. I hate the flu! I bet it's the flu. Yep, it's the flu."

If the sensation was more severe, your thoughts may have sounded more panicked and stressed: "This headache is killing me! Will this agony ever end? I knew I should have told them to hold the MSG." If your thoughts were of this nature, they may have actually made your experience more painful than it had to be. Notice the thoughts that stirred up fear: "I hope it's not the flu," "Will the agony ever end?" Notice the ones rooted in regret and blame: "I should have told them to hold the MSG." Notice the exaggeration: "This is killing me!" None of these thoughts contribute in the least bit to easing the hurt, and they may do a great deal to aggravate the experience. Next time, try to minimize the negative commentary to see if that helps. See if you can take yourself to the point where you do not even label the sensation as "pain." The word "pain," after all, is a thought, a name we give to feelings we regard as unpleasant. Imagine experiencing the sensation without labeling it as "pain." How do you think that would change your experience?

The exercises we've just concluded were designed to give you an experiential acquaintance with the basic techniques for working with pain mindfully. You may or may not find these particular techniques helpful, but I hope they will at least motivate you to consider novel perspectives as you work out your own methods. Reflect on whether turning toward painful sensations in complete awareness might serve as a better approach than turning away from it. See if allowing yourself to feel the pain fully eases some of the distress and removes some of the aversion you may have for it.

Try to locate the place in your awareness where you are observing a person with pain rather than being a person with pain. Consider the role your conditioned thinking plays in your experience of pain. Think about the ways fear and hatred of pain may exacerbate your situation. Examine the lessons pain can teach us. In many instances, pain tells us to seek medical attention to alleviate a physiological problem. This is not always the case, however. The indicative value of pain is greatly diminished with intense chronic pain. Chronic pain can persist long after medical attention has been given. For chronic pain, medication is often ineffective or undesirable because of its side-effects. Meditation, then, may become the best alternative to medication.

As someone who lives with chronic pain, I can personally vouch for the value of meditative practices in easing the suffering associated with pain and, on occasion, the pain itself. My particular malady is cluster headaches, a form of vascular headache similar to, but more intense than, migraines. Cluster headaches usually occur daily for many months each year. The pain lasts about an hour and is totally incapacitating. The cause is of the headaches is unknown, and there is no cure. But fortunately, there are some medicines that can sometimes prevent the headaches and mitigate the painful sensations. But despite the chemical intervention, I must frequently cope by using the techniques I've learned in mindfulness practice. Mindfulness has helped me to become less fearful of the pain. In the past, especially before I had any medicines for treatment, I'd become panicked by the onset on the headaches, knowing I was facing the prospect of an hour of excruciating agony.

The fear, of course, only compounded my suffering. But mindfulness practice helped me to relinquish the fear by allowing me to calm myself and recognize the pain would not last. Pain, like everything else, is transient. The practice also helped me release my anger toward the headaches. I got furious because I knew the pain would interrupt my plans, and there was nothing I could about it. I felt helpless. And I was mad because this was happening to me. When the headaches begin, I am better able now to accept my situation in that moment and release my attachment to my plans. And because of the practice, I'm less inclined to feel pity for myself by thinking my situation is unfair. It's not unfair. I am not so special that I should be exempt from pain. Throughout the world, at every moment of every hour, millions endure great pain. I am no different from anyone else. Pain is a fact of life.

Grief—Learning to Accept Loss
Lecture 22

Mindfully working with grief essentially means removing any obstacles that might impede the natural course of grieving. In other words, grief is an invitation to welcome our experience with equanimity—without fear or aversion. It is to be open to whatever grief brings to us and to allow ourselves to experience that fully. Grief is not always predictable, and it doesn't follow a set timetable or path. It has to be allowed to happen on its own, taking its own good time.

Grief and Loss

- **Grieving** is the process of coming to terms with loss in our lives. Almost from the very moment we're born, we have to deal with loss. Newborns come into the world having lost the warmth and comfort of their mothers' wombs, and from that instant onward, life can seem like a string of losses.

- Some losses, of course, are greater than others. Losing a loved one to death is more significant and more distressing for most people than losing a mere material object, but the loss of anything can cause suffering and can require the process of grieving to help us adjust.

- Take a moment to reflect on the losses in your own life. Almost certainly, you've lost someone close to you to death—a parent or grandparent, a spouse, a friend, or a relative.

- We endure loss through means other than death, of course. We can lose our jobs and our life savings. We can see cherished possessions stolen or accidentally broken. Our friends may leave because of a quarrel, or we may leave them when we move away to embark on a new career.

- In the American courtship system, one can undergo a series of romantic breakups before finding a spouse. Even after marriage, one faces a 50% chance of divorce. As we age, we may begin to recognize that the youthful dreams we had long held are unlikely to materialize.

- These losses can cause us to suffer greatly, but for the significant losses in our lives, we need to grieve, and mindfulness practice can help facilitate our grief skillfully.

- Grief is a natural healing process that has several identifiable dimensions. Often, these aspects of the process are referred to as stages, a notion that suggests that grief follows a predictable, linear course as we come to terms with our loss.

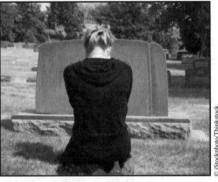

- The typology of grief proposed by Elisabeth Kübler-Ross notes that grief sequentially progresses through the stages of denial, anger, bargaining, depression, and acceptance. While

Practice breathing meditation in a graveyard. Notice and appreciate the way the idea of death affects you.

grief certainly can include these phases and experiences, it may be misleading, and potentially harmful, to suggest that grief is predictable or follows a specific timetable.

- Each person grieves in different ways. There may be times when grief includes anger and sadness and other experiences, but the experiences may not come in a predictable sequence, and there may be no sharp divisions between these stages.

- The mindfulness approach to grief is not to usher us through various stages so that we might hasten onward to the final goal of acceptance. Rather, mindfulness practice can be used to ensure that we accept and fully experience whatever the process of grief brings us.

- Mindfulness assists the grieving process by helping us acknowledge and accept the universality and inevitability of loss. Having to give up what we have is unavoidable. Throughout our lives, things are taken away from us—sometimes with our consent and sometimes without.

- Resisting necessary losses, of course, can cause us to suffer. The mindfulness insight into the impermanence of all reality helps ease our resistance to living in a world where ultimately everything we hold dear will have to be relinquished.

Easing the Suffering of Grief

- Being aware of the universality and inevitability of loss—and realizing your solidarity with everyone else—implies that we are all well advised to begin to prepare for grief now. Why wait?

- Throughout our lives, almost on a daily basis, we are given ample opportunities to practice mindfully coping with loss. These occasions are chances to remind ourselves of the nature of impermanence and of the potential hazards of becoming attached to transient things.

- Remembering the transience of all life helps us to avoid developing unhealthy attachments that can cause us to suffer, but how does mindfulness help us cope with the loss of those things to which we have already become attached?

- Quite simply, it's no different from the way we handle any other unwanted experience we might have, including anger and pain. It involves acknowledging, accepting, and letting go.

- Mindfulness is of greatest benefit in the grieving process in keeping us focused in the present moment, the place we can fully feel the pain of loss. Loss of something important in our lives almost inevitably provokes us to worry about how to fill that void and to face the future. These are absolutely legitimate concerns, and they must be faced.

- Inordinate attention to apprehensions about the future, however, can also hinder the process of grieving, which requires momentarily setting aside these anxieties and being completely aware of our experience in the present.

- During the period of grief, mindfulness meditation can provide a deliberate opportunity for attending to the present. As we discovered in our conversations about anger and pain, fully experiencing what we find in each moment is the precondition for thinking and acting wisely.

- Practicing deliberate acts of self-compassion is also essential to grieving. Being self-compassionate during these periods not only means relaxing our usual tendencies toward self-judgment and criticism, but it also means being open to the expressions of compassion from others.

The Beloved Teacup

Even Zen masters have to be reminded of our attachment to objects and how to cope with loss.

In a Zen monastery several centuries ago, a young monk accidently broke his master's favorite antique teacup while cleaning. When he heard his master approach, he quickly gathered the pieces and put them behind his back. Then, he cleverly asked the master, "Sir, why must people die?" The master answered, "It's natural. Everything has a finite lifespan, and everything must die." Then, the novice produced the broken teacup and told his master, "It was time for your cup to die."

- Bearing in mind one's solidarity with others in grief is one way to ease our suffering; another is to bear in mind the serendipitous nature of life.

- **Serendipity** is the word for the phenomenon of discovering pleasant things not sought for. Part of the surprising and unpredictable quality of existence is the way that, sometimes, things can turn out better than we imagined or hoped.

- Because our foresight is so greatly limited, we're well advised not to rush to judgments about the events that happen to us. Remembering that we really do not know what the future holds for us, except the certainty of death, can often ease the anxieties we have about the future. We fear the worst, but often what turns out is for the best.

Dealing with Staggering Losses

- What do we do with losses that seem staggering, altogether outside the realm of normal human experience? There are times when people lose almost everything. One only has to think of earthquakes, tsunamis, hurricanes, genocides, and terrorist events—disasters whose horrors are difficult to comprehend and to integrate into our ordinary experience of life.

- Perhaps you may be able to understand such staggering events by appealing to the providence of a God or to the belief in rebirth or reincarnation—in which cases such massive suffering can somehow be redeemed and ameliorated.

- If you are hesitant to make such metaphysical claims, it makes it more difficult to put such losses in a comprehensive framework. Sometimes it seems that the only thing these disasters are good for is giving the survivors some perspective—which is of course no consolation to the victims—and perhaps the motivation to be more compassionate.

- These are times when ritual may come to our aid. Whatever our faith or culture, joining with others to share our grief—moving through the familiar elements of a ceremony and sharing words that have been spoken by others in our situation for generations—can help us keep in mind that this is part of our human lot and always has been.

- Here's where your own suffering can be of use to you: Many people find it's not until they have had to cope with setbacks of their own that they are truly able to have compassion for others.

- For as long as we're met with nothing but success—warm friendships, loving family, rewarding job—we're likely to think that all good things have come to us because we deserve them.

- Only when we experience some losses ourselves do we realize we had less control over events than we had believed. It's humbling and disillusioning, in the best sense of the word; it helps us rid ourselves of whatever illusions of permanence and control we may have been holding.

- Many mindfulness practitioners eventually come to see such losses as supports for meditation. It may be going too far to say these problems are actually welcomed, but once you have begun to use the tools of mindfulness in your daily life, it's almost certainly true that you will at least see your problems as opportunities for gaining a more intimate knowledge of the way your mind works.

- If you practice developing skillful means with life's everyday challenges, you'll be able to react more skillfully when the greater losses come to you, as they inevitably will. You'll understand that you're not being singled out for suffering—you're just having a life.

grieving: The process of coming to terms with loss in life.

serendipity: The word for the phenomenon of discovering pleasant things not sought for. Part of the surprising and unpredictable quality of existence is the way that, sometimes, things can turn out better than imagined.

Questions to Consider

1. Reflect on your experiences with grief. Did they follow a particular, specifiable pattern? What losses have caused you the greatest grief? Are there losses you still grieve?

2. Throughout the day, notice the times you experience loss—no matter how small. It may be staining your favorite shirt, losing the perfect parking spot, or being outbid on eBay. Notice your reactions to these losses. Use these experiences to deepen your practice with grief and your acceptance of impermanence.

Grief—Learning to Accept Loss
Lecture 22—Transcript

Bodhidharma was an Indian monk who is credited with transmitting Zen Buddhism to China in the 5th or 6th century. Traditionally, he is depicted as a wild character. Paintings and images of him accent his bulging eyeballs, suggesting a deep intent to see through to the core of reality. The stories about him indicate that he had only that single purpose; everything else was inconsequential. According to one legend, he was so committed to gaining enlightenment that he gazed at a wall for nine years in quest of awakening.

When I came across a delicate ceramic statue of Bodhidharma in a small shop in Hong Kong, I knew I had to have it for my collection. The wild-eyed Bodhidharma was one of my heroes. I carefully packed the image for my return trip and was delighted that he made journey across the Pacific intact. I immediately put the statue on display.

There he stood for years looking out over my office with those serene but bulging eyes—until the day my daughter asked if she could hold my precious ceramic image. She was four years old at the time, and to say I was apprehensive about giving her the image would be an understatement. But she cried and she begged and cried some more. I finally relented, but not until I had thoroughly explained to her the deep affection I had for the statue and pleaded with her to be exceedingly careful with it. She promised she would. I gingerly handed him over to her, and she mindfully took him from me. She was absolutely delighted with the strange-looking character in her hands.

Then she dropped him. Yes, she did. She dropped my beloved Bodhidharma, and he was gone. I was angry. I was crushed. The centerpiece of my collection of Buddhist images was now a pile of glazed rubble. I couldn't believe it. Fortunately, I had the presence of mind not to take my anger out on her. But I was angry, and I felt the loss. It took a bit of time for me to recover my equanimity, but of course I did. Once again, I recognized the irony of my attachment to an image of a person who embodied radical non-attachment. I reminded myself of the words of the Buddha shortly before his death, "All compounded things," he said, "are impermanent." This statue of

Bodhidharma was certainly a "compounded thing," as was now clear by the mound of ceramic fragments.

I mentioned in an earlier lecture about my attachment to another statue and about how I decided to give the image away to a friend who admired it. But that was different. Earlier, I had given away the statue voluntarily. This time the loss came against my will. Previously, I had been able to relinquish my attachment before letting the statue go. The Bodhidharma image was gone before I was prepared, and it hurt. Now I had to relinquish my attachment after the fact. In other words, I had to grieve.

Grieving is the process of coming to terms with loss in our lives. Almost from the very moment we're born, we're having to deal with loss. Newborns come into the world having lost the warmth and comfort of their mothers' womb, and from that instant onward, life can seem like a string of losses. Some losses, of course, are greater than others. Losing a loved one to death is more significant and more distressing for most people than losing a mere material object like a ceramic statue. But the loss of anything can cause suffering and can require the process of grieving to help us adjust.

Take a moment to reflect on the losses in your own life. Almost certainly you've lost someone close to you to death—a parent or grandparent, a spouse, a friend, or a relative. My own maternal grandmother died recently, just a few months shy of her 100th birthday. I thought about how many friends and relatives she had watched come and go during that century. Certainly, one of the difficult aspects of a long life would have to be witnessing and coping with the loss of so many loved ones.

We endure loss through means other than death, of course. We can lose our jobs, our life savings. We can see cherished possessions stolen or accidentally broken. Our friends may leave because of a quarrel, or we may leave them when we move away to embark on a new career. In the American courtship system, one can undergo a series of romantic break-ups before finding a spouse. And even after marriage, one faces a 50 percent chance of divorce. As we age we may begin to recognize that the youthful dreams we had held for so long are unlikely to materialize. These losses can cause us to suffer greatly.

For the significant losses in our lives, we need to grieve, and mindfulness practice can help facilitate our grief skillfully. Grief is a natural healing process that has several identifiable dimensions. Often, these aspects of the process are referred to as "stages," a notion that suggests that grief follows a predictable, linear course as we come to terms with our loss. The typology of grief proposed by Elisabeth Kubler-Ross is perhaps the most widely known of these schemes. Kubler-Ross argued that grief is characterized first by denial, then anger, followed by bargaining, depression, and finally acceptance. While grief certainly can include these phases and experiences, it may be misleading, and potentially harmful, to suggest that grief is predictable or follows a specific timetable.

Each person grieves in different ways. There may be times when grief includes anger and sadness and other experiences. But the experiences may not come in a predictable sequence, and there may be no sharp divisions between these stages. The mindfulness approach to grief is not to usher us through various stages so that we might hasten onward to the final goal of acceptance. Rather, mindfulness practice can be used to ensure that we accept and fully experience whatever the process of grief brings us. Mindfully working with grief essentially means removing any obstacles that might impede the natural course of grieving.

Mindfulness assists the grieving process by helping us acknowledge and accept the universality and inevitability of loss. Having to give up what we have is unavoidable. Throughout our lives things are taken away from us, sometimes with our consent, and sometimes without. Resisting necessary losses, of course, can cause us to suffer. The mindfulness insight into the impermanence of all reality helps ease our resistance to living in a world where ultimately everything we hold dear will have to be relinquished.

Kisagotami was a young woman of wealth and high status who lived during the time of Buddha. She was married and gave birth to a son, who died as a toddler. She was devastated. In her grief, she carried the lifeless body of her son from house to house, and village to village, begging for medicine to bring the boy back to life. One wise man advised her to see the Buddha, who, he said, had the medicine that she needed. Pressing the lifeless boy against her heart, she began the journey. The Buddha told her to find a mustard seed from a household that had not been touched by death. Thinking the seed would be used to make the medicine she wanted, Kisagotami carried her dead child from house to house, making her request. Everyone was willing to help, but she couldn't find a single family untouched by death. Soon she realized that hers was not the only family that had faced death. At last, she brought the corpse to the forest and made a bed of leaves.

Just as she placed his remains upon it, she realized the dead body was no longer her son, and her attitude towards his death immediately changed. She was then able to begin to make peace with his passing, and she returned to the Buddha to share her experience. The Buddha said, "Kisagotami, you thought that you were the only one who had lost a son. As you've now realized, death comes to all beings before their desires are satisfied." On hearing this, Kisagotami fully realized the impermanence of life, and understood how her refusal to accept the death of her son kept her in a state of suffering.

The story of Kisagotami reminds us that loss and grieving are universal experiences. No one is exempt. The Buddha's object lesson allowed Kisagotami to discover how her refusal to acknowledge the inevitability of loss compounded her pain. She realized this truth and was then able to let her son go. I have a deep empathy with the plight of Kisagotami. She not only had to cope with the loss of her son, which of course was painful enough, but she had to face the shock that this event was happening to her. In my early thirties, I too had to face a similar shock. It's a shock that all of us past a certain age probably experience. It's the awareness that we are aging. For the first two decades of your life, you're usually looking forward to getting older and the new privileges and freedom that brings—getting to drive a car, staying out later with friends, dating, going to college, getting married, and having children. During these decades, you actually look forward to getting older, but you don't give a single thought to aging.

Then one day, you look in the mirror and see evidence that that not only have you gotten older, you've actually begun to age. You can see it on your face. And when you do, it can be quite a shock. I clearly remember it happening to me. I also remember experiencing the dimension of grief known as denial. "Wait, a minute! This isn't supposed to be happening to me. Aging is what happens to other people." It took me quite a while to accept the fact that

I was getting older and that my body and appearance were reflecting that process. I recall the many fears I had, particularly the strange fear that if I appeared older, somehow people would no longer like me. Realizing my solidarity with everyone else—that is, recognizing that we are all getting older—helped immensely to ease that fear. We don't often recognize it, but grieving our lost youth is an experience many of us will have to face.

Being aware of the universality and inevitability of loss implies that we are well-advised to begin to prepare for it now. Why wait? All throughout our lives, almost on a daily basis, we are given ample opportunities to practice mindfully coping with loss. These occasions are chances to remind ourselves of the impermanent nature and of the potential hazards of becoming attached to transient things. I was able to come to terms with my shattered Bodhidharma by turning my material loss into a spiritual gain. I recognized just how foolish I had been to become so attached to a mere object, a thing that I knew could not last. That's a lesson we have to relearn again and again.

Even Zen masters have to be reminded of it. In a Zen monastery several centuries ago, a monk, no more than ten, accidently broke his master's favorite antique tea cup while he was cleaning. When he heard his master approach, he quickly gathered the pieces and put them behind his back. Then he cleverly asked the master, "Sir, why must people die?" The master answered, "It's natural. Everything has a finite lifespan and everything must die." Then the novice produced the broken tea cup and told his master, "It was time for your cup to die."

Remembering the transience of all life helps us to avoid developing unhealthy attachments that can cause us to suffer. But how does mindfulness help us cope with the loss of those things to which we have already become attached? It's fine and good to say "avoid attachments," but on this side of enlightenment, we still get attached. And the suffering it causes is very real. What is the mindfulness approach to grieving these losses? Quite simply, it's no different from the way we handle any other unwanted experience we might have, including anger and pain. It involves acknowledging, accepting, and letting go. In other words, grief is an invitation to welcome our experience with equanimity, without fear or aversion. It is to be open to whatever grief brings us and to allow ourselves to experience that fully. As we noted, grief is not always predictable and doesn't follow a set timetable. It has to be allowed to happen on its own, taking its own good time.

I recall going through a grief experience many years ago and being advised by a wise friend who had been through the very same experience to take every opportunity I could to cry. He wasn't suggesting that I force my tears, just to let them come whenever I felt the need. As a man who had always thought that holding back the expressions of sadness was courageous and manly, I greeted his advice with skepticism.

But I also trusted him a great deal and decided to try what he said. I found it easiest to let the tears flow when I was alone, in part because my solitude prompted them and in part because the lack of an audience meant I didn't have to pretend to be courageous and manly. Over a period of several months, I cried a river of tears. Then one day, I simply observed that I had stopped crying. I hadn't shed a tear for a long time. It was then that I realized that my grief was essentially over. I still felt twinges of sadness on occasion, but the intensity of the experience had dissolved.

Mindfulness is of greatest benefit in the grieving process in keeping us focused in the present moment, the place we can fully feel the pain of loss. Upon losing something or someone, our minds can race ahead and begin to worry about the future. The loss of a spouse might bring fears of loneliness and anxieties about how to cope with the day-to-day affairs of living. Divorce might arouse concerns about our worthiness as a person and fears about ever finding meaningful love. Loss of something important in our lives almost inevitably provokes us to worry about how to fill that void and to face the future. These are absolutely legitimate concerns, and they must be faced. But inordinate attention to apprehensions about the future can also hinder the process of grieving, which requires momentarily setting aside these anxieties and being completely aware of our experience in the present. During the period of grief, I can think of no better practice than mindfulness meditation, which provides us a deliberate opportunity for attending to the present. As we discovered in our conversations about anger and pain, fully experiencing what we find in each moment is the precondition for thinking and acting wisely.

Practicing deliberate acts of self-compassion is also essential to grieving. I can think of no time when we might need compassion more. Being self-compassionate, during these periods not only means relaxing our usual tendencies toward self-judgment and criticism, it means being open to the expressions of compassion from others. During the same period of grief that I mentioned earlier, I finally permitted myself to let others reach out and befriend me, something that I had always had difficulty doing. Letting others show me kindness was surprisingly comforting for a young man who had always thought of himself as self-sufficient. When I allowed others to befriend me, it suddenly seemed as if the whole world had gone through the same experience that I had. Like Kisagotami, knowing I was not alone in my grief was immeasurably consoling.

Bearing in mind one's solidarity with others in grief is one way to ease our suffering; another is to bear in mind the serendipitous nature of life. Serendipity is the word for the phenomenon of discovering pleasant things not sought for. Part of the surprising and unpredictable quality of existence is the way that, sometimes, things can turn out better than we imagined or hoped. An old tale claimed by many traditions, including the Daoists and the Sufis, helps make this point.

The tale concerns an old farmer in China who tilled his land with his son. One day their horse ran away and all their neighbors exclaimed about their bad luck. The farmer was philosophical. "Maybe it's bad luck," he said, "maybe not." The next day, the horse came back with six wild horses, and the neighbors changed their tune, now congratulating the farmer for his good luck. "Maybe," he said again. A few days later when the son was riding one of the wild horses, he fell and broke his leg. Now that seemed inarguably like bad luck, but the day after that, the king's agents came to recruit able-bodied young men to go off to war. Because of his broken leg, the farmer's son was left behind. All the other young men were killed in battle, but the farmer's son eventually healed and went back to tilling the fields with his horse. The point of the story is clear: Because our foresight is so greatly limited, we're well advised not to rush to judgments about the events that happen to us.

One of my friends and colleagues was denied tenure about 20 years. It was an unfair decision, and he was crushed. But somehow he picked up the pieces, found another job in another country and began to flourish. He poured his grief and anger into his writing and he became prolific and greatly respected.

He recently retired, highly honored by his university. I sometimes tell Philip that not getting tenure was the best thing that ever happened to him. Remembering that we really do not know what the future holds for us, except the certainty of death, can often ease the anxieties we have about the future. We fear the worst, but often what turns out is for the best.

But what do we do with losses that seem staggering, altogether outside the realm of normal human experience, even more unexpected than the loss of a child? There are times when people lose almost everything. One only has to think of the earthquakes, tsunamis, hurricanes, genocides, and terrorist events of recent years, disasters whose horrors are difficult to comprehend and to integrate into our ordinary experience of life. Perhaps you may be able to understand these events by appealing to the providence of God or the belief in rebirth or reincarnation, in which cases such massive suffering can somehow be redeemed and ameliorated.

I confess that my hesitancy to make such metaphysical claims makes it difficult for me to put such losses in a comprehensive framework. I don't know if there is a heaven or an afterlife where the victims of such suffering will find paradise or perhaps another chance at life. I don't know if God is waiting on the other side of death to welcome us with open arms. Sometimes it seems that the only thing these disasters are good for is giving the survivors some perspective—which of course is no consolation to the victims. And perhaps, they may provide us with some motivation to be more compassionate.

These are times when ritual may come to our aid. Whatever our faith or culture, joining with others to share our grief—moving through the familiar elements of a ceremony and sharing words that have been spoken by others in our situation for generation after generation—can help us keep in mind that this is part of our human lot and always has been.

And here's where your own suffering can be of use to you: Many people find that it's not until they have had to cope with setbacks of their own that they are able to be truly compassionate for others. For as long as we meet with nothing but success—warm friendships, loving family, rewarding job—we're likely to think that all good things have come to us because we deserve them. Only when we experience some losses ourselves, do we realize we had less control over events than we had believed. It's humbling, and disillusioning in the best sense of the word—it helps us rid ourselves of whatever illusions of permanence and control we may have been holding.

Many mindfulness practitioners eventually come to see such losses as "supports for meditation." It may be going too far to say these problems are actually welcomed, but once you have begun to use the tools of mindfulness in your daily life, it's almost certainly true that you will at least see your problems as opportunities for gaining a more intimate knowledge of the way your mind works. If you practice developing skillful means with life's everyday challenges, you'll be able to react more skillfully when the greater losses come to you, as they inevitably will. You'll understand that you're not being singled out for suffering, you're just having a life. In the next lecture, we'll look more closely at one more thing that comes to all of us—having a death.

Finitude—Living in the Face of Death
Lecture 23

There is great value in fully confronting our fear of death and contemplating it deliberately as a way to free ourselves from its bonds and to live our lives with greater appreciation for every moment we have. It is difficult to face our deaths—to imagine our lives ending—but it is precisely because of its impermanence that we value life so dearly. If we are able to live the present moment completely, accepting that all things are impermanent, we can have fulfillment in this moment, right now.

Death and Life

- We've all encountered death in some form, but few of us have actively thought about our own deaths. You might even think the idea sounds morbid. If you do, you're in good company. Most of us spend a lot of energy to avoid thinking about death.

- When death comes close, we have a variety of means at our disposal to prevent it from disturbing us too much. Our minds often function in strange ways to help keep us from thinking much about death.

- These clever psychological dynamics dovetail with the way society itself treats death. Our primary approach as a culture is to stave it off for as long as possible. We try to mask any signs of the aging process that might suggest to ourselves and others that we are inching closer to our inevitable end.

- As the inevitability of death draws nearer, we attempt to keep death at bay by prolonging life artificially with advanced medical technology, often choosing to ignore the diminished quality of life such technology brings.

- When at last death arrives, we often experience it as a defeat rather than as a natural stage of living. Then, to further estrange us from the reality of death, we turn over the dead to a commercial funeral home, which takes care of every aspect of disposing of the body so we don't have to.

- Long gone are the days when families brought the dead into their own homes where they themselves cared for the remains of their loved ones and came to terms with death in their individual ways.

- Removing death from of our midst and disguising its approach has further contributed to our fear of this reality, thus mystifying death and leaving us unprepared for it. What's more, our inordinate fear of death has taken away one of our greatest teachers for living life.

Reflecting on Death

- Contrary to the prevailing attitudes of the modern Western culture, the mindfulness tradition suggests that reflecting on death is not only liberating, but it's essential to living a full, satisfying life.

- Buddhism is by no means the only tradition to encourage the practice of contemplating death. Meditation on death and dying has a long history in the world's wisdom traditions.

- Reflecting on death, especially our own, makes us so familiar with it that we no longer fear it. In addition, when we no longer fear death, we can live more freely. To remove this terror helps bring us equanimity, which allows us to see the world and ourselves more clearly and to accept the fact of impermanence more completely.

- By fully accepting the inevitability of death with a calm mind, we come to greater clarity about what is really important in life. In the light of death, trivialities begin fall away.

- Because we forget that our lives are transitory, we are prone to conflict over matters that are of little consequence. When we hold before our minds the inevitability of our death, we recognize that such inconsequential things are not worth the fight.

- As we've noted many times, intellectually agreeing with the idea of impermanence is not sufficient. To take away the fear of death and enable us to live our life joyously in the face of it, we need specific practices that help us to embrace this wisdom on a deep and unqualified level.

Death Awareness Meditation

- There are a variety of different forms of mindfulness exercises that will allow you to bring awareness to the fact of your own finitude and clear the way for the insights that awareness provides.

- You may not find each of the following exercises equally valuable. Some you might find too frightening to practice at this stage of your journey. You are certainly free to choose which exercises are most meaningful to you.

- We've all been conditioned to live within a culture that is terribly fearful of death, so please extend compassion to yourself and engage those offerings that you feel you can reasonably handle.

- Perhaps the easiest and least intimidating form of meditating on death is the Buddhist practice of reciting the Five Remembrances. These recitations are straightforward observations about life's fragility, and simply contemplating them can help open us to the deeper acceptance of our impermanence and the great benefits that acceptance confers.

- If you wish, you may recite each of the following statements.

    o I am subject to aging. Aging is unavoidable.

    o I am subject to illness. Illness is unavoidable.

o I am subject to death. Death is unavoidable.

o I will be separated and parted from everyone and everything that is dear to me.

o Whatever I do, for good or for ill, that will I reap.

- Another series of statements known as the Nine Meditations on Death makes many of the same points as the Five Remembrances but puts them in different language and elaborates some of their insights.

- If you wish, you may recite each of the following statements.

o There is no possible way to escape death. No one ever has, not even Jesus or the Buddha.

o Life has a definite limit, and each moment brings us closer to our death.

o We are dying from the moment we are born.

o Death comes in a moment, and its time is uncertain. All that separates us from death is one breath.

o The duration of our lifespan is uncertain. The young can die before the old, and the healthy can die before the sick.

o There are many causes and circumstances that lead to death.

o The weakness and fragility of one's physical body contribute to life's uncertainty. The body can be easily destroyed by disease or accident.

- o Worldly possessions such as wealth, position, and money cannot help us with the reality of death. Our relatives and friends cannot help us.

- o Even our own precious body is of no help. We will leave it behind like an empty shell.

- Like the Five Remembrances, the Nine Meditations can be memorized or written down and recited each day. You're free to vary the language to make these reflections more personally meaningful.

- While our culture encourages us to avoid death, traditional Asian societies tend to keep the face of death in open view. In India, for example, the most common funeral is an open-air cremation preceded by a procession through the town or village where the body of the deceased is easily visible.

- Buddhist monastics and Hindu holy men and women would take this exposure to death even further by going to the funeral grounds to practice meditation. The practice was intended, of course, to teach these ascetics to become familiar with death and thus help eliminate their fear of it.

- In some countries in South and Southeast Asia, Buddhist monks were directed to go to secluded fields where corpses had been left in the open rather than buried or burned. There, they would go each day to observe the body in a gradual state of decomposition. They were encouraged to think of the decaying corpses as their own.

- If you're inclined, you might try a variation of this exercise. Go to a graveyard, find a spot to sit, and begin breathing meditation. When your mind is clear and focused, deliberately think about the graves around you. Imagine yourself in such a grave. Imagine your body slowly combining with the soil.

- Take your time with this practice, and try to think of every aspect you can of the physical and chemical changes that will occur to your body after your death. If you feel fear or other emotions arising while you do this, be sure to pay attention. Feel your emotions as completely as you can, and then let them go. Notice and appreciate the way that the idea of your own death affects you.

A Guided Meditation for Death Awareness

- The final example of death awareness meditation is a guided reflection in which you are invited to participate by imagining the described experiences. You can practice this meditation sitting or lying down in *shavasana*, the corpse pose we used in the body scan meditation.

- When you're prepared, sit or lie down on your back in a supine position. Take a few deep breaths, and become attentive to the inhalation and exhalation as the breath returns to its natural rhythm. Focus your attention for a few moments on the sensation of breathing.

- As you breathe, imagine a large box beside you. Picture the box as empty. Now, think of your loved ones, your family and friends, one at a time. Hear each person's voice; think of them laughing and seeing them smile. Imagine embracing each one of them. Summon the love you feel for each person.

- Now, put each person in the box beside you. Imagine that he or she disappears upon stepping into the box. There is room for every friend and every family member—and yet the box is empty. Notice that you are alone. Reflect on how you feel when you realize that your friends and family are all gone.

- Now, picture all the rooms where you live. In your mind, look at what's on the walls and on the tables. See your bed, your books, and your other possessions. Put all the furniture in the box. Now, put all your favorite clothes and jewelry in the box. Watch the box become empty.

- Imagine that you are in your house. Take the walls, the doors, and the windows—the entire house itself—and put them in the box. If you have a car, put it in the box. See the box become empty.

- Notice everything in your neighborhood. Imagine the sounds you hear when you step outside. Imagine how it feels to have the air on your face as you move. Take a good look at everything you see, and put it in the box. See the box become empty.

- Now, search for memories of places you have been and people you have known. As you think of them, cherish them, and then put them in the box. Put everything in the box—memories, music, trees, grass, and even the sky. All that is left is you and the box.

- See the box become empty. Now, put yourself in the box. See the box become empty. See the box disappear. See only emptiness. Be with this moment. Notice what you feel. Feel it fully. Death will come in an ordinary moment just like this one.

- Now, return your awareness to the breath. Feel your heart beating. Notice how wonderful it is to be alive.

- When you are ready to end the meditation, slowly move your fingers and toes and then your arms and legs. Feel the floor beneath you. Open your eyes and gently stretch. Notice how your body feels. Give yourself ample time before you get up.

- Now is a good time to remember the importance of treating yourself with compassion, and be compassionate with yourself if you found this meditation hard to practice. Take a few moments to be grateful for where you are and who you are—right now.

1. What was your first experience with death? When did you come to know that you will one day die? How have those experiences affected your outlook on death today?

2. Assess how comfortable you are with your own impermanence.

Finitude—Living in the Face of Death
Lecture 23—Transcript

A friend told me recently of three times in her life when she became consumed by the fear of death. The first time, she was only six. She's from a big family but still had many times when she was left alone in a large, old house. Each time this happened, she thought about dying.

It was distressing for her to think about, of course, but she couldn't help it. She thought about not being able to walk or move her arms; about not being able to hug her parents, her brothers, or her dog. She thought about not breathing. She would hold her breath and imagine that she couldn't take another. She thought about being under the ground and worms eating her body until it had turned to dirt. My friend had a vivid imagination.

Finally, she thought about death so thoroughly that she simply stopped fearing it. She realized that it was going to happen no matter how many times she thought about it or cried about it. She decided—with the simple wisdom that kids sometimes have—that the best thing she could do would be to pay attention to everything around her and enjoy life while she could. Then, quite literally, she went out to play.

The second time the fear of death grasped my friend, she was in her 40s and in a difficult marriage that she was trying to keep alive. She began waking up in the middle of the night, terrified of dying. Her grandmother and a beloved aunt had died recently, and she would often think of them and wonder if they were in heaven. She thought about how she didn't feel good enough to join them and how disappointed they would be that she was failing in her second marriage. For several months she woke up in terror, and she decided to face her fear and deliberately meditate on her own death. To think intentionally about death, of course, is decidedly different from just feeling afraid of it. Before long, her fear of death dissolved again, just as it had when she was six.

The third time, my friend was in her 50s, and her son had left to fight in the war in Afghanistan just a few days after his best friend had died. She was working seven days a week, and yet the fear of her son's death and the grief for his friend permeated her every waking moment. This time, she began a practice of drawing, which she did weekly for nearly a year, until she felt that all her sorrow, fear, and anger had poured out onto the paper. She wasn't drawing pictures. She was simply picking a crayon that matched her feelings and doodling with it while imagining everything she could about her son's possible death, his friend's death, and her own mortality. Once again, her deliberate effort to face her feelings about death allowed her to come to terms with its inevitability and sharpened her focus on the business of living.

What my friend learned, and what I wish to discuss today, is the great value of fully confronting our fear of death and contemplating it deliberately, as a way to free ourselves from its bonds and to live our lives with greater appreciation for every moment we have. You may not have experienced any of the situations that my friend did, but you have surely looked at death in some way. You may have lost a loved one or a cherished pet. You may know someone who will be taking leave of this life very soon. Perhaps at this very moment you yourself are facing an illness that you know to be terminal. Or perhaps you have come close to dying but lived to see another day. We've all encountered death in some form, but few of us have actively thought about our own deaths. You might even think the idea sounds morbid. If you do, you're in good company. Most of us spend a lot of energy to avoid thinking about death.

When death comes close, we have a variety of means at our disposal to prevent it from disturbing us too much. Leo Tolstoy's novella, *The Death of Ivan Ilyich*, studies the psychological mechanisms we have for preventing our personal demise from coming to full consciousness. When word of Ivan Ilyich's death reaches his associates, his close friend Pyotr Ivanovich momentarily lets the news upset him and then quickly reasons it away.

> Pyotr Ivanovich was overcome with horror as he thought of the suffering of someone he had known so well, first as a carefree boy, then as a schoolmate, later as a grown man, his colleague. ... "Three terrible days of suffering and death," he thought and for a moment felt panic-stricken. "Why, the same thing could happen to me at anytime now." But at once—he himself did not know how—he was rescued by the customary reflection that all this happened to Ivan Ilyich, not to him, that it could not and should not happen to him;

and that if he were to grant such a possibility, he would succumb to depression. … With this line of reasoning, Pyotr Ivanovich set his mind at rest and began to press for details about Ivan Ilyich's death, as though death were a chance experience that could only happen to Ivan Ilyich, never to himself.

Tolstoy's work masterfully reveals the way our minds often function to help keep us from thinking much about death. These clever psychological dynamics dovetail with the way society itself treats death. Our primary approach as a culture is to stave it off for as long as possible. We try to mask any signs of the aging process that might suggest to ourselves and others that we are inching closer to our inevitable end. But as that inevitability draws nearer, we attempt to keep death at bay by prolonging life artificially with advanced medical technology, often choosing to ignore the diminished quality of life that such technology brings. When at last death arrives, we often experience it as a defeat rather than as a natural stage of living. Then, to further estrange us from the reality of death, we turn over the dead to a commercial funeral home, which takes care of every aspect of disposing of the body so we don't have to.

Long gone are the days when families brought the dead into their own homes where they themselves cared for the remains of their loved ones and came to terms with death in their individual ways. Removing death from our midst and disguising its approach has further contributed to our fear of this reality, thus mystifying death and leaving us unprepared for it. What's more, our inordinate fear of death has taken away one of our greatest teachers for living life.

Contrary to the prevailing attitudes of our modern Western culture, the mindfulness tradition suggests that reflecting on death is not only liberating, but essential to living a full, satisfying life. "Of all footprints," said the Buddha, "that of the elephant is supreme. Of all mindfulness meditations, that on death is supreme." Buddhism is by no means the only tradition to encourage the practice of contemplating death. Meditation on death and dying has a long history in the world's wisdom traditions. In the *Phaedo*, Socrates famously defined the practice of philosophy as "training for death." In more recent times, the French essayist Montaigne wrote,

> Let us deprive death of its strangeness, let us frequent it, let us get used to it, let us have nothing more often in mind than death. … [W]e do not know where death awaits us, so let us wait for it everywhere. To practice death is to practice freedom. … A man who has learned to die has unlearned how to be a slave.

Montaigne's admonition gets to the very heart of the value of meditating on death. Reflecting on death, especially our own, makes us so familiar with it we no longer fear it. And when we no longer fear death, as my friend found out, we can live more freely. To remove this terror, helps bring us equanimity, which allows us to see the world and ourselves more clearly and to accept the fact of impermanence more completely. Philip Kapleau, the author of *The Zen of Living and Dying*, says that "Unless this fear and terror is replaced by comfort and hope, a tranquil mind state is impossible. The unwillingness to think of death is itself a kind of death, for the poignancy of life is inseparable from the knowledge of its decay."

By fully accepting the inevitability of death with a calm mind, we come to greater clarity about what is really important in life. One of my closest friends died about 15 years ago, after a long struggle with an immune disorder. About a year before he died, he told me that his illness had been the best thing that had ever happened to him. I was shocked by his claim. I had watched him degenerate from a healthy young man to a frail shadow, little more than a breathing corpse. He explained that knowing his death was imminent and certain freed his mind from playing its usual games and permitted him to concentrate his attention on appreciating the beauty of life and the warmth of his friends. Had it not been for his disease, he would have easily frittered away his existence bit by bit, squandering the precious gift of life he had been given. Now, though the length of his days had been greatly foreshortened, he could die knowing his existence had not been a waste.

In the light of death, trivialities begin to fall away. The Buddha once said, "Those who fight with one another have forgotten that we all die; but for the wise, who know this fact, there are no quarrels."

Because we forget that our lives are transitory, we are prone to conflict over matters that are of little consequence. When we hold before our minds the inevitability of our death, we recognize that such inconsequential things are not worth the fight.

As we've noted many times in this course, intellectually agreeing with the idea of impermanence is not sufficient. To take away the fear of death and enable us to live our life joyously in the face of it, we need specific practices that help us to embrace this wisdom on a deep and unqualified level. To that end, I will offer a variety of different forms of mindfulness exercises to allow you to bring awareness to the fact of your own finitude and to clear the way for the insights that that awareness provides.

You may not find each of the exercises equally valuable. Some you might find too frightening to practice at this stage of your journey. You are certainly free to choose which exercises are most meaningful to you. We've all been conditioned to live within a culture that is terribly afraid of death, so please extend compassion to yourself and engage those offerings that you feel you can reasonably handle.

Perhaps the easiest and least intimidating form of meditating on death is the Buddhist practice of reciting the Five Remembrances. These recitations are straightforward observations about life's fragility, and simply contemplating them can help open us to a deeper acceptance of our impermanence and the great benefits that acceptance confers. If you wish, you may recite each statement after me: 1) I am subject to aging. Aging is unavoidable. 2) I am subject to illness. Illness is unavoidable. 3) I am subject to death. Death is unavoidable. 4) I will be separated and parted from everyone and everything that is dear to me. 5) Whatever I do, for good or for ill, that will I reap.

I find these declarations to be so helpful that at the end of my course on Buddhism, I give every student a printed copy and invite them to frame it and place it somewhere they can see it every day.

Another series of statements known as the Nine Meditations on Death makes many of the same points as the Five Remembrances but puts them in different language and elaborates some of their insights. If you wish, you may simply close your eyes right now and contemplate on my words as I recite these nine meditations. 1) There is no possible way to escape death. No one ever has, not even Jesus or the Buddha. 2) Life has a definite limit and each moment brings us closer to death. 3) We are dying from the moment we are born. 4) Death comes in a moment and its time is uncertain. All that separates us from death is one breath. 5) The duration of our lifespan is uncertain. The young can die before the old, and the healthy can die before the sick. 6) There are many causes and circumstances that lead to death. 7) The weakness and fragility of one's physical body contribute to life's uncertainty. The body can be easily destroyed by disease or accident. 8) Worldly possessions such as wealth, position, and money cannot help us with the reality of death. Our relatives and friends cannot help us. 9) Even our own precious body is of no help. We will leave it behind like an empty shell.

Like the Five Remembrances, the Nine Meditations can be memorized or written down and recited each day. You're free to vary the language to make these reflections more personally meaningful. You might even record these statements on a media player and play them back during a sitting or lying practice. The reflections will be most effective when they are recited in your own voice.

While our culture encourages us to avoid death, traditional Asian societies tend to keep the face of death in open view. In India, for example, the most common funeral is an open-air cremation preceded by a procession through the town or village where the body of the deceased is easily visible. Buddhist monastics and Hindu holy men and women would take this exposure to death even further by going to the funeral grounds to practice meditation. The practice was intended, of course, to teach these ascetics to become familiar with death and thus help eliminate their fear of it.

In some countries in South and Southeast Asia, Buddhist monks were directed to go to secluded fields where corpses had been left in the open rather than buried or burned. There, they would go each day to observe the body in a gradual state of decomposition. For months, they would go to the same location and watch the same body being reclaimed by nature. They were encouraged to think of the decaying corpses as their own.

If you're inclined, you might try a variation of this exercise. Go to a graveyard, find a spot to sit, and begin breathing meditation. When your mind is clear and focused, deliberately think about the graves around you. Imagine yourself in such a grave. Imagine your body slowly combining with the earth. Take your time with this practice and try to think of every aspect you can of the physical and chemical changes that will occur to your body after your death. If you feel fear or other emotions arising while you do this, be sure to pay attention. Feel your emotions as completely as you can, and then let them go. Notice and appreciate the way that the idea of your own death affects you.

Now, we'll conclude our discussion with a final example of a death awareness meditation. This will be a guided meditation in which you are invited to participate by imagining the experiences I describe to you. You can practice this meditation sitting or lying down in *shavasana*, the corpse pose we used in the body scan meditation.

When you're prepared, sit or lie down on your back in a supine position and follow my instructions. Take a few deep breaths and become attentive to the inhalation and exhalation as the breath returns to its natural rhythm. Focus your attention for a few moments on the sensation of breathing.

As you breathe, imagine a large box beside you. Picture the box as empty. Now think of your loved ones, your family and friends, one at a time. Hear each person's voice; think of them laughing and seeing them smile. Imagine embracing each one of them. Summon the love you feel for each person.

Now put each person in the box beside you. Imagine that he or she disappears upon stepping into the box. There is room for every friend, every family member, and yet the box is empty. Notice that you are alone. Reflect on how you feel when you realize that your friends and family are all gone.

Now, picture all the rooms where you live. In your mind, look at what's on the walls, on the tables. See your bed, your books, your other possessions. See your favorite chair. Put all the furniture in the box. Now put all your favorite clothes and jewelry in the box. Watch the box become empty.

Imagine that you are in your house. Take the walls, the doors, and the windows, the entire house itself, and put them in the box. If you have a car, put it in the box. See the box become empty.

Notice everything in your neighborhood. Imagine the sounds you hear when you step outside. Imagine how it feels to have the air on your face as you move. Imagine how the sun feels on your face. Imagine the feeling of rain on your body. Take a good look at everything you see, and put it in the box. See the box become empty.

Now search for memories of places you have been and people you have known. As you think of them, cherish them, and then put them in the box. Put everything in the box, memories, music, trees, grass, and even the sky. All that is left is you and the box.

See the box become empty. Now put yourself in the box. See the box become empty. See the box disappear. See only emptiness. Be with this moment. Notice what you feel. Feel it fully. Death will come in an ordinary moment just like this one. Now return your awareness to the breath. Feel your heart beating. Notice how wonderful it is to be alive.

When you are ready to end the meditation, slowly move your fingers and toes, and then your arms and legs. Feel the floor beneath you. Open your eyes and gently stretch. Notice how your body feels. Give yourself ample time before you get up.

We have talked throughout this series about the importance of treating yourself with compassion. Now is a good time to remember that lesson. Be compassionate with yourself if you found this meditation hard to practice. Take a few moments to be grateful for where you are and who you are, right now.

It is difficult to face our deaths, to imagine our lives ending. But it is precisely because of its impermanence that we value life so dearly. If we are able to live the present moment completely, accepting that all things are impermanent, we can have fulfillment in this moment, right now.

Life—Putting It All in Perspective
Lecture 24

T he Buddha always encouraged his followers to take a critical eye toward anyone claiming to present the truth and to judge the veracity of any claim or practice for themselves. In a famous statement, he urges them never to accept anything as true simply because it is said to be revelation, because it is traditional, because it comes from sacred texts, or because the teacher seems competent. Rather, he said, when you know for yourself that something is wholesome, blameless, and leads to benefit and happiness, then you should accept it and abide in it.

Putting Mindfulness in Perspective

- In this course, we have looked at the fundamental components of the practice of mindfulness and have discussed a great many areas of life in which these practices can be beneficially exercised.

- If there is anything about that practice that remains unclear, return to the lectures and read them again. Reading the lectures again—and still again—may prove valuable.

- It might be helpful to find a couple of books on basic mindfulness practice and read those as well. You'll readily see that different meditation teachers teach the discipline in slightly—and sometimes substantially—different ways.

- You may find that what other teachers have to say about mindfulness practice is more meaningful to you than what has been taught in this course. The practice is simple but extremely rich.

- A word of caution: Beware of spending too much time with the lectures or reading too many books about meditation. These activities can easily become ends in themselves—to the point that you're studying the practice of meditation rather than practicing the practice of meditation.

- Once you've understood the essential features of the discipline and have become comfortable doing them, begin to trust yourself to customize the practice to suit your own individual qualities.

- In this series, we've discussed and demonstrated a wide range of exercises. Not all of them, certainly, were equally appealing. Take as much as you can from each of them. Some you'll want to practice just as explained, others you may want to vary a bit, and still others may have no appeal at all.

- However, resist dismissing any exercise immediately. If a practice carries little meaning for you now, revisit it later. The practices we dislike the most are often the ones from which we gain the greatest benefit.

- If you have the opportunity to study with a reputable teacher of mindfulness meditation, try to take to take advantage of it. A good teacher can answer questions or concerns you may have in ways that are not possible with a series of lectures.

- The trick is to ensure that a potential teacher is a good one, which is not always an easy thing to do. As you may know, there are many teachers, sages, preachers, evangelists, missionaries, and gurus out there who are eager to tell you what to believe and how to live your life.

Following Up with Mindfulness

- As you proceed with your daily practice, you may consider at some point to intensify your meditation experience with a retreat. There are many types of retreats, and each can be very beneficial for your practice. Perhaps the simplest is to dedicate a day to mindfulness in the comfort of your own home.

- Try to arrange to be alone and quiet for four to eight hours—more if you're able—where you do nothing other than practice. You can design this self-retreat in any way that suits you, but it ought to include alternating sitting and walking practice.

- If you choose, you can add a body scan, mindful eating, and listening to a recorded talk on mindfulness. There are many locations on the Internet where you can download such talks.

- If you search the Internet, you'll also find plenty of listings for other kinds of retreats. There are a growing number of retreat centers across the country and throughout the world that offer retreats lasting from a weekend to three months to the traditional three-year, three-month, three-day retreat taken by some very committed practitioners.

- A very popular type of retreat in the mindfulness tradition lasts for ten days. In a ten-day retreat, you're usually with other practitioners, sitting and walking for as much as 16 hours a day—all in silence. A retreat of this length will benefit your practice (and the rest of your life) enormously.

- The most important thing about practicing mindfulness is: Just do it. It's difficult to get started sometimes, and it's difficult to continue, but the rewards are immeasurable.

Mindfulness and Life

- Meditation, of course, does more than just provide a quiet refuge. It also profoundly alters the way you view yourself, the world, and your place in it.

- When you study a lot of traditions, it is hard not to take away something from each one that impacts the way you live and view the world. Even for a viewpoint or practice that you would never dream of adopting wholesale, you should always find something worth affirming.

- In addition, views sometimes change, and you should always remain open to that change. Being firmly attached to beliefs and perspectives, as mindfulness practice suggests, can lead to great confusion and quarreling.

- The Buddha even cautioned his students not to become attached to his teachings. He told his students that his teachings are a raft. When you use a raft to get from one side of the lake to the other, you don't pick it up and carry it around with you. You leave it on the shore.

- Subverting the notion of a fixed identity is one of the things a mindfulness practice will do for you. And best of all, it can help you be comfortable without having a fixed identity.

- Gaining insight into the transience of the self enables you to think of yourself as a fluid reality, unable to be adequately named by conventional labels.

- Underneath the words you might use to identify yourself lies a reality that is a genuine mystery—at once conscious and self-aware, interrelated with the rest of the cosmos, and yet unfathomable in its depth.

- Likewise, the practice of mindfulness can alter your understanding of ultimate reality—the underlying nature of the universe and the ultimate power that governs the universe—to allow you to feel at home with its mystery.

- Mindfulness can encourage you to feel immense awe and happiness at being able to marvel at this world and our lives in it without having to provide a comprehensive and systematic explanation for the entire universe.

Lessons from Mindfulness

- Within the joyous mystery that surrounds and permeates our lives, mindfulness practice allows us to affirm some very simple things about living that has struck many individuals as being true.

- One simple realization is the acknowledgement that our control over life, like our knowledge of it, is very limited indeed. Mindfulness permits us to see clearly how little control we really have over the events that profoundly affect us.

- Much of our suffering, we realize, is caused by our dogged efforts to try to command these things over which we have no authority, but the practice also allows us to recognize that we have a capacity to shape our minds in ways that are wholesome for us and for others.

- With the training that mindfulness practice provides, we can learn to develop our minds in ways that allow us to relinquish the need to control and to accept reality as it is in this very moment.

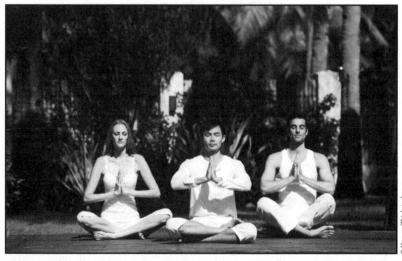

© Hemera/Thinkstock.

One of the central insights of mindfulness practice is seeing the interrelatedness of reality.

- Mindfulness practice also teaches us that everything we do, think, and say has an important effect—particularly on our own character, but also in the lives others. With that recognition comes a responsibility to tend to our minds with great care.

- All we do and think shapes the quality of our character, and for that reason, it vitally important to be attentive to what we put in our minds and allow them to dwell on.

Mindfulness and Compassion

- Our species is at a critical juncture in its evolution. Perhaps because of our fragility, we always seem to be at a critical juncture.

- Today, we face a great number of global crises: addressing the great inequities between rich and poor, providing adequate food and health care to all people, dealing with serious environmental issues, coping with acts of terrorism, and coming to terms with a religious pluralistic world in which misunderstandings often lead to hatred.

- If there was ever a time that we needed to practice compassion, it's now. The problem is that many of us are not yet convinced of its importance, or if we are, we are insufficiently trained in how to practice it.

- The mindfulness discipline offers one very compelling way for us to grasp the importance of compassion and to learn how to implement it in our everyday life.

- A growing number of people around the world are beginning to see the necessity for us to devote more deliberate attention to the study and practice of compassion as a way to help address these massive issues that face us.

- Exercising compassion and kindness is one practice that the core of every religious tradition affirms. Religions may not be able to agree about the nature and existence of God, or they may have differing views of the soul and the ultimate destiny of human life. Religions certainly profess different doctrines and perform different rituals and ceremonies, but about the importance of being kind to others and oneself they seem to be in accord.

- One of the central insights of mindfulness practice is seeing the interrelatedness of reality. Once you see how your life is closely connected with that of others, you recognize that it is only with their support that you are able do anything at all.

- May each and every person—and, indeed, may all beings—be well and happy.

Questions to Consider

1. Which mindfulness exercises discussed in the series seem to have the most and the least appeal to you? Why?

2. What are the advantages and disadvantages of resisting fixed labels to define your identity?

Life—Putting It All in Perspective
Lecture 24—Transcript

It is the nature of reality for all things to come to an end. Just so, the time has come for us to bring this series to a close. Before we part, I'd like to share some final remarks. I have a few things I'd like to say about mindfulness practice; a few things I'd like to say about myself, and a few things I'd like to say about others.

At this point, there is little more I can say to add substance to what I've already said about the practice of mindfulness. We've looked at the fundamental components of the discipline and discussed a great many areas of life in which these practices can be beneficially exercised. If there is anything about that practice that remains unclear, let me urge you to return to the lectures and listen to them again. I don't usually invite students to retake one of my courses after they've taken it once, but the study and practice of mindfulness is different. Listening to the lectures again and still again may prove valuable. After over 25 years of meditation practice, I still return to the meditation manuals I started with, and each time, I seem to find a new insight that somehow I overlooked before or was simply not ready to receive in earlier readings. One of the things that I've appreciated about the opportunity to put together this course has been the chance to return to the fundamentals of the practice with what Suzuki Roshi called "beginner's mind." I can genuinely say that I have learned more in composing this course than any other I've ever done.

I'd encourage you to find a couple of books on basic mindfulness practice and read those as well. You'll readily see that different meditation teachers teach the discipline in slightly—and sometimes substantially—different ways. You may find that what other teachers have to say about mindfulness practice is more meaningful to you than what I've said or the way I've said it. The practice is simple but extremely rich. The Buddha himself taught for 45 years and tailored his lessons in different ways for different individuals. Since recorded lectures prevent us from fashioning the course to each person's individual needs and temperaments, as the Buddha did, much of that work will be up to you.

But just a word of caution: Beware of spending too much time with the lectures or reading too many books about meditation. These activities can easily become ends in themselves, to the point that you're studying the practice of meditation rather than practicing the practice of meditation. The bookshelf in my office is loaded with books on Zen, the tradition that insists, more than any other, that true reality can never be grasped through words.

Once you've understood the essential features of the discipline and have become comfortable doing them, begin to trust yourself to customize the practice to suit your own individual qualities. In this series, we've discussed and demonstrated a wide range of exercises. Not all of them, I'm sure, were equally appealing. Take as much as you can from each of them. Some you'll want to practice just as explained; others you may want to vary a bit; and still others may have no appeal at all. But resist dismissing any exercise out of hand. If a practice carries little meaning for you now, revisit it later. The practices we dislike the most are often the ones from which we can gain the greatest benefit. I was initially repelled by the idea of loving-kindness meditation, but ultimately incorporated it into my practice and discovered it to be immensely important.

If you have the opportunity to study with a reputable teacher of mindfulness meditation, try to take to take advantage of it. A good teacher can answer questions or concerns you may have in ways that are not possible with a recorded series of lectures. The trick is to ensure that a potential teacher is a good one, which is not always an easy thing to do. As you know, there are lots of teachers, sages, preachers, evangelists, missionaries, and gurus out there who are eager to tell you what to believe and how to live your life. The Buddha always encouraged his followers to take a critical eye toward anyone claiming to present the truth and to judge the veracity of any claim or practice for themselves. In a famous statement he urges them never to accept anything simply because it is said to be revelation; because it is traditional; because it comes from sacred texts; or because the teacher seems competent. Rather, he said, when you know for yourself that something is wholesome, blameless, and leads to benefit and happiness, then you should accept it and abide in it. The Buddha even insisted that his own teachings be subjected to this same rigorous test.

As you proceed with your daily practice, you may consider at some point to intensify your meditation experience with a retreat. There are many types of retreats, and each can be very beneficial for your practice. Perhaps the simplest is to dedicate a day to mindfulness in the comfort of your own home. Try to arrange to be alone and quiet for four to eight hours—more if you're able—where you do nothing other than practice. You can design this self-retreat in any way that suits you, but it ought to include alternating sitting and walking practice. If you choose, you can add a body scan, mindful eating, and listening to a recorded talk on mindfulness. There are many locations on the Internet where you can download such talks for free.

If you search the Internet, you'll also find plenty of listings for other kinds of retreats. Just Google "mindfulness or meditation retreat." There are a growing number of retreat centers across the country and throughout the world that offer retreats lasting from a weekend to three months, and even to the traditional three year, three month, three day retreat taken by some very committed practitioners. A very popular type of retreat in the mindfulness tradition lasts for ten days. In a ten day retreat, you're usually with other practitioners, sitting and walking for as much as 16 hours a day, all in silence. A retreat of this length will benefit your practice (and the rest of your life) enormously.

My final word and most important word about practicing mindfulness is: Just do it. It's difficult to get started sometimes, and it's difficult to continue, but the rewards, I believe, are immeasurable. I'm confident that you'll find dedicating yourself to this discipline to be one of the most significant things you've ever done. I've learned many things in life, and I've had many experiences, but nothing has been more important to me as learning this practice.

Because the practice of meditation is intensely personal, I thought that perhaps one of the best things I could do to wrap up this series would be to tell you a bit about my own experiences with this discipline. Unlike other things I teach, it's difficult to maintain an air of objectivity in teaching mindfulness. It's relatively easy to keep my personal experiences out of the discussion when I'm talking about an ancient text like the *Upanishads* or the scholarly debate about the life of the historical Confucius. But when the topic is something like anger and grief and fear, my own subjectivity necessarily comes into view.

You've noticed, I'm sure, the many personal anecdotes that I've used throughout these lectures to help make my points. But even beyond those anecdotes, in ways not so obvious, my own experiences have shaped this course. The topics I chose to discuss, for example, have all been subjects that have had a personal bearing on my life. I wanted to talk about mindful driving because a few years ago a dear uncle of mine was killed in a senseless car accident caused by another driver not paying attention. I wanted to speak about eating mindfully because I have a hard time doing it, and I needed to be reminded of its importance. I wanted to discuss anger, not because I necessarily thought you needed to hear about it, but because I did. And I rewrote the lecture on perfectionism four times because I was not satisfied with it—and I'm still not. Teaching this course has put me in the odd position of being both a lecturer and an auditor. I hope that in my case the old saying is true: "that you teach best what you most need to learn."

I share this information to let you know that I'm a fellow struggler. I have been on this path for a good while and have gained some insights that I think might be worth sharing. So let me tell you some of what I've learned.

Although I dabbled with meditation as a teenager, I didn't begin a serious practice until I had come to an important crossroad in my life. I had just finished my Ph.D. in the philosophy of modern Western religion, and I was finding my personal life in quite a shambles. I wasn't completely certain that I wanted to become a professor, and I wasn't even sure if I'd be able to find a job. At a time in my life in which little seemed certain, I was extended an opportunity to study meditation with a group of Tibetan monks. I had studied Buddhism in graduate school but never actually tried the very practice that is the centerpiece of the tradition. When the opportunity arose, I jumped at the chance, thinking that meditative skills might somehow provide direction out of the disarray that had become my life. Looking back, I now realize that it took a serious crisis to break open the armor that I had been wearing for years, to allow me to entertain the possibility of seeking help and trying something novel.

My first real experience with mindfulness practice was a weekend retreat with these monks. I found the whole occasion to be very challenging and yet oddly refreshing. I still have vivid recollections of the whole experience.

With the encouragement of a friend who had already traveled the same road I was on, I continued with the practice. Trying to meditate every day was extremely hard for me, and often I simply couldn't manage it. But even when the resistance to meditating was too great, I knew that I could always return to it and find a place of serenity. Even today, I think of meditation as an island of refuge, a place where I can go to be tranquil. What appealed to me so much was that meditation did not require me to speak, think, or perform for others. After eight years of graduate school, I was finding those activities to be extremely toilsome. And after 30 years of teaching, I still find them so. The first thing I do when I finish a class is run up to my office and shut the door, so I don't have to speak to anyone. I'm not asocial; I just find words to be a burden.

I was grateful for the way meditation helped me craft a new relationship with my thoughts. For much of my life, I was very anxious about finding the truth about myself and the world. And by truth, what I meant was correct beliefs, metaphysical propositions that corresponded with what I then called the "really real." What I found in meditation was relief from this anxiety about getting my beliefs in order. I learned that to live a happy, fulfilled life, it wasn't necessary to find the correct metaphysical viewpoint or to have the right opinion on every issue. It was a tremendous relief to discover that I didn't have to have everything figured out.

Although I didn't always practice meditation consistently for many years, I always knew that it would be an important part of my life. At times, I could become extremely enthusiastic about the discipline and even considered for a while becoming a Buddhist monk so I could practice all the time. But instead, I used the opportunities afforded me by my teaching position to travel to various places in the world where I could study the discipline with meditation masters. Back home, I began teaching the practice to undergraduates as part of my courses in comparative religion, and I started a sitting group in the city where I lived.

A dozen years ago, a young woman from Sri Lanka called me, inquiring about my meditation group. She had recently come to Memphis and was looking for place to practice the discipline that was such an important part of her Buddhist religion. She and I met at 6:30 in the morning twice a week to sit together in silence. The group was open to anyone, but there were few takers at that early hour. Usually it was just the two of us. For months we hardly spoke a word to one another, except to greet and say goodbye. But eventually we came to discover that sitting in silence had established a deep bond between us. Now the woman from Sri Lanka is my wife. We didn't go to movies or restaurants; our courtship took place on meditation cushions.

Meditation, of course, has done more than just provide me with a quiet refuge and a loving spouse. It has also profoundly altered the way I view myself, and the world, and my place in it. I could spend a lot time discussing those transformations, but I can only mention a few things that at this moment seem most significant.

As a teacher of comparative religion, people are always interested in knowing what religion I follow. It's one of the first questions I'm asked by students on the first day of class. I think it's a fair question, but I have a difficult time answering it.

My "religion" doesn't fall under a particular category. I can't offer them a tidy label that they can use to identify my religious and philosophical commitments. Even as much as I've been influenced by practicing Buddhist meditation, I'm still reluctant simply to adopt the label "Buddhist."

Part of the reason I have no specific label to offer is that my outlook on life has been greatly influenced by a wide range of religions and philosophies. When you study a lot of traditions, it's hard not to take away something from each one that impacts the way you live and view the world. Even for a viewpoint or a practice that I would never dream of adopting wholesale, I would always find something worth affirming. The other reason I resist identifying with a single religion or philosophy is that my views sometimes change, and I like to stay open to that change. Being firmly attached to beliefs and perspectives, as mindfulness practice suggests, can lead to great confusion and quarreling. The Buddha even cautioned his students not to become attached to his teachings. My teachings are a raft, he told them. When you use a raft to get from one side of the lake to the other, you don't pick it up and carry around with you. You leave it on the shore.

In recent years I've begun to post a tongue-in-cheek compositional analysis outside my office door to assist those who think they might benefit from knowing my theological and philosophical identity. On a given day, one might find that I am 55 percent Theravada Buddhist, 18 percent Orthodox Christian, 12 percent Sufi, 7 percent Agnostic, 4 percent American Pragmatist, and 3 percent Rice Krispies Treats—with traces of Hegelianism and Texas redneck. Of course, I have to change the various elements and percentages from time to time. It's about the best I can do to assess my worldview and quietly subvert the belief that one's identity is fixed and monolithic.

Subverting the notion of fixed identity is one of the things a mindfulness practice will do for you. And best of all, it can help you be comfortable without having a fixed identity. Gaining insight into the transience of the self has enabled me to think of myself as a fluid reality, unable to be adequately named by conventional labels. It has helped me to see that underneath the words that I might use to identify myself—husband, father, son, professor, man, American, and so on—lies a reality that is a genuine mystery, at once conscious and self-aware, interrelated with the rest of the cosmos, and yet unfathomable in its depth. And that is true for every one of us.

Likewise, the practice of mindfulness has altered my understanding of ultimate reality and allowed me to feel at home with its mystery. By ultimate reality, I'm referring to the underlying nature of the universe, the reality that is indicated by terms such as God, the absolute, and Brahman. After years of trying to understand and experience the reality these terms signify, I've come to the point where I've recognized my utter inability to do so. I have, in other words, accepted this limitation on my knowledge and feel at ease with saying I don't really know about the ultimate power that governs the universe or whether there even is one. I'm also comfortable acknowledging my inability to answer such questions as what happens to us when we die or why the universe even exists. Taking refuge in the category of "mystery" does not mean I'm uninterested in these questions or that I'm indecisive; rather it means that after years of study and thought, and struggling to be honest with myself, I can come up with no better answer than mystery. And I put that forth as an answer—if it is an answer—with great joy. I feel immense awe and happiness at being able to marvel at this world and our lives in it without having to provide a comprehensive and systematic explanation for the entire universe.

But within the joyous mystery that surrounds and permeates our lives, mindfulness practice has also allowed me to affirm some very simple things about living that strike me as being true. The first thing that comes to mind is the acknowledgement that our control over life, like our knowledge of it, is very limited indeed. Mindfulness permits us to see clearly how little control we really have over the events that profoundly affect us. Much of our suffering, we realize, is caused by our dogged efforts to try to command those things over which we have no authority. But the practice also allows us to recognize that we have a capacity to shape our minds in ways that are wholesome for us and for others. With the training that mindfulness practice provides, we can learn to develop our minds in ways that allow us to relinquish the need to control and to accept reality as it is in this very moment.

I'm also persuaded by mindfulness practice, that everything we do, everything we think, and everything we say has an important effect, particularly on our own character, but also in the lives others. With that recognition comes a responsibility to tend to our minds with great care.

I didn't always think this way. As a youth, especially, I used to believe that doing, saying, and thinking unwholesome things was perfectly fine as long as I didn't hurt anyone else. Today, I think differently. I believe that all we do and think shapes the quality of our character, and for that reason it is vitally important to be attentive to what we put in our minds and allow them to dwell on.

Now, I want to say a word about compassion. It's cliché to use this phrase, but I think our species is at a critical juncture in its evolution. Perhaps because of our fragility, we always seem to be at a critical juncture.

Today, we face a great number of global crises: addressing the inequities between rich and poor, providing adequate food and healthcare to all persons, dealing with serious environmental issues, coping with acts of terrorism, and coming to terms with a religious pluralistic world in which misunderstandings often lead to hatred. If there was a time that we needed to practice compassion, it's now. The problem is, many of us are not yet convinced of its importance or, if we are, we are insufficiently trained in how to practice it. The mindfulness discipline offers one very compelling way for us to grasp the importance of compassion and to learn how to implement it in our everyday life.

A growing number of people around the world are beginning to see the necessity for us to devote more deliberate attention to the study and practice of compassion as a way to help address issues that face us today. Exercising compassion and kindness is one practice that the core of every religious tradition affirms. Religions may not be able to agree about the nature and existence of God; they may have differing views of the soul and the ultimate destiny of human life; they certainly profess different doctrines and perform different rituals and ceremonies. But about the importance of being kind to others and oneself they seem to be in accord.

One of the central insights of mindfulness practice is seeing the interrelatedness of reality. Once you see how your life is closely connected that with of others, you recognize that it is only with their support that you are able do anything at all. Accordingly, I cannot conclude these lectures without thanking some very important people who made them possible. First and foremost, I am grateful to my wife, Dhammika, and my daughter, Ariyana, who continue to be my dearest companions and my greatest teachers. I'm thankful for the good work of the many people of the august company that produces these lectures, especially those who have worked most closely with me on this and other projects.

Finally, let me express my gratitude to those of you who have accompanied me on this journey through mindfulness. May each and every one of you—and indeed may all beings—be well and happy.

Glossary

anger: The feeling of displeasure, usually accompanied by antagonism; it encompasses a wide range of experiences from simple irritation and annoyance to rage and fury.

attachment: The way in which people cling to the various items of their experiences as if they can't live without them.

bhavana: Most accurately translated as "cultivation," this is what Buddhism calls meditation. It does not mean deep thinking but, rather, the awareness and discipline that allow one to shape the mind in ways conducive to happiness and well-being.

Burmese style: In this position, one sits on a cushion, crossing the legs at the ankles without having to place the feet on opposite thighs—as when sitting on the floor.

compassion: The desire to alleviate suffering.

conditioning: The process of habitual thinking that significantly determines what people think, feel, and perceive. The more people entertain a particular thought or a particular kind of thought, the more their minds are prone to generate thoughts of that nature.

courage: The ability to accept suffering rather than flee from it; the determination to look at difficulty straight in the eye.

dana: The Buddhist word for generosity.

dukkha: A Buddhist term that basically means "suffering" and that denotes the fundamental frustrating, insatiable quality of the mindless existence of human beings.

Eightfold Path: In Buddhism, mindfulness is a component of this path, which leads to enlightenment and freedom from the cycle of continual rebirth.

ekgrata: The term that Hindu yogis use for concentration, or one-pointedness.

gatha: A short verse from the Buddhist tradition that focuses the mind on a wholesome thought.

generosity: The willingness to give to others; on a deeper level, it is the eagerness to relinquish anything that one might feel is a possession.

greed: The self-centered desire for unnecessary things; it is considered to be a poison of the mind because it distorts one's view of reality and leaves one unhappy.

grieving: The process of coming to terms with loss in life.

harsh speech: Speech that may be hurtful without any real intent to be so; the use of language that shows little or no regard for the feelings of others. It is usually thoughtless and includes profanity, sarcasm, and shouting.

idle chatter: Generic, inessential language whose basic purpose is to fill airspace; it is the verbal equivalent of unnecessary material possessions.

karma: The belief of many Hindus, Buddhists, and Jains that thoughts, deeds, and words from people's previous lives profoundly influence the mental states they have at birth.

labyrinth: Intricate structures or patterns that define a pathway; it has twists and turns but only a single route.

lotus position: In this traditional pose, one sits on the bare floor or a thin cushion and places the right foot on top of the left thigh and the left foot on top of the right thigh.

malicious speech: The Buddhist term for the practice of making hurtful assertions under the veil of truth. A malicious statement may be either true or false, but its objective is to harm.

mantra: A short saying or set of syllables that a meditator repeats to him- or herself.

maze: A kind of puzzle with many pathway options; one can get lost in a maze, and the goal is to find a way out.

meditation: Refers to certain exercises that can be used to enlarge and refine mindfulness. Not all forms of meditation, however, intend to cultivate mindfulness.

metta meditation: An ancient practice that has long been the cornerstone for cultivating compassion in the Buddhist tradition. "Metta" is a Buddhist term that usually translates as "loving-kindness."

mindfulness: The process of attentively observing an experience as it unfolds in a moment-by-moment awareness; it is devoid of the constant comparing and assessing that ordinarily occupies our mental functioning.

mindlessness: A mental state in which the mind generates a constant swirl of remarks and judgments that create a barrier of words and images that separate people from their lives. This condition makes it difficult to be mindful—or attentive—to life's experiences.

nirvana: A state of bliss; in Buddhism, it transcends suffering and karma.

not-knowing: A beginning practice that starts with an honest assessment of what one really knows and what one really can know.

not-self: A term that is sometimes compared to "insubstantiality." This is the third mark of existence that is central to the Buddhist worldview—and the most difficult to grasp both by intellect and by insight, even for those within the tradition.

pity: Feeling sorry for someone who has to endure suffering.

pleasure principle: A term introduced by Sigmund Freud that describes the way in which people grasp for the things they enjoy and evade the things they don't.

sati: A special form of heightened awareness that promotes the end of suffering and fosteres happiness and well-being for all; it is the Buddha's word that is translated into English as "mindfulness."

seiza: A posture that involves sitting on one's calves with the knees, shins, and feet resting on the ground. This manner of sitting is very common throughout Japan, even among those who do not practice meditation.

serendipity: The word for the phenomenon of discovering pleasant things not sought for. Part of the surprising and unpredictable quality of existence is the way that, sometimes, things can turn out better than imagined.

shavasana: This position is known as the corpse pose and is practiced in hatha yoga.

Upanishad: One of the earliest Hindu documents in which instructions in contemplative practice were recorded.

vipassana: The Buddhist word for "insights" or "clear gazing," these are unmistakable moments when a person sees things differently.

Bibliography

Armstrong, Karen. *Twelve Steps to a Compassionate Life*. New York: Alfred A. Knopf, 2011. Karen Armstrong is a popular religious writer who has called for greater attention to the study and practice of compassion. This work, strongly influenced by the mindfulness traditions, provides her outline for the development of compassion.

Bacovcin, Helen. *The Way of a Pilgrim and the Pilgrim Continues His Way: Spiritual Classics from Russia*. Garden City, NY: Image Books, 1978. I love this book. It's a memoir of a Russian peasant who learns the Jesus Prayer—part of the mindfulness tradition in Eastern Orthodoxy—and puts it into practice as he wanders through 19th-century Russia.

Batchelor, Stephen. *Buddhism without Beliefs: a Contemporary Guide to Awakening*. New York: Riverhead Books, 1998. A former Tibetan and Zen monk, Batchelor presents an understanding of Buddhism that attempts to make the tradition more accessible to modern sensibilities. Recommended.

Beck, Charlotte Joko, and Steve Smith. *Everyday Zen: Love and Work*. New York, NY: HarperOne, 2007. Charlotte Beck was a Zen teacher in San Diego. This is a surprising and lucid collection of her essays on a variety of subjects. Recommended.

Berger, K. T. *Zen Driving*. New York: Ballantine, 1988. Tips on how to incorporate mindfulness practice into your experience of driving.

Bernhard, Toni. *How to Be Sick: A Buddhist-Inspired Guide for the Chronically Ill and Their Caregivers*. Boston: Wisdom Publications, 2010. This moving book is a memoir of one woman's coming to terms with chronic illness and pain using the techniques of mindfulness practice. Recommended.

Bodhi, Bhikkhu. *The Noble Eightfold Path: Way to the End of Suffering*. Seattle, WA: BPS Pariyatti Editions, 2000. One of the clearest short presentations of the Buddha's path to awakening. Scholarly, yet very accessible to the lay audience.

Boyce, Barry Campbell. *The Mindfulness Revolution: Leading Psychologists, Scientists, Artists, and Meditation Teachers on the Power of Mindfulness in Daily Life.* Boston: Shambhala, 2011. This anthology is an excellent introduction to the concept and practice of mindfulness and the way it informs and transforms every aspect of life. Recommended.

Carroll, Michael. *Awake at Work: Facing the Challenges of Life on the Job.* Boston: Shambhala Publications, 2004. Practical advice for incorporating mindfulness practice in the work environment. Helpful for people with jobs!

Chah, Achaan. *Food for the Heart: The Collected Teachings of Ajahn Chah.* Boston: Wisdom Publications, 2002. An insightful collection of essays by a Thai Buddhist monk who was a teacher to many American meditators in the latter part of the 20th century.

Chödrön, Pema. *Start Where You Are: A Guide to Compassionate Living.* Boston: Shambhala, 2004. Pema Chödrön is a nun in the Shambhala Buddhist tradition and one of the most popular writers on mindfulness practices today. Any of her works are worth reading. This one on developing compassion is a good place to start.

Dermond, Susan Usha. *Calm and Compassionate Children: A Handbook.* Berkeley: Celestial Arts, 2007. One of the best resources for introducing mindfulness practices to children. Recommended.

Feldman, Christina. *Compassion: Listening to the Cries of the World.* Berkeley: Rodmell Press, 2005. A thorough and accessible study of the idea and practice of compassion. Contains useful exercises for developing this virtue.

Fetzer Institute Website. Accessed August 18, 2011. http://www.fetzer. org. This website is devoted to encouraging the practice of forgiveness and compassion.

Germer, Christopher K. *The Mindful Path to Self-Compassion: Freeing Yourself from Destructive Thoughts and Emotions*. New York: Guilford Press, 2009. A comprehensive analysis and practical guidebook for learning to extend compassion to one's self.

Goenka, S. N. Vipassana Meditation Website. Accessed August 18, 2011. http://www.dhamma.org/. Website for the organization that teaches mindfulness practices in the tradition of S. N. Goenka.

Goldstein, Joseph. *The Experience of Insight: A Simple and Direct Guide to Buddhist Meditation*. Boston: Shambhala Publications, 1987. As the subtitle rightly indicates, this guide to mindfulness meditation is both simple and direct.

Gunaratana, Henepola. *Beyond Mindfulness in Plain English: An Introductory Guide to Deeper States of Meditation*. Boston: Wisdom Publications, 2009. This guide is for those who have gained experience in the basic practices of mindfulness and are interested in taking the practice to the next level.

———. *Eight Mindful Steps to Happiness: Walking the Path of the Buddha*. Boston: Wisdom Publications, 2001. A comprehensive and understandable account of the Buddha's path to awakening. Helps to explain the relationships among the many components of the path.

———. *Mindfulness in Plain English*. Boston: Wisdom Publications, 2002. In my opinion, this book is by far the best written guide on how to practice mindfulness meditation. Highly recommended.

Hanson, Rick, and Richard Mendius. *Buddha's Brain: The Practical Neuroscience of Happiness, Love & Wisdom*. Oakland, CA: New Harbinger Publications, 2009. An accessible overview of the neuroscience of mindfulness practice.

Hart, William. *The Art of Living: Vipassana Meditation as Taught by S. N. Goenka*. San Francisco: Harper & Row, 1987. S. N. Goekna is a highly regarded Indian teacher of *vipassana* (insight) meditation. He learned his practice in Burma and has taught it throughout the world. This book explains his approach.

Kabat-Zinn, Jon. *Full Catastrophe Living: Using the Wisdom of Your Body and Mind to Face Stress, Pain, and Illness*. New York, NY: Delacorte Press, 1990. Jon Kabat-Zinn is a popular American physician, writer, and meditation instructor. This is one of his best books. It focuses on his specialty: using mindfulness to ease physical pain and suffering.

Kaza, Stephanie. *Hooked!: Buddhist Writings on Greed, Desire, and the Urge to Consume*. Boston: Shambhala, 2005. An informative anthology containing essays written from a variety of Buddhist perspectives on consumerism and greed in the modern world. Recommended.

Khema, Ayya. *Who Is My Self?: A Guide to Buddhist Meditation*. Boston: Wisdom Publications, 1997. Ayya Khema was a German who ordained as a Buddhist nun in the 20th century. Her writings on meditation and mindfulness practices are very lucid.

Kornfield, Jack. *A Path with Heart: A Guide through the Perils and Promises of Spiritual Life*. New York, NY: Bantam Books, 1993. Jack Kornfield is a highly respected American meditation teacher and an engaging storyteller. This is a good book for getting acquainted with mindfulness practices. Recommended.

Leloup, Jean-Yves, and M. S. Laird. *Being Still: Reflections on an Ancient Mystical Tradition*. Leominster, Herefordshire, UK: Gracewing, 2003. A fascinating book on mindfulness practice in the Eastern Orthodox tradition of Christianity.

McDonald, Michele. *Awake at the Wheel: Mindful Driving*. CD. More Than Sound Productions, 2011. This is an excellent audio CD for driving practice. I'm indebted to McDonald for her insights on mindful driving.

Mindful Website. Accessed August 18, 2011. http://mindful.org. Accessible website devoted to the practice of mindfulness in a wide range of areas.

Muesse, Mark W. "Cultivating a Quiet Mind." Explorefaith.org . Accessed August 18, 2011. http://www.explorefaith.org/prayer/meditation/questions_ and_answers_about_meditation.php?ht=. This is one of my own articles about the basics of meditation practice and its relationship to other contemplative practices in the world's religions.

Nhat Hạnh, Thich. *Guide to Walking Meditation.* Parallax Press, 2005. One of the few books dedicated solely to the practice of walking meditation. Like all of Thich Nhat Hanh's works, this book is highly accessible and easy to understand.

———. *Peace Is Every Step: The Path of Mindfulness in Everyday Life.* Shambhala Pubns, 2009. Another highly readable book by Thich Nhat Hanh.

Nhat Hạnh, Thich, and Mai Vo-Dinh. *The Miracle of Mindfulness: A Manual on Meditation.* Boston: Beacon Press, 1987. Probably the most accessible introduction to the concept and practice of mindfulness meditation. Recommended.

Phra, Thēpwisutthimēthī, and Santikaro Bhikkhu. *Mindfulness with Breathing: A Manual for Serious Beginners.* Boston: Wisdom Publications, 1997. Buddhadasa Bhikkhu (Phra Thēpwisutthimēthī) was a highly regarded Thai Buddhist monk. This text is a very clearly written and well-translated meditation manual. Recommended.

Rosenberg, Larry, and David Guy. *Breath by Breath: The Liberating Practice of Insight Liberation.* Boston: Shambhala, 1998. Rosenberg's clear explanation of the *Anapanasati Sutta*, one of the classic ancient texts on meditating on the breath. Recommended.

———. *Living in the Light of Death: On the Art of Being Truly Alive.* Boston: Shambhala, 2001. Larry Rosenberg is an excellent meditation teacher. This book focuses on his engagement with death awareness practices.

Salzberg, Sharon. *Loving-kindness: The Revolutionary Art of Happiness*. Boston: Shambhala, 1995. An easy-to-read guide to the basic loving-kindness meditation for the development of compassion.

Shaw, Sarah. *Introduction to Buddhist Meditation*. London: Routledge, 2009. More of a scholarly study of meditation in the Buddhist tradition focused on the ancient texts and manuals.

Siegel, Daniel J. *Mindsight: The New Science of Personal Transformation*. New York: Bantam Books, 2010. An integrative study of neuroscientific research on mindfulness and its application in psychotherapy.

Sīlānanda, U, and Ruth-Inge Heinze. *The Four Foundations of Mindfulness*. Boston: Wisdom Publications, 2002. The scripture on the four foundations of mindfulness are believed to represent the Buddha's basic teaching on meditation. This book by a Burmese monk is an effort to explain those teachings for a modern audience. The writing style can be difficult at times.

Snyder, Stephen, and Tina Rasmussen. *Practicing the Jhānas: Traditional Concentration Meditation as Presented by the Venerable Pa Auk Sayadaw*. Boston: Shambhala, 2009. This work is for those who are ready to begin more advanced mindfulness practices.

Sogyal, Patrick Gaffney, and Andrew Harvey. *The Tibetan Book of Living and Dying*. San Francisco, CA: HarperSanFrancisco, 2002. This work has become a modern classic on the Tibetan Buddhist understanding of mindful living. Recommended.

Somov, Pavel G. *Eating the Moment: 141 Mindful Practices to Overcome Overeating One Meal at a Time*. Oakland, CA: New Harbinger Publications, 2008. Very practical guide for learning to eat mindfully. Highly recommended.

Sumedho, Ajahn. *The Mind and the Way: Buddhist Reflections on Life*. Boston: Wisdom Publications, 1995. Ajahn Sumedho is one of my favorite Buddhist writers. This is a clear and highly insightful collection of his essays. Recommended.

———. *The Sound of Silence: The Selected Teachings of Ajahn Sumedho*. Boston: Wisdom Publications, 2007. Another excellent collection of Sumedho's essays.

Suzuki, Shunryu. *Zen Mind, Beginner's Mind.* Shambhala Pubns, 2011. A classic modern Zen text. Highly recommended.

Thera, Nyanaponika. *Satipatthāna: The Heart of Buddhist Meditation*. San Francisco, CA: Weiser Books, 2007. Well-informed and erudite explanation of mindfulness meditation based on the earliest Buddhist texts. Recommended for those with an academic interest in the practice.

Thubten, Chodron. *Working with Anger*. Ithaca, NY: Snow Lion Publication, 2001. A good work for learning how to cope with anger.

Tonkinson, Carole. *Wake Up and Cook: Kitchen Buddhism in Words and Recipes*. New York: Riverhead Books, 1997. This is both an anthology on mindful eating and a cookbook. Recommended.

Wallis, Glenn. *The* Dhammapada*: Verses on the Way*. New York: Modern Library, 2004. The *Dhammapada* is a classic wisdom text of Buddhism. It is written in an accessible, aphoristic form. Wallis's translation is one of the best. Highly recommended.

Walpola, Rāhula. *What the Buddha Taught.* New York: Grove Press, 1987. A classic in the field, this book remains one of the best introductions to the basic teachings of the Buddha over 50 years after its publication. Highly recommended.

Young, Shinzen. The Science of Meditation in Action. Accessed August 18, 2011. http://www.shinzen.org/. Website for Shinzen Young, a popular mindfulness teac

Notes

Notes

Notes

Notes

Notes

Notes

Notes